Management Considerations in Beef Heifer Development and Puberty

Editors

DAVID J. PATTERSON
MICHAEL F. SMITH

VETERINARY CLINICS OF NORTH AMERICA: FOOD ANIMAL PRACTICE

www.vetfood.theclinics.com

Consulting Editor
ROBERT A. SMITH

November 2013 • Volume 29 • Number 3

ELSEVIER

1600 John F. Kennedy Boulevard • Suite 1800 • Philadelphia, Pennsylvania, 19103-2899

http://www.vetfood.theclinics.com

VETERINARY CLINICS OF NORTH AMERICA: FOOD ANIMAL PRACTICE Volume 29, Number 3
November 2013 ISSN 0749-0720, ISBN-13: 978-0-323-26136-4

Editor: John Vassallo; j.vassallo@elsevier.com
Developmental Editor: Susan Showalter

Veterinary Clinics of North America: Food Animal Practice (ISSN 0749-0720) is published in March, July, and November by Elsevier Inc., 360 Park Avenue South, New York, NY 10010-1710. Subscription prices are $235.00 per year (domestic individuals), $326.00 per year (domestic institutions), $110.00 per year (domestic students/residents), $265.00 per year (Canadian individuals), $430.00 per year (Canadian institutions), $335.00 per year (international individuals), $430.00 per year (international institutions), and $165.00 per year (international and Canadian students/residents). To receive student/resident rate, orders must be accompanied by name of affiliated institution, date of term, and the signature of program/residency coordinator on institution letterhead. *Clinics* subscription prices. All prices are subject to change without notice. **POSTMASTER:** Send address changes to *Veterinary Clinics of North America*: *Food Animal Practice*, Elsevier Health Sciences Division, Subscription Customer Service, 3251 Riverport Lane, Maryland Heights, MO 63043. Customer Service (orders, claims, online, change of address): Elsevier Health Sciences Division, Subscription Customer Service, 3251 Riverport Lane, Maryland Heights, MO 63043. Tel: 1-800-654-2452 (U.S. and Canada); 314-447-8871 (ouside U.S. and Canada). Fax: 314-447-8029. E-mail: journalscustomerservice-usa@elsevier.com (for print support); journalsonlinesupport-usa@elsevier.com (for online support).

Reprints. For copies of 100 or more, of articles in this publication, please contact the Commercial Reprints Department, Elsevier Inc., 360 Park Avenue South, New York, NY 10010-1710. Tel.: 212-633-3874; Fax: 212-633-3820; E-mail: reprints@elsevier.com.

Veterinary Clinics of North America: Food Animal Practice is covered in *Current Contents/Agriculture, Biology and Environmental Sciences, MEDLINE/PubMed (Index Medicus), and Excerpta Medica.*

Printed and bound by CPI Group (UK) Ltd, Croydon, CR0 4YY

Transferred to digital print 2012

Contributors

CONSULTING EDITOR

ROBERT A. SMITH, DVM, MS
Diplomate, American Board of Veterinary Practitioners; Veterinary Research and Consulting Services, LLC, Greeley, Colorado

EDITORS

DAVID J. PATTERSON, PhD
Professor, Division of Animal Sciences, Animal Sciences Research Center, University of Missouri, Columbia, Missouri

MICHAEL F. SMITH, PhD
Professor, Division of Animal Sciences, Animal Sciences Research Center, University of Missouri, Columbia, Missouri

AUTHORS

JACQUELINE A. ATKINS, PhD
Director of Science and Educational Operations, American Simmental Association, Bozeman; Embryologist, Progenesis Embryo Transfer, Belgrade, Montana

D. SCOTT BROWN, PhD
Research Assistant Professor, Department of Agricultural and Applied Economics, University of Missouri, Columbia, Missouri

ROBERT CUSHMAN, PhD
Research Physiologist, ARS, USDA, U.S. Meat Animal Research Center, Clay Center, Nebraska

JARED E. DECKER, PhD
Assistant Professor, Division of Animal Sciences, University of Missouri, Columbia, Missouri

RICHARD N. FUNSTON, PhD
Professor, Department of Animal Science, Beef Reproductive Physiology Specialist, West Central Research and Extension Center, University of Nebraska – Lincoln, North Platte, Nebraska

JOHN B. HALL, PhD, PAS
Professor, Department of Animal and Veterinary Science, University of Idaho, Moscow; Extension Beef Specialist and Superintendent, Nancy M. Cummings Research, Extension, and Education Center, University of Idaho, Carmen, Idaho

HARLAN HUGHES, PhD
Professor Emeritus, North Dakota State University, Fargo, North Dakota

SANDY K. JOHNSON, PhD
Associate Professor, Livestock Specialist, Department of Animal Sciences and Industry, Northwest Research and Extension Center, Kansas State University, Colby, Kansas

G. CLIFF LAMB, MS, PhD
Assistant Director and Professor, North Florida Research and Education Center, University of Florida, Marianna, Florida

BRIAN VANDER LEY, DVM, PhD
Diplomate, American College of Veterinary Preventive Medicine; Assistant Professor, Department of Food Animal Medicine & Surgery, University of Missouri College of Veterinary Medicine, Columbia, Missouri

NEAL T. MARTIN, MS
College of Veterinary Medicine, University of Missouri, Columbia, Missouri

JUSTIN M. NASH, MS
College of Veterinary Medicine, University of Missouri, Columbia, Missouri

DAVID J. PATTERSON, PhD
Professor, Division of Animal Sciences, Animal Sciences Research Center, University of Missouri, Columbia, Missouri

CRAIG A. PAYNE, DVM, MS
Director, Associate Professor and Extension Assistant Professor, Department of Veterinary Extension and Continuing Education, College of Veterinary Medicine, University of Missouri, Columbia, Missouri

GEORGE A. PERRY, PhD
Professor, Department of Animal Science, South Dakota State University, Brookings, South Dakota

KY G. POHLER, MS
Graduate Research Assistant, Division of Animal Sciences, Animal Sciences Research Center, University of Missouri, Columbia, Missouri

SCOTT E. POOCK, DVM
Diplomate, American Board of Veterinary Practitioners; Associate Professor, Veterinary Extension and Continuing Education, Department of Medicine and Surgery, College of Veterinary Medicine, University of Missouri, Columbia, Missouri

GEORGE E. SEIDEL Jr, PhD
Animal Reproduction and Biotechnology Laboratory, Colorado State University, Fort Collins, Colorado

W. JUSTIN SEXTEN, PhD
Assistant Professor, Division of Animal Sciences, University of Missouri, Columbia, Missouri

MICHAEL F. SMITH, PhD
Professor, Division of Animal Sciences, Animal Sciences Research Center, University of Missouri, Columbia, Missouri

ADAM F. SUMMERS, PhD
Post Doctoral Research Associate, Department of Animal Science, University of Nebraska – Lincoln, Lincoln, Nebraska

JORDAN M. THOMAS
Graduate Research Assistant, Division of Animal Sciences, University of Missouri, Columbia, Missouri

ALISON L. VAN EENENNAAM, PhD
Cooperative Extension Specialist, Animal Biotechnology and Genomics, Department of Animal Science, University of California, Davis, California

Contents

> Use of existing and emerging management technologies enable beef pro-
> ducers to improve breeding performance of heifers during the first breed-
> ing season and during subsequent calving and rebreeding periods as
> 2 year olds. These practices ensure that heifers that enter the herd as
> raised or purchased replacements contribute to the general performance
> and productivity of an entire cowherd immediately, and cumulatively
> long-term. Rebuilding the US cowherd requires careful consideration
> and use of these newer management technologies. Veterinarians will
> play a crucial role in influencing the technologies used during the rebuild-
> ing process.

> When it comes to development of beef heifers, the importance of maximiz-
> ing the proportion of heifers that are born early in the calving season
> cannot be overemphasized. Because early onset of puberty is of critical
> importance to heifer development, the purpose of this article was to
> describe the physiological and endocrine maturation that control the onset
> of puberty in beef cattle. These concepts will be helpful in understanding
> the physiological and endocrine changes that take place in a heifer as
> she approaches puberty and in understanding how specific estrous syn-
> chronization products are able to induce and synchronize estrus and
> ovulation.

> This article reviews the literature on breed, biological type, and breeding
> system and their impact on female fertility, especially as they relate to
> heifer development. The attributes of different breeding systems and their
> appropriate use is discussed. In addition, the extant and emerging selec-
> tion tools that are available for replacement heifer selection are reviewed.

> In beef cattle, the main factors influencing nutrient partitioning between
> the dam and fetus include age of the dam, number of fetuses, production
> demand, and environmental stress. These factors play a critical role in
> programming the fetus for its future environment and available resources.

Fetal programming reportedly affects neonatal mortality and morbidity, postnatal growth rate, body composition, health, and reproduction. Two main mechanisms responsible for fetal programming include DNA methylation and histone modifications. Alterations in the genome can be passed through multiple generations. Maternal environment (nutrition, age, physiologic status) can program progeny heifer growth and reproductive performance.

Postnatal nutrition has immediate and long-lasting effects on beef heifer reproductive efficiency, longevity, and productivity. This article reviews the effects of nutrients and nutritional management on reproduction in developing heifers. In addition, the current debate on the preferred target weight for heifers at breeding is discussed.

This article discusses some of the aspects of heifer development that contribute to long-term health and productivity, such as disease prevention and control. Nutrition is also an important component of long-term health, and body condition score is discussed as a way to determine whether the nutrient demands of heifers are being met.

At weaning, heifers should be considered for replacements based on their dam's previous performance; heifer calving date, age, and weight; and previous exposure to implants. Before breeding, heifers should be selected as replacements based on whether they have attained puberty (determined by a prebreeding examination), do not have abnormal pelvic areas, or fail to meet temperament standards. After breeding, heifers should be selected as replacements if they conceive early in the breeding season, are capable of achieving 85% of their mature weight by calving, and calve at a body condition of 5.5 to 6.0.

Age at puberty is a critical trait, because pregnancy success during the breeding season is correlated with the percentage of heifers that reach puberty before or early in the breeding season. A negative genetic correlation between age at puberty and heifer pregnancy rate indicate that selection to decrease age at puberty would increase heifer pregnancy rates. Calving late has been reported to increase the chance of calving late or not calving the following year, and heifers need to wean 3 to 5 calves to pay for development costs. Therefore, puberty is important to the sustainability and profitability of beef operations.

Expanded use of artificial insemination (AI) and/or adoption of emerging reproductive technologies for beef heifers and cows require precise methods of estrous-cycle control. New protocols for inducing and synchronizing a fertile estrus in replacement beef heifers and postpartum beef cows in which progestins are used provide new opportunities for beef producers to synchronize estrus and ovulation and to facilitate fixed-time AI. This article reviews the various estrous synchronization protocols currently available for use in replacement beef heifers. New methods of inducing and synchronizing estrus now create the opportunity to significantly expand the use of AI in the United States cowherd.

The only practicable method for sexing mammalian sperm is by measuring DNA content with a flow cytometer/cell sorter. Although many other methods have been tried and patented, they either are inaccurate, damage sperm severely, or otherwise are unsuitable for practical application. Procedures for sexing sperm damage them slightly, and fewer sperm are packaged per straw than with unsexed semen. These 2 characteristics result in lower fertility with sexed than unsexed semen. Incremental improvements of current sexing procedures are being developed constantly.

Rebreeding performance of the first-calf heifer has major economic consequences for cow-calf producers. Management systems that allow heifers to cost-effectively achieve a body condition score of 5 to 6 at calving and maintain this through rebreeding have a higher probability of pregnancy success.

This article lays out the recommended procedure for determining the economic cost of developing a proposed set of replacement heifers. In particular, a 6-step process that calculates the economic cost of developing a raised pregnant replacement heifer is described.

This article provides an overview of the Missouri Show-Me-Select Replacement Heifer Program, and is included to provide an example of a working model for the collective considerations that relate to beef heifer development presented in this issue. This program expanded services provided by veterinarians to cow-calf producers, making veterinary practitioners a more integral part of the overall reproductive management of beef herds in their practice areas.

Scott E. Poock and Craig A. Payne

Veterinarians play an important role in reproductive management of dairy herds across the United States; however, in many cases, their involvement in reproductive management of beef herds has been limited. The reasons for this vary; however, there are ways for veterinarians to become more actively involved in reproductive management of US beef herds. Veterinarians can have an impact on producers' profits by implementing their skills and knowledge to beef heifer development programs. This article provides an overview of the services veterinarians can provide to beef cattle producers that pertain to reproductive management of replacement beef heifers.

VETERINARY CLINICS OF NORTH AMERICA: FOOD ANIMAL PRACTICE

FORTHCOMING ISSUES

March 2014
Bovine Orthopedics
David E. Anderson, DVM, MS, DACVS and
André Desrochers, DMV, MS, DACVS,
DECBHM, *Editors*

July 2014
Fluid and Electrolyte Therapy
Geof Smith, DVM, MS, PhD and
Allen Roussel, DVM, MS, *Editors*

RECENT ISSUES

July 2013
Metabolic Diseases of Dairy Cattle
Thomas H. Herdt, DVM, MS, *Editor*

March 2013
Pain Management
Johann (Hans) Coetzee, BVSc,
Cert CHP, PhD, *Editor*

November 2012
Diagnostic Pathology
Vicky L. Cooper, DVM, MS, PhD, *Editor*

RELATED INTEREST

Veterinary Clinics of North America: Equine Practice
April 2011 (Vol. 27, No. 1)
Endocrine Diseases
Ramiro E. Toribio, DVM, MS, PhD, *Editor*

VETERINARY CLINICS OF
NORTH AMERICA:
FOOD ANIMAL PRACTICE

FORTHCOMING ISSUES

March 2015
Bovine Orthopedics
David E. Anderson, DVM, MS, DACVS and
Andre Desrochers, DMV, MS, DACVS,
DECBHM, Editors

July 2014
Fluid and Electrolyte Therapy
Geof Smith, DVM, MS, PhD and
Allen Roussel, DVM, MS, Editors

RECENT ISSUES

July 2014
Metabolic Diseases of Dairy Cattle
Thomas H. Herdt, DVM, MS, Editor

March 2013
Pain Management
Johann (Hans) Coetzee, BVSc,
Cert CHP, PhD, Editor

November 2012
Digestive Pathology
Robert J. Callan, DVM, MS, PhD, Editor

RELATED INTEREST

Veterinary Clinics of North America: Equine Practice
Month 2014, Vol. 12, No. 5
Infectious Diseases
Author J. Author, DVM, MS, PhD, Editor

Preface

Management Considerations in Beef Heifer Development and Puberty

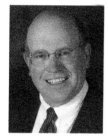 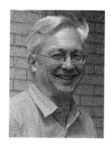

David J. Patterson, PhD   Michael F. Smith, PhD
Editors

The US beef industry finds itself confronted with a significant long-term decline in cattle numbers driven in part by record input costs and severe drought conditions in many of our nation's major cattle-producing states. These recent challenges only add to long-term issues the industry has faced, which include an aging producer population, increased global competition, weaker domestic demand for beef, increased competition from other meat proteins, and a perceived lack of economic incentives to expand the cattle herd. Coincident with the downturn in cattle numbers, there now exists an array of technologies currently available or emerging that offer the potential to expedite genetic progress, enhance efficiencies of production, and add value to beef cattle produced in the United States. As the US cattle industry moves to rebuild its declining numbers, the focus of much of the industry will turn to heifer retention and appropriate practices related to beef heifer development. Veterinarians can and should contribute to this process.

Dr Scott Poock, contributing author in this issue, encourages the veterinary community to consider opportunities related to incorporation of heifer development programs (scheduled vaccination programs; pre-breeding reproductive examinations, including reproductive tract scoring and pelvic measurement; estrous synchronization and artificial insemination; early pregnancy diagnosis with ultrasound, including fetal aging and fetal sexing, etc) into a veterinary practice. These services afford veterinarians the opportunity to interact with clients beyond pulling calves or treating sick animals. Collectively, these skills create avenues for veterinarians to become more actively involved in management and resulting profitability of beef cattle operations. Likewise, training of veterinary students will be enhanced by supporting students in developing these skills as part of the veterinary curriculum. Veterinary colleges will be well served by establishing a large enough client base (especially

Vet Clin Food Anim 29 (2013) xiii–xiv
http://dx.doi.org/10.1016/j.cvfa.2013.07.014
0749-0720/13/$ – see front matter © 2013 Published by Elsevier Inc.

vetfood.theclinics.com

given the increased class size at many of our nation's veterinary colleges) or through cooperative relationships, with progressive veterinary clinics in ways that expand training opportunities for students intent on serving the beef industry.

This issue provides a comprehensive overview of the various considerations involved with successful development of replacement beef heifers and is intended to serve as a resource for veterinarians to support beef producers in better managing their herds.

David J. Patterson, PhD
Division of Animal Sciences
132 Animal Sciences Research Center
920 East Campus Drive
University of Missouri
Columbia, MO 65211, USA

Michael F. Smith, PhD
Division of Animal Sciences
160A Animal Sciences Research Center
920 East Campus Drive
University of Missouri
Columbia, MO 65211, USA

E-mail addresses:
PattersonD@missouri.edu (D.J. Patterson)
smithmf@missouri.edu (M.F. Smith)

Rebuilding the US Beef Herd
Rethinking the Way Industry Develops Replacements

David J. Patterson, PhD[a],*, D. Scott Brown, PhD[b]

KEYWORDS

- Beef heifer development • Cattle inventory • Reproductive management

KEY POINTS

- The US beef industry finds itself confronted with a significant long-term decline in cattle numbers driven in part by record input costs and severe drought conditions in many of the nation's major cattle-producing states.
- Increased global competition in beef markets requires that US beef producers identify key strengths, recognize the intense global competition in producing beef on a commodity basis, and focus breeding programs directed to production of higher-quality beef products.
- Focus within the beef industry will turn to heifer retention and appropriate practices related to beef heifer development as the US cattle industry moves to rebuild numbers.
- Most factors related to reproductive performance in cattle are influenced almost entirely by management, because most components of fertility that influence calving and subsequent reproductive performance are not highly heritable.

INTRODUCTION

The US beef industry finds itself confronted with a significant long-term decline in cattle numbers driven in part by record input costs and severe drought conditions in many of the nation's major cattle-producing states. These recent challenges only add to long-term issues the industry has faced, which include an aging producer population, increased global competition, weak domestic demand for beef and increased competition from other meat proteins, and a perceived lack of economic incentives to expand the cattle herd.

Coincident with the downturn in cattle numbers, however, there now exist an array of technologies currently online or emerging that offer the potential to expedite genetic

Disclosures: The authors have nothing to disclose.
[a] Division of Animal Sciences, University of Missouri, Columbia, MO 65211, USA; [b] Department of Agricultural and Applied Economics, University of Missouri, Columbia, MO 65211, USA
* Corresponding author.
E-mail address: pattersond@missouri.edu

Vet Clin Food Anim 29 (2013) 469–477
http://dx.doi.org/10.1016/j.cvfa.2013.07.004
0749-0720/13/$ – see front matter © 2013 Elsevier Inc. All rights reserved.

progress, enhance efficiencies of production, and add value to beef cattle produced in the United States. Improvements in reproductive technologies have enabled beef producers to use artificial insemination without the need to detect estrus, existing and emerging genetic and genomic technologies enable beef producers to make more rapid strides toward improving the quality of beef they produce, and producers' ability to access and target individual marketing grids enable them to be rewarded for specific quality end points. As cattle prices and input costs increase, traits of efficiency and quality will become bigger drivers of profitability than ever before, and the commodity model of US beef production in all likelihood will no longer be viable.[1] Beef producers in the United States have the tools to maintain the country's ranking as the leading global supplier of high-quality beef. As US beef producers look to the future, the challenge most will face centers on determining which if any of these tools will be adopted and used to the extent that enables current and future generations to compete in a global arena, and if so, how effectively.

In comparison with other domestic livestock species produced and marketed in the United States, tradition and segmentation within the US cattle industry has hindered the adoption of newer production and marketing strategies. Coordinating the various industry segments (cow-calf, stocker, feed yard, processor) with allied industry (artificial insemination companies, seed stock suppliers, feed and pharmaceutical industries) offers the potential to enhance technology adoption and contribute to increases in production efficiency. As the US cattle industry moves to rebuild its declining numbers, the focus of much of the industry will turn to heifer retention and appropriate practices related to beef heifer development. Veterinarians can and should contribute to this process.

CURRENT SITUATION

Fig. 1 illustrates the significant decline in number of US beef cows in production, a decline that began in the mid-1970s.[2] The decline in cattle inventories during the 1980s and 1990s is equated by many in the industry to coincide with the period of extreme weakness in beef demand. The more recent acceleration in cattle inventory decline coincides with the difficult combination of drought and record feed prices. The weakness in beef demand provided the impetus for the industry to begin the

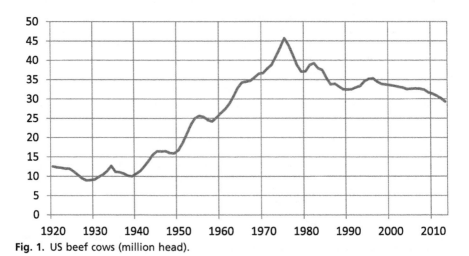

Fig. 1. US beef cows (million head).

Beef Quality Assurance program. Although the industry has experienced more consistency in beef products during the last three decades, there are major strides left to be made when today less than 5% of cattle grade prime.

Two factors are largely responsible for the lack of traction in increasing the industry trend of beef quality during the past three decades. First, market segmentation made it difficult for consumer signals asking for higher quality to reach cow-calf producers. The industry has provided better signal transmission to support the production of higher-quality beef through available marketing grids, yet these grids generally require cow-calf producers to maintain some ownership stake in their cattle through the feed yard.

Second, producers that invested in developing higher-quality cattle and beef often found genetic improvement to be slow and inconsistent, which often eliminated or reduced economic incentives for the quality focus. The technologies that came online over the past few years and new genomic advances on the horizon seem poised to rapidly increase genetic improvement and consistency. The combination of better market signals and incentives for higher-quality beef coupled with technologies that allow producers to more easily invest in genetics focused on quality provide the industry a unique opportunity to increase the cow herd with a more refined focus on the genetic potential of the herd as it relates to efficiency and higher quality. It seems these technologies have the added value of reducing producer risk by providing more consistency in the beef produced.

The decline in beef cow inventory was accelerated by an increase in cow slaughter and a decrease in beef heifer retention as illustrated in **Fig. 2**.[2] This figure calculates beef heifer retention by looking at the change in beef cow inventory each year, the amount of beef cow slaughter as reported by the US Department of Agriculture, and an assumed 2% death loss in beef cow inventory each year. As seen from this graph, nearly 7 million beef heifers entered the US cowherd in the mid-1970s, whereas in recent years it has dropped to roughly 3 million replacements based on recent US Department of Agriculture data. The opportunity for an increase in retention of beef heifers to exceed 5 million head remains a possibility as the herd attempts to recover

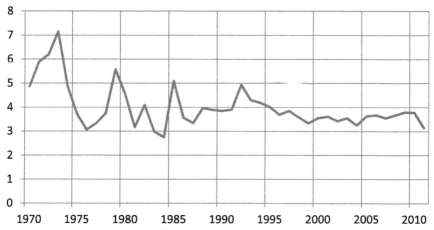

Fig. 2. US retained beef heifers (million head). (*Data from* United States Department of Agriculture, National Agricultural Statistics Service. Quick stats. Available at: http://quickstats. nass.usda.gov. Accessed May 20, 2013.)

from the long-term inventory decline. **Fig. 2** shows that nearly 5 million head of beef heifers were retained in years where beef cow inventories grew.

Long-term survival and prosperity of the US beef industry depends on its economic viability, which is best served by its competitiveness, profitability, and economic efficiency.[3] The effective management of an enterprise requires the fundamental ability to make informed decisions. A range of procedures are available to cow-calf producers to aid in reproductive management of replacement beef heifers and determine the outcome of a development program. These procedures, when viewed collectively as a "program," assist producers in more effectively managing reproduction in their herds.[4,5] Producers that use these procedures are able to use data generated on their own farms and with their own heifers to plan, execute, and accomplish reproductive, genetic, and economic goals for their herds. These procedures facilitate improvements in breeding performance of replacement heifers during the first breeding season and during subsequent calving and rebreeding periods as 2 year olds. Adoption of specific procedures for an operation depends on factors including current level of performance, availability of facilities and labor, and economic return. Not to be overlooked in this discussion includes services and procedures available through local veterinary practices that contribute to this process.

In recent years it was estimated that approximately 12% of beef heifers in the United States are purchased as bred replacements on an annual basis.[6] As the beef industry begins an expansion phase, this percentage will undoubtedly increase. One can assume that a very small percentage of either raised or purchased replacement heifers are "programmed" per se in terms of reproductive procedures currently available. The expertise to develop and market programmed heifers exists, but requires a team approach to managing heifers from the perspectives of health, nutrition, reproduction, genetics, and emerging management practices.[4,5]

Effecting change in reproductive management of the US cowherd requires a fundamental change in the approach to management procedures and development practices being used on heifers retained for breeding purposes.[4] A point has been reached concerning reproductive management of the nation's beef cow herd in which the tasks of development and transfer of technology must be emphasized equally and progress parallel to one another for the United States to maintain a strong beef cattle sector in the agricultural economy. Unless efforts are taken to implement change and incentives in the US beef cattle industry, many of the products of research and technology will be exported to more competitive international markets.[4,7]

As one looks to the future, increased global demand for beef stemming from an expanding middle class with a preference for beef and the means to afford it raises the question as to where higher-quality beef supplies will originate.[7] It is clear that the US beef industry faces growing challenges from major global competitors. The Brazilian beef industry, along with other international players, is investing heavily in the adoption of reproductive and genetic technologies to increase productivity in their countries. The challenge the US beef industry faces is whether educators, veterinarians, and beef producers in this country will optimize the transfer and adoption of technology that ensures the country's position as the global leader in the production of high-quality beef, or whether that role will be relinquished to more technically astute and competitively advantaged international players.[4,7]

Although cattle inventories have been in long-term decline, the effect on beef production has been muted as a result of an increase in the pounds of beef produced per beef cow as shown in **Fig. 3**.[2] Investment in development of technologies by the cattle industry over time has led to an increase in slaughter weights, reductions in death loss, and an increase in the number of calves produced per cow. To

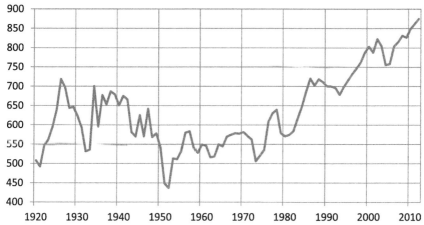

Fig. 3. US beef produced per beef cow (pounds, carcass weight basis). (*Data from* United States Department of Agriculture, National Agricultural Statistics Service. Quick stats. Available at: http://quickstats.nass.usda.gov. Accessed May 20, 2013.)

maintain this growth in economic efficiency, further adoption of technology is essential. The fixed overhead cost associated with the inventory of US beef cows is a critical component that must be managed when compared with other livestock industries. Technology that reduces the overhead per pound of beef produced provides the means for beef producers to compete more effectively with other livestock industries.

The beef industry must continue to recognize that one of the major areas of growth in consumption of US beef products lies outside the borders of the United States. As other countries experience economic growth and their consumers begin to realize income levels that allow for the purchase of higher-valued meat proteins, the United States is the source often turned to for higher-quality beef. The United States currently dominates this portion of the global beef market sees more competitors are entering the quality arena. The value of US beef exports is currently approaching $7 billion (**Fig. 4**).[8]

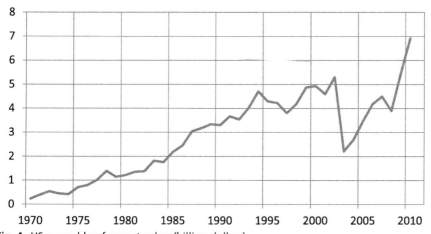

Fig. 4. US annual beef export value (billion dollars).

The role of the newer technologies in maintaining the US position in higher-quality international markets cannot be overlooked. High-quality US beef is in short supply. The ability as an industry to grow supplies of higher-quality beef products through the adoption of technology provides users of the technology with an insurance policy in terms of maintaining a competitive position in higher-quality international beef markets.

THE US BEEF INDUSTRY AND REPRODUCTIVE TECHNOLOGY

Table 1 provides a summary of the 700,000 beef operations in the United States with regard to herd size.[9] These statistics indicate that 90% of beef operations in the United States are involved with herds of less than 100 cows. However, the cumulative number of cows on these operations accounts for 46% of the total number of cows in production nationwide.

Larger-size herds make use of more of the technologies currently available.[9] There is also indication of regional differences in use of reproductive technologies in cow-calf herds. In general, operations in the East and South Central regions of the United States are less likely to use any reproductive procedures, because only 22% and 32% of operations in the East and South Central regions, respectively, use any of the reproductive procedures currently available including estrous synchronization, artificial insemination, pregnancy diagnosis, ultrasound, pelvic measurement, body condition scoring, semen evaluation, or embryo transfer. This compares with 55% of operations in the West and 49% of operations in the Central regions. Perhaps more troubling is that 55% of beef operations in the United States report having no defined breeding season, representing 34% or more than one-third of all beef cows in the United States.[10] The demographics of US beef production that include large numbers of operations with small numbers of cows in production, low adoption rates of technology, and failure to adopt technology because of limited time and labor point to an industry destined to concede its competitive position worldwide.[4]

Moving forward the veterinary community and allied industry will be required to take on larger roles in supporting beef producers in understanding the benefits of incorporating improved technologies into management schemes on the farm or ranch, and that benefits derived from these technologies outweigh their costs.[9]

DEVELOPING A PLAN FOR EXPANSION

As one considers beef production in broad terms, the reproductive phase of this production to consumption process is characterized by the breeding, conception, birth,

Table 1
Number of beef cow operations and herd size

	Number of Head			
	1–49	50–99	100–499	≥500
Percent of US beef operations				
By herd size	79.1	11.2	8.9	0.8
Percent of US beef cow				
Inventory by herd size	28.7	17.2	38	16.1

Percentages represent beef operations in the United States for 2007.
Data from NAHMS. Beef 2007-2008. Part II. Reference of cow-calf management practices in the United States. p. 50.

and early nurturing of an animal.[3] Increased weaning rate represents the greatest time-adjusted economic value to commercial cow-calf producers, simply because without a calf to sell no other characteristic has much meaning.[3] Reproductive failure or loss within a herd occurs primarily as a result of cows failing to become pregnant or the loss of calves at or near birth.[11,12] Puberty in the heifer and resumption of estrous cyclicity after calving in the postpartum cow are the critical reproductive events that determine if and when pregnancy occurs.

Production of forage and the reproductive process in beef cattle are cyclical events (**Fig. 5**).[13] The broad general categories that describe this cycle include developing the replacement heifer and rebreeding the lactating dam. Heifers bred to calve as 2 year olds should be exposed for breeding before mature herd mates and early calving periods can be used as a means of increasing production efficiency.[14] The timing of puberty is critical in determining whether a heifer remains in the herd and the extent to which lifetime productivity is achieved.[15]

In 1996 extension specialists, veterinarians, beef producers, and allied industry in Missouri linked arms to develop and implement a plan that would impact long-term sustainability of beef herds across the state. Their plan was focused on the aforementioned cyclical reproductive process and involves five basic steps:

1. Create an understanding of the importance of heifer development based on reproductive outcomes.
2. Implement changes in heifer development that will eventually spill over into the cow herd.
3. Emphasize the importance of reproductive management, which becomes apparent as changes are implemented.
4. Expand producer focus to genetic improvement.
5. Emphasize to participating herds that creation of a value-added product requires a re-evaluation of marketing strategies.

These five steps have built equity in herds that embraced the plan, and 16 years later the Missouri Show-Me-Select Replacement Heifer Program has impacted the cattle industry state wide. The program incorporates all available tools to support long-term health, reproduction, and genetic improvement of replacement beef heifers and includes provisions for ownership; health and vaccination schedules; parasite control; implant use; weight, pelvic measurement and reproductive tract score; estrous

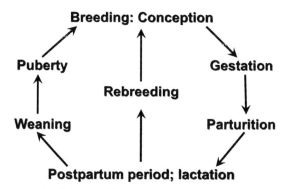

Fig. 5. Reproduction cycle of the beef female. (*Adapted from* Bellows RA. Physiologic relationships that limit production of range beef cattle. In: Achieving efficient use of rangeland resources. Fort Keogh Research Symposium. Proc. Miles City (MT): 1987. p. 50–3.)

synchronization and artificial insemination; service-sire requirements for BW- or CE-EPD; and early pregnancy diagnosis, fetal aging, fetal sexing, and body condition score.[5]

As beef producers in the United States move to expand numbers, veterinarians are positioned to play a key role in the process of rebuilding the US cowherd. Veterinary practitioners are critical components in the implementation of the five-point plan previously described. Veterinarians serve as a key information source for US beef producers and are essential in facilitating the adoption of reproductive procedures.[16] Just over one-half (53%) of beef operations in the United States cited their veterinarian as a "very important" source of information for their cow-calf operation including health, breeding and genetics, nutrition, or questions pertaining to production or management.

On-farm development programs that involve local veterinarians, state, regional, or county livestock specialists, and individual farm and ranch operators provide the structure from which change within the industry can occur.[5] In these programs evaluation has an impact in itself, because meaningful assessment of these programs builds in evaluation as part of the design. Data collection is part of the delivery process and reinforces the development of sound management practices on individual farms and ranches regardless of their size.[17] Producers use data generated on their own farms or ranches to focus on action alternatives based on the data that are generated. Methods flow from issues through a "program" that involves veterinarians, livestock specialists, beef producers, and allied industry.

This issue provides a comprehensive overview of the various considerations involved with successful development of replacement beef heifers. The articles that follow are intended to serve as a resource for veterinarians to support beef producers in better managing their herds and to rethink the way in which heifers are developed as they enter herds across the United States.

REFERENCES

1. Marshall T. The quality revolution awakens. In: Beef Cow Calf Weekly. 2011.
2. United States Department of Agriculture, National Agricultural Statistics Service. Quick stats. Available at: http://quickstats.nass.usda.gov. Accessed May 20, 2013.
3. Melton BE. Conception to consumption: the economics of genetic improvement. In: Proceedings of the Beef Improvement Federation. Sheridan (WY): 1995. p. 40–87.
4. Patterson DJ, Wood SL, Randle RF. Procedures that support reproductive management of replacement beef heifers. Proc Am Soc Anim Sci 1999. Available at: http://www.asas.org/jas/symposia/proceedings/0902.pdf. Accessed August 3, 2000.
5. Patterson DJ, Mallory DA, Parcell JL, et al. The Missouri Show-Me-Select Replacement Heifer Program. In: Proceedings, Applied Reproductive Strategies in Beef Cattle. August 31–September 1. Joplin (MO): 2011. p. 237–51.
6. NAHMS. Part IV. Changes in the U. S. beef cow-calf industry, 1993-1997. 1998; p. 1–48.
7. Pohler KG, Mallory DA, Patterson DJ, et al. Reproductive technology and global production of beef: Why beef producers in the US need to pay attention. In: Proceedings, Applied Reproductive Strategies in Beef Cattle. August 31–September 1. Joplin (MO): 2011. p. 379–96.
8. United States Department of Agriculture, Foreign Agriculture Service. Global Ag. Trade Atlas (GATS). Available at: http://www.fas.usda.gov/gats/ExpressQuery1.aspx. Accessed May 20, 2013.

9. NAHMS. Beef 2007-2008. Part II. Reference of cow-calf management practices in the United States. p. 1–122.
10. NAHMSb. Beef 2007-2008. Part III. Changes in the U.S. beef cow-calf industry, 1993-2008. p. 1–79.
11. Wiltbank JN. Challenges for improving calf crop. In: Proceedings of the 39th Annual Beef Cattle Short Course. Gainesville (FL): University of Florida; 1990. p. 1–22.
12. Bellows RA, Short RE. Reproductive losses in the beef industry. In: Proceedings of the 39th Annual Beef Cattle Short Course. Gainesville (FL): University of Florida; 1990. p. 109–33.
13. Bellows RA. Physiological relationships that limit production of range beef cattle. In: Achieving efficient use of rangeland resources. USDA-ARS Fort Keogh Research Symposium. Proc. Miles City (MT): 1987. p. 50–3.
14. Wiltbank JN. Research needs in beef cattle reproduction. J Anim Sci 1970;31:755–62.
15. Patterson DJ, Perry RC, Kiracofe GH, et al. Management considerations in heifer development and puberty. J Anim Sci 1992;70:4018–35.
16. APHIS. U. S. beef cow-calf producers' consultation with veterinarians and use of other sources of information. 2011. Available at: http://www.aphis.usda.gov/animal_health/nahms/beefcowcalf/downloads/beef0708/Beef0708_is_InfmSources.pdf.
17. Randle RF. The Missouri Show-Me-Select Replacement Heifer Program: production summary from the first two years. In: Proc. reproductive tools and techniques. Columbia (MO): University of Missouri; 1999. p. 1–9.

Physiology and Endocrinology of Puberty in Heifers

Jacqueline A. Atkins, PhD[a,b], Ky G. Pohler, MS[c],
Michael F. Smith, PhD[c],*

KEYWORDS

- Heifer • Puberty • Physiology • Endocrinology

KEY POINTS

- Puberty is defined as the first ovulatory estrus and should not be confused with nonpubertal estrus (estrus not followed by a luteal phase) or an ovulation without estrus (ie, silent ovulation), which normally occurs before the pubertal estrus.
- The pubertal estrus is preceded by a progressive increase in uterine development, length of follicular waves, and size of the dominant follicle.
- A reproductive tract score is a subjective measurement of pubertal development that is performed 4 to 6 weeks before breeding and can be used to determine whether heifers are good candidates for an estrous synchronization program.
- Onset of puberty is preceded by a progressive decrease in the sensitivity of the hypothalamic/anterior pituitary axis to the negative feedback of estradiol.
- The pubertal estrus is preceded by a silent ovulation followed by a short luteal phase. Progestin treatment (eg, MGA or CIDR) during the peripubertal period can induce the establishment of normal estrous cycles in a large proportion of heifers.

INTRODUCTION

When it comes to development of beef heifers, the importance of maximizing the proportion of heifers that are born early in the calving season cannot be overemphasized. Data from the University of Nebraska reported that heifers born during the first 20 days compared with the second or third 20 days of the calving season had greater weaning weights, prebreeding weights, and precalving weights; more heifers cycling by the start of the breeding season; and higher pregnancy rates.[1,2] Breeding heifers to calve at 2 years of age is generally thought not to be a problem for *Bos taurus* breeds.

The authors have nothing to disclose.
[a] Progenesis Embryo Transfer, 4990 E Baseline Rd, Belgrade, MT 59714, USA; [b] American Simmental Association, 1 Simmental Way, Bozeman, MT 59715, USA; [c] Division of Animal Sciences, Laboratory 160, ASRC, University of Missouri, 920 East Campus Drive, Columbia, MO 65211, USA
* Corresponding author.
E-mail address: smithmf@missouri.edu

However, when you consider that the breeding season for heifers frequently begins 2 to 3 weeks before the cows and that the fertility of heifers bred at their pubertal estrus is 15% lower than the third estrus,[3] heifers need to reach puberty at least 6 to 10 weeks before you begin breeding the cows to increase the proportion of heifers that conceive early. Because early onset of puberty is of critical importance to heifer development, the purpose of this article is to describe the physiological and endocrine maturation that controls the onset of puberty in beef cattle. These concepts will be helpful in understanding the physiological (eg, uterine and ovarian development) and endocrine (eg, decrease in negative feedback of estradiol) changes that take place in a heifer as she approaches puberty and in understanding how specific estrous synchronization products (eg, progestins) are able to induce and synchronize estrus and ovulation in heifers.

DEFINITION OF PUBERTY

The onset of puberty coincides with the first opportunity for a heifer to conceive and should be defined as the first ovulatory estrus followed by a luteal phase of normal duration. Although the pubertal estrus is the first opportunity for a heifer to conceive, fertility is not optimal at this time.[3] It is important to remember that expression of estrus and ovulation can occur independently in peripubertal heifers. Ovulation without expression of estrus normally occurs 7 to 10 days before the first ovulatory estrus and secretion of progesterone during the short luteal phase following the first ovulation is important for establishing normal estrous cycles (discussed later in this article). In addition, it is not uncommon for heifers to display a nonpubertal estrus, which is defined as standing estrus without subsequent luteal function.[4] The incidence of nonpubertal estrus can vary from 17% to 63%,[4,5] and the mechanisms associated with nonpubertal estrus are not known. Expression of nonpubertal estrus can be affected by breed, age, season, or photoperiod.[4] Detection of estrus should not be the only criterion for establishing the onset of puberty in heifers.

PHYSIOLOGICAL CHANGES IN REPRODUCTIVE ORGANS

Although sexual differentiation begins during fetal life, development of the reproductive organs (eg, uterus) continues well after the pubertal estrus. The following sections briefly describe the physiological changes in the uterus and ovaries, as well as a management tool (reproductive tract score [RTS]) that can be used to assess the sexual maturity of a heifer before the first breeding season.

UTERINE GROWTH

The diameter of the uterus increases rapidly from 2 to 10 weeks of age (from 9 to 14 mm), then continues to grow more slowly until 24 weeks of age (16 mm), at which time uterine diameter plateaus.[6] The uterine diameter begins to increase again from 32 to 60 weeks of age (up to 21 mm). This biphasic growth pattern has a strong positive correlation with the size of the largest follicle,[6] suggesting that increased estradiol from the larger follicles drives the growth and development of the uterus. The length and weight of the uterus increase from birth (7.7 cm and 6 g, respectively) to 12 months of age (24.3 cm and 150 g, respectively).[7] There is a rapid increase in uterine weight, RNA, and protein content after 6 months of age in heifers, but the amount of DNA (suggesting number of cells) remains unchanged.[7] The uterine weight, RNA, and protein content reaches a plateau after 10 months of age, which may mark the end of the rapid prepubertal development of the uterus. Uterine glands were detected after 5 months of age and the glands became progressively larger after 6 months. Uterine glands, which produce histotroph for early embryonic development, were detected after 5 months of age and the glands became progressively larger after 6 months. However, uterine gland development was inhibited by 65% in heifers that received implants containing progesterone and estradiol at birth[8] and administration of growth-promoting implants between birth and 30 days of age decreased pregnancy rates in heifers during the first breeding season (see section on RTSs for more information[9]).

OVARIAN DEVELOPMENT

Desjardins and Hafs[7] reported a period of rapid increase in ovarian weight during the first 5 months in heifers followed by a plateau until 8 months and a resumption of growth (although not as rapid) until 12 months of age. Honaramooz and colleagues[6] also reported a biphasic pattern of growth for ovarian diameter and length. The length and diameter increased from 2 to 14 weeks of age and the length grew again from 34 to 60 weeks while the diameter increased from 30 to 44 weeks of age.

During the first 2 or 3 months of age, there is an increase in the number of follicles greater than or equal to 3 mm present on the ovaries followed by little change in the number of total antral follicles.[6,7,10] The size of the follicles and number of large antral follicles increases as heifers mature (see the section on follicle waves later in this article). In B taurus cattle, there is a positive correlation between the ovarian reserve (total number of follicles) and antral follicle count.[11,12] In addition, antral follicle count ($\geq$3 mm) is repeatable within an animal but highly variable among animals.[13] Factors affecting antral follicle count are not clear; however, there is evidence to support an effect of the maternal environment. Heifers born to dams that were restricted to 60% of maintenance requirements during the first trimester had an antral follicle count that was 60% lower than heifers born to dams receiving 100% of their maintenance requirements.[13] Therefore, antral follicle count in heifers may be affected by maternal nutrition during gestation.

Antral follicle count has been positively associated with fertility in B taurus cattle.[14,15] For example, heifers with a low antral follicle count (<15 antral follicles) had a lower pregnancy rate at the end of the breeding season compared with heifers with a high antral follicle count (>25 antral follicles).[14] Furthermore, pregnancy rates of in vitro–produced (IVP) embryos were increased when oocytes were recovered from calves with larger pools of follicles (before gonadotropin stimulation).[16] In the future, antral follicle count, as measured by ultrasonography, may be incorporated into the reproductive tract scoring system (see later in this article) and become an additional criterion for selecting replacement heifers before the breeding season or selecting juvenile donor calves for IVP embryos.

Follicular Waves

Early studies in cattle described cyclical growth of antral follicles and noted the presence of a large follicle inhibited the growth of subordinate follicles.[17,18] In the late 1980s, the use of transrectal ultrasonography expanded our understanding of follicular waves (**Fig. 1**).[19–23] The first stage of a follicular wave is recruitment. At recruitment, a cohort of small follicles (4–6 mm in diameter) begin their final growth. Recruitment is initiated by a transient rise in follicle-stimulating hormone (FSH)[24] and the recruited follicles are dependent on gonadotropins for survival. The second stage of a follicular wave is selection, which occurs approximately 36 to 48 hours after the initiation of recruitment. The recruited cohort of follicles secrete estradiol and inhibin, which in turn decrease the circulating concentrations of FSH. During selection, one follicle

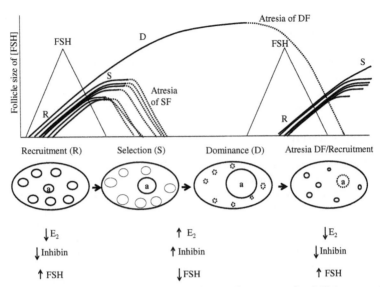

Fig. 1. Diagram of changes in follicle growth during the stages of a follicle wave. Recruitment is initiated by a transient rise in FSH. Increased estradiol (E_2) and inhibin from the recruited follicles causes a reduction in concentrations of FSH. During selection, one follicle has a competitive advantage (*bold line*) over the subordinate follicles (SF). The selected follicle acquires LH receptors in the granulosa cells and more free IGF-1, both of which make the selected follicle capable of producing E_2 and inhibin in a low-FSH environment. During dominance, the SF are atretic (*dotted line*) while the dominant follicle (DF, *bold line*) continues to grow. While healthy, the DF secretes E_2 and inhibin, which keeps FSH at nadir levels and prevents initiation of a new wave. In the absence of an LH surge, the DF eventually becomes atretic (*dotted line*). Once atretic, concentrations of E_2 and inhibin drop, FSH increases, followed by the emergence of the next follicular wave (represented by the *double-lined circles*).

becomes larger than the others in the cohort. The selected follicle is equipped to survive in a low FSH environment, whereas the subordinate follicles are not. The third stage of a follicle wave is dominance and is characterized by the growth of typically one large follicle and atresia of the subordinate follicles. The dominant follicle suppresses FSH, and the gonadotropin-dependent subordinate follicles become atretic. The dominant follicle grows approximately 1 to 2 mm per day[21,22] until reaching its maximum diameter of 10 to 20 mm.[20,22,25,26] In cycling cattle, the dominant follicle will either ovulate in the absence of a corpus luteum (CL) or become atretic during the luteal phase of the cycle. Typically, *B taurus* cows have 2 or 3 waves per cycle but *Bos indicus* cattle frequently have 4 waves.[27]

Heifer calves as young as 2 weeks old have follicles that mature and grow in periodic patterns similar to the follicular waves of adult cows.[10] Similar to cycling cows, recruitment of follicles is preceded with a rise in FSH.[10] The positive feedback mechanism between estradiol and luteinizing hormone (LH), which leads to an LH surge and ovulation in cycling cows is not established in prepubertal heifers (see endocrinology section later in this article). Therefore, the dominant follicle becomes atretic and a new follicular wave emerges. The maximum diameter of the dominant follicle[6,10,28] and the duration of dominance[10,29] increase as heifers mature (reviewed in Ref.[30]). This poses a challenge when synchronizing follicular waves in heifers as the period of time when a dominant follicle can be induced to ovulate with exogenous gonadotropin-releasing hormone (GnRH) agonists is shorter in heifers than cows. Pre-synchronization of heifers to be in the early part of the estrous cycle at the beginning of a GnRH-PGF$_{2\alpha}$-GnRH synchronization system is one way to improve the proportion of heifers able to respond to the initial GnRH injection.

Oocyte Competence

Using in vitro technologies, it is possible for an oocyte from calves as young as 2 months of age to be fertilized, form an embryo, and when transferred into a recipient, result in the birth of a live calf.[16] This process is less efficient using calf oocytes compared with oocytes from adult cows[31] (reviewed in Ref.[32]); however, using heifer calves as oocyte donors offers an opportunity to decrease generation interval and use the large pool of follicles present after birth that become atretic before puberty. Therefore, there is a large research focus aimed at understanding the competence of calf oocytes and overcoming inefficiencies of IVP embryos from prepubertal donors.

Oocytes from calves are smaller, have thinner zonae pellucidae, exhibit delayed migration and redistribution of the cortical granules, have abnormal chromatin and microtubule configurations, and irregular calcium oscillations (an important second messenger during fertilization) compared with cows. Calf oocytes have different protein and metabolic profiles compared with cow oocytes, and the machinery for oocyte activation is compromised in calf oocytes.[32] Given the previous list of abnormalities and strong evidence from nuclear transfer experiments,[33] it is commonly argued that the cytoplasm of calf oocytes is inadequately developed. A study using prepubertal lamb oocytes suggests that prepubertal oocytes also have nuclear immaturities[34] and the investigators caution against a conclusion of simply cytoplasmic problems associated with juvenile oocyte donors.

Another research area in juvenile oocyte retrieval aims to understand the gonadotropin stimulation in prepubertal heifers. Gonadotropin stimulation before oocyte recovery improved embryo production with oocytes from 5-month-old, 7-month-old, and 9-month-old heifers compared with age-matched heifers with no stimulation; however, embryo development was similar in oocytes from 11-month-old heifers regardless of gonadotropin stimulation before oocyte retrieval.[35] This suggests that younger heifers require gonadotropin support before oocyte retrieval, not only to improve the number of oocytes collected but also to improve the ability of the oocyte to result in an embryo capable of transfer.

Short Luteal Phase

Heifers often have a short luteal phase preceding the onset of puberty,[36–38] similar to short luteal phases observed in postpartum cows.[39] In the late 1970s, research groups noticed a rise in progesterone before the first estrous cycle that was shorter than a normal luteal phase.[36,37] Berardinelli and colleagues[37] reported the rise in progesterone is from luteal tissue that was not palpable or visible by gross inspection but detected after microscopic examination of the ovary. During the short luteal phase, there is a premature release of the uterine luteolytic agent, prostaglandin F$_{2\alpha}$ (PGF$_{2\alpha}$), causing premature luteal regression (reviewed in Ref.[40]).

The short luteal phase preceding puberty has an important biologic role in the timing of luteal regression for the next cycle. Should a heifer conceive but have an early release of PGF$_{2\alpha}$, the embryo secretion of interferon τ (the signal for maternal recognition of pregnancy in cattle) will not be able to prevent luteolysis and the pregnancy will fail. A period of progesterone followed by a rise in estradiol is necessary for the appropriate timing of PGF$_{2\alpha}$ release from the uterus for a normal luteal life span during the subsequent cycle.[41] Therefore, it is important to include a progestin source in synchronization systems designed for peripubertal heifers not only to induce cyclicity but also to establish the timing for $PGF_{2\alpha}$ release during the period of maternal recognition of pregnancy.

RTS: A SUBJECTIVE ASSESSMENT OF PUBERTAL DEVELOPMENT

An RTS is a subjective measurement of the sexual maturity of a heifer that is normally performed approximately 4 to 6 weeks before the breeding season, a convenient time to administer prebreeding vaccinations. The score is obtained by palpation per rectum of the uterus and ovaries and is based on the degree of uterine development and ovarian status (size of dominant follicle and presence or absence of a CL). Each heifer is assigned a score of 1 to 5 and the uterine and ovarian dimensions for each of the RTSs are described in **Table 1**.[42] An RTS of 1 refers to a prepubertal heifer that has an infantile tract, based on small uterine horns that have no tone and very little follicular development. A heifer with an RTS of 2 is closer to puberty than one with an RTS of 1 based on larger uterine horns and more ovarian activity. A heifer with an RTS of 3 has larger uterine horns and ovaries than a heifer with an RTS of 2 and is relatively close to reaching puberty. A heifer assigned an RTS of 4 is considered to have reached puberty based on size and tone of the uterine horns (horns are frequently coiled and have a lot of tone) and the presence of a preovulatory-size follicle. Some heifers assigned an RTS of 4 may have a CL that is not easily detectable by palpation per rectum. A heifer with an RTS of 5 is similar to a heifer with an RTS of 4 except for the presence of a palpable CL. RTSs were reported to be an accurate assessment of pubertal status and were repeatable within and between veterinarians.[43] In addition, RTS was positively associated with pregnancy rate during a 50-day artificial insemination (AI) season and with pregnancy rate during the subsequent breeding season and negatively associated with days to calving.[44] A general recommendation is that a minimum of 50% of heifers should have an RTS of 4 or more approximately 6 weeks before the start of breeding. Therefore, RTS is a good predictor of the pubertal status of a heifer and of a heifer's response to an estrous synchronization protocol.

Growth-promoting implants are extensively used during various stages of beef production and normally contain anabolic agents, such as estrogen or zeranol, progesterone, or a synthetic androgen (eg, trenbolone acetate). As previously mentioned,[9]

			Ovarian	Ovarian	Ovarian	
RTS	Classification	Uterine Horn Diameter (mm)	Length (mm)	Height (mm)	Width (mm)	Ovarian Structures
1	Prepubertal	<20 mm, no tone	15	10	8	No palpable follicles
2	Prepubertal	20–25 mm, no tone	18	12	10	8-mm follicles
3	Peripubertal	20–25 mm, slight tone	22	15	10	8–10-mm follicles
4	Pubertal	30 mm, good tone	30	16	12	>10-mm follicles, CL possible
5	Pubertal	>30 mm	>32	20	15	CL present

Table 1
Uterine and ovarian measurements and descriptions for reproductive tract scores

Data from Holm DE, Thompson PN, Irons PC. The value of reproductive tract scoring as a predictor of fertility and production outcomes in beef heifers. J Anim Sci 2009;87:1935.

treatment of heifers with growth-promoting implants during the neonatal period decreased pregnancy rates during the first breeding season.[9] A study was conducted to examine the effect of a growth-promoting implant (Synovex-C [Zoetis, New Jersey]; contains estradiol and progesterone) on uterine development in neonatal heifers.[8] Heifers that received a Synovex-C implant at birth, day 21, or day 45 had decreased uterocervical weight, myometrial area, endometrial area, and uterine gland density (**Table 2**).[8] Although this study did not measure the fertility of heifers that received Synovex-C during the neonatal period, the dramatic effects on the uterine histoarchitecture, including uterine gland density, suggest that the contributions of uterine tissues and secretions for conceptus development would be compromised. The preceding results are relevant to RTS because the effect of growth-promoting implants on uterine development can frequently be detected via palpation per rectum. Although, the RTS system is a valuable tool for identifying heifers that are ready for the breeding season and good candidates for an estrous synchronization protocol, just over 1% of producers use this management tool.

ENDOCRINE REGULATION OF PUBERTY

During the follicular phase in a cycling cow, estradiol secretion from the dominant follicle stimulates (indirectly) GnRH secretion from the hypothalamus, which causes release of gonadotropins (LH and FSH) from the pituitary. These gonadotropins drive follicle growth, which increases estradiol production and establishes a positive feedback loop among the ovary, hypothalamus, and pituitary (hypothalamic-pituitary-ovarian [HPO] axis). The positive feedback loop culminates in an LH surge, which initiates the cascade of events leading to ovulation and luteinization of the dominant follicle. Given the appropriate stimulus or removal of inhibition, each component of the HPO axis is capable of responding in prepubertal heifers months before the onset of puberty (reviewed in Refs.[38,45,46]). The following section discusses the endocrine development of the HPO axis, including the gonadadostat hypothesis and key changes in the hypothalamus and pituitary.

Table 2
Effects of neonatal exposure to progesterone and estradiol on reproductive tract development of adult beef heifers

Response[a]	Birth	Neonatal Age at Treatment[b] Day 21	Day 45	Control
Uterocervical weight[c] (g)	113.7[d]	123.5[d]	101.3[d]	173.9[e]
Myometrial area (mm²)	123.7[f]	141.8[f]	111.3[f]	162.8[g]
Endometrial area (mm²)	29.9[h]	32.4[h]	37.7[h]	45.4[i]
Gland density (hits/mm²)	172.2[d]	380.3[e]	328.2[e]	486.9[j]
Uterine luminal protein content (mg/flush)	2.8[d]	2.9[d]	2.3[d]	4.9[e]

[a] Treated heifers received a single Synovex-C implant containing progesterone (100 mg) and estradiol benzoate (10 mg). Implants were placed (subcutaneously) on the designated day of neonatal life. Control heifers were untreated.
[b] Data were collected from cyclic adult heifers on day 12 of an induced estrous cycle.
[c] Wet weight.
[d,e,f,g,h,i,j] Means within a row with different superscripts differ (P<.05).
   Data from Bartol FF, Johnson LL, Floyd JG, et al. Neonatal exposure to progesterone and estradiol alters uterine morphology and luminal protein content in adult beef heifers. Theriogenology 1995;43:835–4.

GONADOSTAT HYPOTHESIS

The gonadostat hypothesis[47] suggests an initial inhibitory effect of estradiol on gonadotropin secretion followed by a gradual decrease in the negative effect of estradiol (**Fig. 2**). The decreased sensitivity to estradiol allows for increased gonadotropin secretion, increased follicle growth, increased estradiol concentrations, and eventually an LH surge and ovulation. Although the gonadostat hypothesis may not apply to all animals, it has been supported in the heifer (reviewed in Refs.[38,46,48]). The shift of estradiol feedback on the hypothalamus and pituitary from strongly negative, to less negative, to positive around the time of puberty is discussed in more detail in the following section.

HYPOTHALAMUS

The hypothalamus is the last component in the HPO axis to mature in the prepubertal heifer.[38] If given the appropriate stimulus, juvenile heifers are capable of releasing GnRH in adequate quantities to release gonadotropins and cause ovulation of a follicle and formation of luteal tissue.[38] During the peripubertal time, reduced sensitivity of

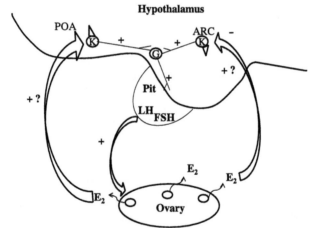

	Pre-pubertal	Peri-pubertal	Peri-pubertal	Pubertal
Hypothalamus ER	High	Medium	Low	Varies
E$_2$ feedback on LH	Strongly negative	Less Negative	Less negative	Positive
LH secretion	Low pulse frequency	Increasing pulse frequency	Increasing pulse frequency	LH surge
[E$_2$]	Low	Low	Medium	High
[Kisspeptin]	Low	Low	Medium	High
Sensitivity of GnRH to kisspeptin	Low	Low	Medium	High
Reproductive tract score	1	2	3	4 or 5

Fig. 2. Theoretical HPO axis and endocrine changes from peripuberty to prepuberty to puberty in heifers. Estradiol (E$_2$) from ovarian follicles binds to its receptor (ER, *triangles*) and may have a negative effect on kisspeptin-secreting neurons (K) in the ARC of the hypothalamus. As heifers approach puberty, the number of ERs in the hypothalamus decreases, which could increase kisspeptin secretion and stimulate GnRH-secreting neurons (G). The GnRH causes the release of LH and FSH from the gonadotroph cells of the pituitary (Pit). The gonadotropins stimulate ovarian follicle growth and E$_2$ production. At the time of puberty, the surge center is also established, which allows for a positive feedback loop between E$_2$, GnRH, and LH/FSH, possibly through special kisspeptin-secreting neurons in the ARC or the POA. (*Data from* Day ML, Anderson LH. Current concepts on the control of puberty in cattle. J Anim Sci 1998;76(S3):1–15.)

GnRH neurons to the negative inhibition of estradiol causes an increase in GnRH pulses followed by an increase in LH pulse frequency (reviewed in Refs.[38,46]). The amount of GnRH present in the hypothalamus does not change during maturation.[38] Morphologic changes in GnRH neurons have been reported in the pubertal rabbit, rat, and hamster, as well as postpartum cows during the resumption of cyclicity (reviewed in Ref.[46]) but no morphologic changes were detected in GnRH neurons of the developing heifer (from 7 to 11 months).[49] Changes in estrogen receptor (ER) and kisspeptin, a relatively new player in the HPO axis, help explain the final maturation of the hypothalamus before puberty.

Estradiol Receptors

The inhibitory effect of estradiol on GnRH secretion is indirect as GnRH containing neurons do not have ER.[50] Neurons with ER are found in several regions of the hypothalamus, including the medial preoptic area (MPOA), anterior hypothalamus (AH), ventrolateral septum, bed nucleus of the stria terminalis, ventromedial hypothalamus (VMN), and the arcuate nucleus (ARC, reviewed in Ref.[46]). Day and others[51] reported a decrease in ER-positive neurons in the AH and the medial basal hypothalamus (MBH) leading up to puberty and this decline was associated with an increase in LH pulse frequency. The investigators argue the decrease in ER receptors may explain the reduced sensitivity to estradiol and thus increase in GnRH and LH secretion. Heifers treated with progesterone to induce puberty had decreased numbers of ER-positive neurons in the MPOA, AH, and VMN and increased LH pulse frequency.[49] Furthermore, there was a negative correlation between the number of ER-positive neurons and LH secretion.

Kisspeptin

Within the past 10 years, kisspeptin has emerged as a likely mediator between steroids and GnRH secretion. Since the link between kisspeptin and reproduction was first reported,[52,53] research into kisspeptin has been extensive in multiple species, including mice, rats, hamsters, sheep, monkeys, and humans. As the scope of kisspeptin research in cattle has been limited, this section reviews kisspeptin's role in puberty in multiple species with the understanding that the information may not apply directly to cattle. Kisspeptin is a potent stimulator of GnRH secretions (reviewed in Refs.[54,55]) acting directly on GnRH neurons.[56-59] There is strong evidence of steroid control of kisspeptin and a role of kisspeptin in the onset of puberty in many species using a variety of models summarized in **Box 1**.

PITUITARY

Heifers as young as 1 month of age begin to secrete LH in pulses.[60] During the first 3 months of age, mean serum concentrations of LH and, to a lesser extent, FSH, increase in the heifer calf.[61] The increase in gonadotropins is thought to stimulate the growing follicle pools, which in turn increase estradiol production. The increase in circulating concentrations of estradiol coupled with increased (negative) hypothalamic sensitivity to estradiol results in the inhibition of GnRH neurons and decreased gonadotropin secretion. Thus, circulating concentrations of gonadotropins drop to basal levels until the peripubertal rise (50–120 days before puberty; reviewed in Ref.[38]). During the peripubertal time, the negative effect of estradiol on GnRH secretion dampens, and the frequency of LH pulses increases (up to 1 pulse/hour by the first ovulation).[51] The increase in LH pulse frequency is the major signal needed for the first ovulation.

Box 1
Evidence for steroidal control of kisspeptin and kisspeptin's role in puberty

Steroidal Control	Controlling Onset of Puberty
• There are gender differences in kisspeptin expression as well as temporal differences during seasonal anestrous and estrous and menstrual cycles.	• Administration of kisspeptin shortened the time to puberty in mice and the use of kisspeptin antagonists delayed puberty in rats.
• In all species studied to date, the ARC (an important site for negative steroidal control of GnRH) contains large numbers of kisspeptin neurons, most of which contain ERα (93% in the sheep).	• Both male and female mice and monkeys had an increase in hypothalamic *kiss1* expression at the time of puberty
• Ovariectomy increases mRNA expression of the kisspeptin gene, *kiss1*, in the ARC and estradiol replacement returns *kiss1* levels to that of control animals.	• The number of kisspeptin immunoreactive fibers associated with GnRH neurons increased after puberty.
• In the ewe, subpopulations of neurons in the ARC and preoptic area are thought to control estradiol's positive feedback on GnRH contain kisspeptins.	• The sensitivity of GnRH neurons to kisspeptin increased after puberty.

Data from Refs.[54,57,59,68–70]

Pituitary GnRH receptors do not change with puberty,[51] and the pituitary is capable of secreting gonadotropins in response to GnRH in heifers as young as 1 month of age.[61] The pituitary has adequate stores of LH and FSH[62] and the amount of LH and FSH released after GnRH stimulus increases with age.[61] The ability of a heifer to have an LH surge in response to external stimulus is established between 3 and 5 months of age.[63] These points support the theory that the pituitary is capable of synthesizing and releasing gonadotropins to promote follicle growth and induce ovulation before puberty, but GnRH secretion is limited by estradiol negative feedback.

PHYSIOLOGIC DIFFERENCES BETWEEN *B INDICUS* AND *B TAURUS* HEIFERS

Genetic makeup is a primary factor affecting the age at puberty in heifers. In general, *B indicus* heifers attain puberty at an older age compared with *B taurus* heifers,[64] and a contributing factor may be the lack of selection pressure on early age at puberty in *B indicus* heifers.[65] *B indicus* heifers have more visible follicles on the ovary,[66] decreased size of the dominant follicle,[67] and decreased ovulation rates[66] compared with *B taurus* and Holstein heifers. In Nelore (*B indicus*) heifers, the proportion of follicles having a diameter of 7.0 to 8.4, 8.5 to 10, and larger than 10 mm that were induced to ovulate in response to exogenous LH heifers was 33.3%, 80.0%, and 90.0%, respectively.[67] Consequently, *B indicus* heifers acquire ovulatory capacity at a smaller diameter compared with *B taurus* females. In general, estrous synchronization protocols that have proven to be effective in *B taurus* heifers are not necessarily transferable to *B indicus* heifers. Although the reason(s) for this observation are not clear, many speculate that *B indicus* females may metabolize exogenous hormones more slowly compared with *B taurus* females. Treating *B indicus* and *B taurus* heifers with a progesterone intravaginal device resulted in *B indicus* heifers having higher circulating concentrations of progesterone independent of body weight.[66] In conclusion, there are physiologic and endocrinologic differences between *B indicus* and *B taurus* heifers that may explain some of the differences in age at puberty and in response to specific estrous synchronization protocols.

SUMMARY

During the peripubertal period, expression of estrus and ovulation can occur independently. Therefore, puberty is defined as the first ovulatory estrus and should not be confused with nonpubertal estrus or an ovulation without estrus. During the prepubertal and peripubertal periods, there is a progressive increase in uterine development and an increase in both the length of follicular waves and size of the dominant follicle associated with a follicular wave. A gradual decrease in the sensitivity of the hypothalamic/anterior pituitary axis to the negative feedback of estradiol occurs during the 50 days preceding the pubertal estrus. In addition, the pubertal estrus is preceded by an ovulation, not accompanied by estrus, that results in a short luteal phase. An RTS is a subjective measurement of the changes in uterine development and ovarian activity that occur before and around the time of puberty. RTS is performed 4 to 6 weeks before breeding and can be used to determine the pubertal status of heifers and whether they are good candidates for an estrous synchronization program.

REFERENCES

1. Larson DM, Funston RN. Estrous synchronization increases early calving frequency, which enhances steer progeny value. In: Proceedings from Western Section American Society of Animal Science. Ft Collins (CO): 2009;60. p. 72–5.
2. Funston RN, Musgrave JA, Meyer TL, et al. Effect of calving period on ADG, reproduction, and first calf characteristics of heifer progeny. In: Proceedings from Western Section American Society of Animal Science. Miles City (MT): 2011;62. p. 231–3.
3. Byerley DJ, Staigmiller RB, Berardinelli JG, et al. Pregnancy rates of beef heifers bred either on pubertal or third estrus. J Anim Sci 1987;65:645–50.
4. Nelson TC, Short RE, Phelps DA. Nonpuberal estrus and mature cow influences on growth and puberty in heifers. J Anim Sci 1985;61:470–3.
5. Rutter LM, Randel RD. Nonpuberal estrus in beef heifers. J Anim Sci 1986;63: 1049–53.
6. Honaramooz A, Aravindakshan J, Chandolia RK, et al. Ultrasonographic evaluation of the pre-pubertal development of the reproductive tract in beef heifers. Anim Reprod Sci 2004;80:15–29.
7. Desjardins C, Hafs HD. Maturation of bovine female genitalia from birth through puberty. J Anim Sci 1969;28:502–7.
8. Bartol FF, Johnson LL, Floyd JG, et al. Neonatal exposure to progesterone and estradiol alters uterine morphology and luminal protein content in adult beef heifers. Theriogenology 1995;43:835–44.
9. Hargrove DD. Use of growth promotants in replacement heifers. In: Fields MJ, Sands RS, editors. Factors affecting calf crop. Boco Raton (FL): CRC Press; 1994. p. 91–104.
10. Evans AC, Adams GP, Rawlings NC. Follicular and hormonal development in prepubertal heifers from 2 to 36 weeks of age. J Reprod Fertil 1994;102:463–70.
11. Erickson BH. Development and senescence of the postnatal bovine ovary. J Anim Sci 1966;25:800–5.

12. Cushman RA, Hedgpeth VS, Echternkamp SE, et al. Evaluation of numbers of micro- and macroscopic follicles in cattle selected for twinning. J Anim Sci 2000;78:1564–7.

13. Evans AC, Mossa F, Fair T, et al. Causes and consequences of the variation in the number of ovarian follicles in cattle. In: Lucy MC, Pate JL, Smith MF, et al, editors. Proceedings VIII International Symposium on Reproduction in Domestic Ruminants. Nottingham (United Kingdom): Nottingham University Press; 2010. p. 421–9.

14. Cushman RA, Allan MF, Kuehn LA, et al. Evaluation of antral follicle count and ovarian morphology in crossbred beef cows: investigation of influence of stage of the estrous cycle, age, and birth weight. J Anim Sci 2009;87:1971–80.

15. Mossa F, Walsh SW, Butler ST, et al. Low numbers of ovarian follicles less than or equal to 3 mm in diameter are associated with low fertility in dairy cows. J Dairy Sci 2012;95:2355–61.

16. Taneja M, Bols PE, Van de Velde A, et al. Developmental competence of juvenile calf oocytes in vitro and in vivo: influence of donor animal variation and repeated gonadotropin stimulation. Biol Reprod 2000;62:206–13.

17. Rajakoski E. The ovarian follicular system in sexually mature heifers with special reference to seasonal, cyclical, and left-right variations. Acta Endocrinol Suppl (Copenh) 1960;52:1–68.

18. Ireland JJ, Coulson PB, Murphree RL. Follicular development during four stages of the estrous cycle of beef cattle. J Anim Sci 1979;49:1261–9.

19. Pierson RA, Ginther OJ. Follicular populations during the estrous cycle: influence of day. Anim Reprod Sci 1987;124:165–76.

20. Savio JD, Keenan L, Boland MP, et al. Pattern of growth of dominant follicles during the oestrous cycle of heifers. J Reprod Fertil 1988;83:663–71.

21. Sirois J, Fortune JE. Ovarian follicular dynamics during the estrous cycle in heifers monitored by real-time ultrasonography. Biol Reprod 1988;39:308–17.

22. Knopf L, Kastelic JP, Schallenberger E, et al. Ovarian follicular dynamics in heifers: test of two-wave hypothesis by ultrasonically monitoring individual follicles. Domest Anim Endocrinol 1989;6:111–9.

23. Ginther OJ, Kastelic JP, Knopf L. Composition and characteristics of follicular waves during the bovine estrous cycle. Anim Reprod Sci 1989;20:187–200.

24. Adams GP, Matteri RL, Kastelic JP, et al. Association between surges of follicle-stimulating hormone and the emergence of follicular waves in heifers. J Reprod Fertil 1992;94:177–88.

25. Fortune JE, Sirois J, Quirk SM. The growth and differentiation of ovarian follicles during the bovine estrous cycle. Theriogenology 1988;29:95–109.

26. Ginther OJ, Knopf L, Kastelic JP. Temporal associations among ovarian events in cattle during oestrous cycles with two and three follicular waves. J Reprod Fertil 1989;87:223–30.

27. Bo GA, Baruselli PS, Martinez MF. Pattern and manipulation of follicular development in Bos indicus cattle. Anim Reprod Sci 2003;78:307–26.

28. Bergfelt EG, Kojima FN, Cupp AS, et al. Ovarian follicular development in prepubertal heifers is influenced by level of dietary intake. Biol Reprod 1994;51:1051–7.

29. Driancourt MA. Regulation of ovarian follicular dynamics in farm animals. Implications for manipulation of reproduction. Theriogenology 2001;55:1211–39.

30. Adams GP. Comparative patterns of follicle development and selection in ruminants. J Reprod Fertil 1999;54:17–32.

31. Revel F, Mermillod P, Peynot N, et al. Low developmental capacity of in vitro matured and fertilized oocytes from calves compared with that of cows. J Reprod Fertil 1995;103:115–20.

32. Armstrong DT. Effects of maternal age on oocyte developmental competence. Theriogenology 2001;55:1303–22.
33. Salamone DF, Damiani P, Fissore RA, et al. Biochemical and developmental evidence that ooplasmic maturation of prepubertal bovine oocytes is compromised. Biol Reprod 2001;64:1761–8.
34. Ptak G, Matsukawa K, Palmieri C, et al. Developmental and functional evidence of nuclear immaturity in prepubertal oocytes. Hum Reprod 2006;21: 2228–37.
35. Presicce GA, Jiang S, Simkin M, et al. Age and hormonal dependence of acquisition of oocyte competence for embryogenesis in prepubertal calves. Biol Reprod 1997;56:386–92.
36. Gonzalez-Padilla E, Wiltbank JN, Niswender GD. Puberty in beef heifers. I. The interrelationship between pituitary, hypothalamic, and ovarian hormones. J Anim Sci 1975;40:1091–104.
37. Berardinelli JG, Dailey RA, Butcher RL, et al. Source of progesterone prior to puberty in beef heifers. J Anim Sci 1979;49:1276–80.
38. Kinder JE, Bergfeld EG, Wehrman ME, et al. Endocrine basis for puberty in heifers and ewes. J Reprod Fertil 1995;49:393–407.
39. Odde KG, Wards HS, Kiracofe GH, et al. Short estrous cycles and associated serum progesterone levels in beef cows. Theriogenology 1980;14:105–12.
40. Garverick HA, Zollers WG, Smith MF. Mechanisms associated with corpus luteum lifespan in animals having normal or subnormal luteal function. Anim Reprod Sci 1992;28:111–24.
41. Kieborz-Loos KR, Garverick HA, Keisler DH, et al. Oxytocin-induced secretion of prostaglandin $F_{2\alpha}$ in postpartum beef cows: effects of progesterone and estradiol-17β treatment. J Anim Sci 2003;81:1830–6.
42. Anderson KJ, Lefever DG, Brinks JS, et al. The use of reproductive tract scoring in beef heifers. Agri-Practice 1991;12:19–26.
43. Rosenkrans KS, Hardin DK. Repeatability and accuracy of reproductive tract scoring to determine pubertal status in beef heifers. Theriogenology 2003;59: 1087–92.
44. Holm DE, Thompson PN, Irons PC. The value of reproductive tract scoring as a predictor of fertility and production outcomes in beef heifers. J Anim Sci 2009; 87:1934–40.
45. Kinder JE, Day ML, Kittok RJ. Endocrine regulation of puberty in cows and ewes. J Reprod Fertil 1987;34:167–86.
46. Day ML, Anderson LH. Current concepts on the control of puberty in cattle. J Anim Sci 1998;76:1–15.
47. Ramirez DV, McCann SM. Comparison of the regulation of luteinizing hormone (LH) secretion in immature and adult rats. Endocrinology 1963;72:452–64.
48. Moran C, Quirke JF, Roche JF. Puberty in heifers: a review. Anim Reprod Sci 1989;18:167–82.
49. Anderson LH, Day ML. Site-specific reductions in the number of hypothalamic estradiol receptor-containing neurons during progestin-induced puberty in heifers [abstract]. Biol Reprod 1996;54(Suppl 1):178.
50. Shivers BD, Harlan RE, Morrell JI, et al. Absence of oestradiol concentrations in cell nuclei of LHRH-immunoreactive neurones. Nature 1983;304:345–7.
51. Day ML, Imakawa K, Wolfe PL, et al. Endocrine mechanisms of puberty in heifers. Role of hypothalamo-pituitary estradiol receptors in the negative feedback of estradiol on luteinizing hormone secretion. Biol Reprod 1987;37: 1054–65.

52. de Roux N, Genin E, Carel JC, et al. Hypogonadotropic hypogonadism due to loss of function of the KiSS1-derived peptide receptor GPR54. Proc Natl Acad Sci U S A 2003;100:10972–6.
53. Seminara SB, Messager S, Chatzidaki EE, et al. The GPR54 gene as a regulator of puberty. N Engl J Med 2003;349:1614–27.
54. Smith JT. Kisspeptin signalling in the brain: steroid regulation in the rodent and ewe. Brain Res Brain Res Rev 2008;57:288–98.
55. Colledge WH. GPR54 and kisspeptins. Results Probl Cell Differ 2008;46:117–43.
56. Irwig MS, Fraley GS, Smith JT, et al. Kisspeptin activation of gonadotropin releasing hormone neurons and regulation of KISS-1 mRNA in the male rat. Neuroendocrinology 2004;80:264–72.
57. Han SK, Gottsch ML, Lee KJ, et al. Activation of gonadotropin-releasing hormone neurons by kisspeptin as a neuroendocrine switch for the onset of puberty. J Neurosci 2005;25:11349–56.
58. Kinoshita M, Tsukamura H, Adachi S, et al. Involvement of central metastin in the regulation of preovulatory luteinizing hormone surge and estrous cyclicity in female rats. Endocrinology 2005;146:4431–6.
59. Clarkson J, Herbison AE. Postnatal development of kisspeptin neurons in mouse hypothalamus; sexual dimorphism and projections to gonadotropin-releasing hormone neurons. Endocrinology 2006;147:5817–25.
60. Anderson WJ, Forrest DW, Goff BA, et al. Ontogeny of ovarian inhibition of pulsatile luteinizing hormone secretion in postnatal Holstein heifers. Domest Anim Endocrinol 1986;3:107–16.
61. Schams D, Schallenberger E, Gombe S, et al. Endocrine patterns associated with puberty in male and female cattle. J Reprod Fertil 1981;30:103–10.
62. Roberson MS, Wolfe MW, Stumpf TT, et al. Steady-state amounts of alpha- and luteinizing hormone (LH) beta-subunit messenger ribonucleic acids are uncoupled from pulsatility of LH secretion during sexual maturation of the heifer. Biol Reprod 1992;46:435–41.
63. Staigmiller RB, Short RE, Bellows RA. Induction of LH surges with 17β estradiol in prepubertal beef heifers: an age dependent response. Theriogenology 1979; 11:453–61.
64. Wiltbank JN, Gregory KE, Swiger L, et al. Effect of heterosis on age and weight of puberty in beef heifers. J Anim Sci 1966;25:744.
65. Eler JP, Silva JA Jr, Feraz JB, et al. Genetic evaluation of the probability of pregnancy at 14 months for Nelore heifers. J Anim Sci 2002;80:951–4.
66. Carvalho JB, Carvalho NA, Reis EL, et al. Effect of early luteolysis in progesterone-based timed AI protocols in Bos indicus, Bos indicus × Bos taurus, and Bos taurus heifers. Theriogenology 2008;69:167–75.
67. Gimenes LU, Sá Filho MF, Carvalho NA, et al. Follicle deviation and ovulatory capacity in Bos indicus heifers. Theriogenology 2008;69:852–8.
68. Lehman MN, Merkley CM, Coolen LM, et al. Anatomy of the kisspeptin neural network in mammals. Brain Res 2010;1364:90–102.
69. Pineda R, Garcia-Galiano D, Roseweir A, et al. Critical roles of kisspeptins in female puberty and preovulatory gonadotropin surges as revealed by a novel antagonist. Endocrinology 2010;151:722–30.
70. Shahab M, Mastronardi C, Seminara SB, et al. Increased hypothalamic GPR54 signaling: a potential mechanism for initiation of puberty in primates. Proc Natl Acad Sci U S A 2005;102:2129–34.

Considerations Related to Breed or Biological Type

Alison L. Van Eenennaam, PhD

KEYWORDS

- Breed • Biological type • Crossbreeding • Heterosis • Complementarity
- Expected progeny difference (EPD) • Genomics

KEY POINTS

- Age at puberty is variable among breeds and biological types (British<Continental<*Bos indicus*–influenced) and is moderately heritable.
- Heterosis (also known as hybrid vigor) occurs when the performance of the crossbred progeny for a specific trait is greater than the average of their parents.
- Heterosis effects are significant and important for fitness and survival traits such as longevity, lifetime production, and reproduction rate.
- Complementarity results from crossing breeds of different but complementary biological types.
- Properly designed crossbreeding systems based on heterosis and complementarity generally out-produce those based on straightbreeding in productivity, but the challenge is to manage the program and to produce progeny that meet market specifications and acceptance.
- Before making a commitment to any breed(s) or breeding system, the logistics, costs (including opportunity costs), benefits, and feasibility should be objectively evaluated in the context of the environment, feed resources, and marketing system.
- Expected progeny difference genetic merit estimates for heifer pregnancy, stayability, and scrotal circumference are available for some breeds and have all been positively associated with female fertility.
- Selection for replacement heifers is based on their readiness and ability to conceive in the proposed breeding season, which places indirect selection on dam fertility, because fertile cows tend to conceive early and generate those early heifers that are selected as replacements.
- Emerging reproductive and genomic technologies offer exciting possibilities for innovative approaches to heifer selection and breeding program design, but as with all new technologies, enthusiasm needs to be tempered with a realistic evaluation of the costs and expected benefits.

Funding: National Research Initiative Competitive Grant no. 2013-68004-20364 from the USDA National Institute of Food and Agriculture.
Department of Animal Science, University of California, One Shields Avenue, Davis, CA 95616, USA
E-mail address: alvaneenennaam@ucdavis.edu

INTRODUCTION

From a heifer development perspective, age at puberty can be an important factor as to whether a heifer conceives and delivers a calf by 2 years of age. Because this trait is variable among breeds and moderately (0.1–0.67) heritable,[1] breed selection and type of breeding system can greatly influence this trait. Many other factors come into play when determining the ideal breed or combination of breeds and breeding program to best match genetic resources to the environment and marketing system.

Biological type is a term used to describe breeds of cattle that share common characteristics. Among beef cattle breeds these include the terms: British (eg, Angus, Hereford, South Devon), Continental European (eg, Charolais, Gelbvieh, Limousin, Maine-Anjou, Simmental), and *Bos indicus*–influenced (eg, Brangus, Santa Gertrudis) breeds. More than 60 breeds of beef cattle are present in the United States; however, a few breeds make up most genetics used in the United States for commercial beef production. The optimal breed, or combination of breeds, for any given location is governed by several factors, including:

- Resources (size of the herd, facilities, labor, management ability)
- Target market
- Quantity and quality of feedstuffs available
- Climate
- Breed complementarity
- Cost and availability of purebred livestock

To optimize reproductive rate in the cow herd, genetic potential for environmental stress, mature size, and milk production should be matched to the environment and available feed resources. The reproduction potential of cows with large size and high milk declines if the environment and feed resources are insufficient to meet the higher requirements for maintenance and lactation.

The US Meat Animal Research Center (MARC) characterized more than 30 sire breeds for a wide variety of economically relevant traits, including growth rate and mature size, percent retail yield, age at puberty, and milk production. The breeds evaluated by MARC grouped by age at puberty are shown in **Table 1**.[2]

Heifers sired by breeds that are heaviest at 400 days of age tend to be the oldest at puberty. Conversely, heifers sired by breeds with smaller mature size tend to reach puberty earlier. However, some large breeds that have been selected for milk production reach puberty at a comparatively young age. Cattle that have some *Bos indicus* influence generally mature at a later age. Correlations between milk production and age at puberty are –0.87 among *Bos taurus* breeds and –0.19 including *Bos indicus* breeds, whereas correlations between mature size and age at puberty are 0.57 and 0.25, respectively.[1]

Purebred Hereford and purebred Angus heifers had greater ages at puberty (389.5 ± 12.9 and 372.2 ± 10.0 days, respectively)[3] than Hereford or Angus heifers derived from dams crossed with Charolais, Jersey, South Devon, Simmental, and Limousin sires, showing that both breed and breeding system contribute to age at puberty. A summary of the literature from a variety of studies on reported ages and weights at puberty by breed is shown in **Table 2**. Heterosis effects can also significantly reduce the interval from calving to first estrus (–2.66 days), average date of conception (–2.8 days), and increase the first-service conception (6.6%), and calf crop weaned (6.4%) to natural service breeding for a 65-day season when comparing straightbred Hereford, Angus, and Shorthorn heifers to reciprocal cross heifers of the same breeds.[4]

Table 1
Breeds classified by 4 economically relevant criteria[a]

Breed Group	Growth Rate and Mature Size	Lean/Fat Ratio (% Retail Product)	Age at Puberty	Milk Production
Jersey	X	X	X	XXXXX
Holstein	XXXX	XXXX	XX	XXXXXX
Red Poll	XX	XX	XX	XXX
South Devon	XXX	XXX	XX	XXX
Tarentaise	XXX	XXX	XX	XXX
Pinzgauer	XXX	XXX	XX	XXX
Braunvieh	XXXX	XXXX	XX	XXXX
Gelbvieh	XXXX	XXXX	XX	XXXX
Piedmontese	XXX	XXXXXX	XX	XX
Hereford × Angus	XXX	XX	XXX	XX
Devon	XX	XX	XXX	XX
Longhorn	X	XXX	XXX	XX
Galloway	XX	XXX	XXX	XX
Shorthorn	XXX	XX	XXX	XXX
Maine-Anjou	XXXXX	XXXX	XXX	XXX
Salers	XXXXX	XXXX	XXX	XXX
Simmental	XXXXX	XXXX	XXX	XXXX
Limousin	XXX	XXXXX	XXXX	X
Charolais	XXXXX	XXXXX	XXXX	X
Chianina	XXXXX	XXXXX	XXXX	X
Brangus	XXX	XX	XXXX	XX
Santa Gertrudis	XXX	XX	XXXX	XX
Sahiwal	XX	XXX	XXXXX	XXX
Brahman	XXXX	XXX	XXXXX	XXX
Nellore	XXXX	XXX	XXXXX	XXX

[a] Increasing number of Xs indicates higher values. These numbers are only generalizations; genetic merit (ie, EPD) should still be the basis of selection decisions within breed.

Data from Cundiff LV, Szabo F, Gregory KE, et al. Breed comparisons in the Germplasm evaluation program at MARC. Presented at: Beef Improvement Federation 25th Anniversary Conference. Asheville (NC), May 26–29, 1993.

CROSSBREEDING

Hybrid vigor (also known as heterosis) occurs when the performance of the crossbred progeny for a specific trait is greater than the average of their parents. Heterosis results from the increase in heterozygosity of a crossbred animal's makeup. It is thought that heterosis is the result of gene dominance and the recovery from accumulated inbreeding depression of pure breeds. Much of this factor occurs by reclaiming losses caused by inbreeding that occurred when the breeds were originally formed. The amount of hybrid vigor varies for different traits and environments, although generally, hybrid vigor and heritability are inversely related.

Heterosis effects are significant and important for fitness and survival traits such as longevity, lifetime production, and reproduction rate. These traits have low heritability

Table 2
Reported ages and weights at puberty by breed

Breed Group	Age at Puberty (d)	Weight at Puberty (kg)
Angus	390–420	300–310
	360–384	309
	349–357	338–350
	410	294
	358–374	288
Belgian Blue	341–353	323–335
Boran	385–407	306–326
Brahman	420–432	352–364
Brahman cross	429	324
Brangus	528	310–338
	480–524	317
Brown Swiss	300–335	280–300
	341–355	305
	317	279
Brown Swiss cross	332	280
Charolais	365–395	320–355
	391–405	355
	388	340
Charolais cross	345–355	320
	384	345
	391–405	318
Chianina	400	340
Chianina cross	384	318
Devon	356	290
Galloway cross	346–353	305
Gelbvieh	341	284
	332–350	283
Gelbvieh cross	330–340	285
	326	283
Hereford	420–450	300–310
	377–403	302
	349–361	354–356
	429	317
	407–423	291
Hereford-Angus	357	283
Holstein	365–395	265–289
Jersey	240–300	160–180
Jersey cross	308	235
	315–329	234
Limousin	391	340
	392–404	308
Limousin cross	384	309
	392–404	307
Longhorn cross	343–355	283
Maine-Anjou	370	305
Maine-Anjou cross	357	305

(continued on next page)

Table 2
(continued)

Breed Group	Age at Puberty (d)	Weight at Puberty (kg)
Nellore	496–610	275–354
Nellore cross	369–394	341
Piedmontese	340–356	293–307
Piedmontese cross	333–339	298
Pinzgauer	334	277
Pinzgauer cross	JJ4 3/2	278
	334	27/
Red Poll	344–360	270
	355	263
Red Poll cross	337	264
Sahiwal cross	414	292
Salers	365	338
Salers cross	352–355	338
Santa Gertrudis	484–531	391–429
Shorthorn	359	260–294
Shorthorn cross	341–348	329
Simmental	335–365	320–330
	360	328
	366–378	340
	348	302
Simmental cross	358	303
	366–378	302
South Devon	364	290
South Devon cross	350	289
	358–370	329
Tarentaise cross	349	283
Tuli	363–379	298–314
Zebu	510–810	330–350

Data from Refs.[2,17,33–48]

(<10%). The effects of heterosis on growth traits are more intermediate and small on carcass and meat traits. Improvements in cow-calf production because of heterosis result from both the improved maternal performance of the crossbred cow and individual performance of the crossbred calf. Cundiff and colleagues[5] reported that the lifetime production of reciprocal-cross and straightbred cows of the Hereford, Angus, and Shorthorn breeds showed that the lifetime production of weight of calves weaned was increased by about 36% by the effects of heterosis. This effect was broken down into direct effects on crossbred calf survival (+4.9%) and growth (+3.8%), and maternal effects on weaning rate (+6.2%), increased weaning weight of progeny because of the crossbred dam (+5.8%), and longevity (+16.2%) of crossbred cows.

Generally, the more different the breeds are, the greater the hybrid vigor obtained. Differing levels of heterosis are generated when different breeds are crossed. Similar levels of heterosis are observed when members of the *Bos taurus* species, including the British and Continental European breeds, are crossed among themselves. Greater levels of heterosis are obtained when *Bos indicus* breeds (eg, Brahman) are crossed with *Bos taurus* breeds.

Complementarity results from crossing breeds of different but complementary biological types. It is exploited to the fullest by terminal crossing systems in which specialized terminal sire breed bulls (with efficiency of growth, and superior carcass characteristics) are joined to crossbred maternal breed females (with high reproductive rate, low feed requirements for maintenance, and optimum milk production) to optimize desired characteristics in the resulting progeny. Antagonism between terminal and some maternal and calving traits means that positive selection on the terminal traits can result in negative selection on the maternal traits. Both male and female progeny of terminal sires should be sold for slaughter rather than kept as replacement heifers.

A well-planned crossbreeding system is required to retain acceptable levels of heterosis and manage breed complementarity over the long-term. Properly designed systems based on crossbreeding generally out-produce those based on straightbreeding in productivity, but the challenge is to manage the program and to produce progeny that meet market specifications and acceptance. Poorly designed crossbreeding programs in which a new breed is introduced periodically in an investigational fashion results in an inconsistent product and a cow herd consisting of a plethora of breeds and biological types.

The Straightbreeding/Crossbreeding Debate

There is some discussion in the beef cattle industry regarding the relative merits of crossbreeding versus straightbreeding. There are pros and cons associated with any breeding system, and no one approach fits all environments and markets. **Table 3** outlines some different breeding systems and when they might be best used. If there really is no cross with another breed that produces superior offspring for a given production and marketing scenario, then it may be that straightbreeding is the appropriate choice. The important point is that the full costs (including the opportunity costs of forgoing breed complementarity and the documented 36% increase in lifetime weight of crossbred calves weaned by crossbred cows[5]) and benefits of the chosen breeding system should be evaluated before making a commitment to any given breed(s) or breeding system.

Arguments have been made that because breed differences have diminished over time, the benefits of complementarity have become less pronounced. Although this claim is undoubtedly true as shown by the convergence of breed averages for certain growth traits, the value associated with increased heterozygosity resulting from crossbreeding remains. It has also been posited that if 1 breed is clearly superior for a given trait, then even in the presence of hybrid vigor, it is possible that neither cross will be superior to the better parent breed for that particular character. A clear example of this is when a high milking breed (eg, Holstein) is mated to a lower milking breed (eg, Jersey). Even although hybrid vigor for milk production will be about 5%, there is no possibility that the crosses will be superior to the purebred Holstein for this trait. The traits that benefit the most from hybrid vigor (eg, reproduction, longevity) tend to be similar between most breeds in any given environment, and so the crosses are normally superior to either parent breed for these low heritability traits.[6]

The expression of heterosis in several reproductive traits suggests that improvements in reproductive efficiency can be realized through crossbreeding. Earlier puberty,[1] increased pregnancy rate,[7,8] and decreased calving interval[9] have all been associated with improvements from crossbreeding. Because many of the

Table 3
Different breeding systems and their appropriate use

System	Description	Appropriate Use	% Hybrid Vigor	
			Calf	Dam
Purebred	Crossing males and females of the same breed	When no cross with another breed produces superior offspring	0	0
2-way/terminal cross	Crossing males and females from 2 different breeds, creating F1 progeny	When direct, but not maternal, heterosis is important	100	0
3-Breed cross/terminal sire over F1 cows	Crossing F1 cows with bulls of a third breed	When direct and maternal heterosis are important or when it is necessary to design the optimal type of cow for a particular environment	100	100
4-Breed cross	Crossing F1 cows (with parental breeds A and B) with F1 bulls (with parental breeds C and D)	When direct, maternal, and paternal heterosis are important	100	100
Backcross	Crossing F1 cows with bulls from 1 of the parent breeds	When there are only 2 good parental breeds available and direct heterosis is not important	38	100
2-Breed rotation	Daughters of bulls of breed A are bred to bulls of breed B, daughters of bulls of breed B are bred to bulls of breed A; can also be used with 3 or 4 breeds	When producing female replacements (F1 cross females) is advantageous	67	67
Open or closed synthetic	Creating a new breed from 2 or more breeds that retains heterosis in future generations without further crossbreeding (closed); or with minimal crossbreeding for improvements (open)	When a consistent level of heterosis is important. Heterosis increases as number of foundation breeds increases and can be maintained if adequate numbers of sires are used in each generation to avoid re-inbreeding. Difficult to find bulls with high-accuracy EPD	50	50
Crossbred/composite sire	Maintain a given level of breed composition by using crossbred bulls (eg, 50% breed A, 50% breed B)	When planned crossbreeding system is not feasible (eg, small herd size). Results in slightly less heterosis than a 2-breed rotation using purebreds. It may be difficult to find crossbred or composite bulls with accurate EPD	50	50

Adapted from Kinghorn B. Breed utilisation and crossbreeding. In: Cottle D, editor. Genetic evaluation and breeding program design. Armidale (Australia): University of New England, School of Environmental and Rural Science; 2011; with permission.

crossbreeding studies were conducted when there were more pronounced differences between the breeds, the old estimates of the heterosis adjustments are no longer valid, because the studies were carried out more than 20 years ago. A 2010 meta-analysis estimating heterosis effects of crossbreeding from studies published in the literature from 1976 to 1996 is summarized in **Tables 4** and **5**.[10] These data do not include heterotic effects on reproduction and longevity estimates for crossbred cows. Older data suggest an increase in calving rate of almost 4%, an increase in longevity of more than 1 year, and a lifetime increase of 272 kg cumulative weaning weight in *Bos taurus* crossbred dams.[11] It is difficult to obtain new estimates in the absence of large controlled research projects to continuously estimate heterosis effects. Some recent industry studies have been conducted showing improved heifer pregnancy (HP) rates in crossbred heifers,[12,13] but these data have not yet been published in the peer-reviewed literature. Heterosis is exploited extensively in other animal protein (eg, poultry, swine) and agricultural (eg, hybrid corn) industries, and there is little doubt that when used in commercial beef production it continues to provide a heterotic boost to reproductive and longevity traits.

There are some logistical considerations associated with crossbreeding that must be addressed in the design of a successful crossbreeding program, which are summarized in **Table 6**. These considerations include the following points

- More difficult in small herds: the smaller the herd, the greater are the problems with systematic crossbreeding and organizing the supply of replacement heifers and bulls.
- Marketing difficulties: supply of a consistent product can be a problem if there is a lot of variation in the calf crop derived from crossbreeding such that it is difficult to put together a load or pen-sized group of similar-type cattle.
- Management requirements: producers who have trouble identifying and managing a straightbred herd are likely to have difficulty managing a crossbreeding system.
- Additional mating groups: many crossbreeding systems have additional mating groups and breed(s) of bulls being run, and good fencing is required to keep the herds separate. The perceived complexity of this approach can be

Table 4
Individual and maternal heterosis adjustments (SD) for birth weight, weaning weight, and postweaning body weight gain by biological type combination

Biological Type Combination	Birth Weight (kg)		Weaning Weight (kg)		Postweaning Body Weight Gain (kg)
	Individual Heterosis	Maternal Heterosis	Individual Heterosis	Maternal Heterosis	Individual Heterosis
British × British	0.90 (0.06)	0.57 (0.07)	8.22 (0.25)	8.33 (0.35)	6.30 (0.42)
British × Continental	0.70 (0.05)	0.83 (0.08)	5.79 (0.25)	7.41 (0.38)	7.90 (0.43)
British × Zebu	2.43 (0.11)	1.53 (0.13)	23.02 (0.54)	22.09 (0.66)	14.68 (1.00)
Continental × Continental	0.63 (0.23)	1.12 (0.69)	3.47 (1.28)	15.63 (3.54)	9.10 (2.04)
Continental × Zebu	2.00 (0.30)	1.10 (0.48)	25.93 (1.20)	10.66 (1.47)	1.49 (2.59)

Data from Williams JL, Aguilar I, Rekaya R, et al. Estimation of breed and heterosis effects for growth and carcass traits in cattle using published crossbreeding studies. J Anim Sci 2010;88:460–6.

Table 5
Individual heterosis adjustments (SD) for carcass weight, Longissimus muscle (LM) area, fat thickness, and marbling score by biological type combination

Biological Type Combination	Carcass Weight (kg)	LM Area (cm²)	Fat Thickness (cm)	Marbling Score[a]
British × British	10.34 (0.48)	2.40 (0.16)	0.11 (0.01)	0.17 (0.01)
British × Continental	13.13 (0.48)	2.62 (0.15)	−0.02 (0.01)	0.06 (0.01)
British × Zebu	42.04 (1.07)	6.57 (0.35)	0.20 (0.01)	0.09 (0.03)
Continental × Continental	16.44 (1.57)	3.18 (0.47)	−0.01 (0.02)	−0.05 (0.06)
Continental × Zebu	24.63 (1.47)	4.43 (0.51)	0.16 (0.02)	0.30 (0.04)

[a] Marbling score was measured from practically devoid (2.0–2.9) to abundant (10.0–10.9).
Data from Williams JL, Aguilar I, Rekaya R, et al. Estimation of breed and heterosis effects for growth and carcass traits in cattle using published crossbreeding studies. J Anim Sci 2010;88:460–6.

avoided by opting for a simple terminal crossing strategy or by using a composite bull.

- Supply of replacements: the supply of female replacements is one of the most challenging issues when crossbreeding. They can be bred within herd or purchased. Purchasing is the easiest option, but heifers of known breeding are not readily available on a consistent basis. Self-replacing systems for systematic crossbreeding are available, such as 2-breed rotation (**Fig. 1**).
- Retention of hybrid vigor: several crossbreeding systems manage to overcome the replacement female dilemma by allowing breeders to produce replacement heifers from their own hybrid populations. However, this convenience comes at a price typically paid in loss of hybrid vigor, breed complementarity, and simplicity. When considering the options, it is worth asking "Why am I crossbreeding?" If it is to combine the attributes of 2 breeds, then a fixed cross using a crossbred bull may well be satisfactory, but if it is to maximize complementarity or hybrid vigor, then a more sophisticated breeding scheme may be required.
- Additional mating groups: many crossbreeding systems have additional mating groups compared with straightbred systems. Additional mating groups and good fencing are required to keep the groups separate. This issue may be overcome by use of a composite bull.
- Social pressures: there may be some stigma associated with crossbreeding in certain communities with a strong tradition of straightbreeding.
- Accuracy of sire selection: the additive genetic value of the crossbred progeny (that which can be passed on to progeny) can only be as good as that of the parents. Selection of parents is just as important when crossbreeding as it is when straightbreeding. It may be difficult to find crossbred or composite bulls with accurate genetic merit estimates or expected progeny differences (EPD).
- Feasibility analysis: before embarking on a crossbreeding program the whole exercise should be evaluated and solutions for problems identified before moving forward with the crossbreeding program.

SELECTING REPLACEMENT HEIFERS

Female fertility cannot be easily defined as a single trait, because it comprises several different factors. Some of these factors are related to the ability of the cow to become

Table 6

Summary of the attributes and problems associated with the main crossbreeding strategies

Primary Objective for Crossbreeding	Crossing System	Ease of Management	Female Replacements	Marketing Problems	Breed Composition (When Herd is Stable)	Expression of Heterosis (When Herd is Stable) (%)
To grade up to a desired breed	**Grading up:** Produce first-cross females and continually backcross the latest generation to bulls of the desired breed	Several generations may be on hand at once but only 1 bull breed is involved	Inbuilt: higher grades replace lower grades	Minimal, and should be restricted to first few years	100% of genes from the desired breed	None
Use the complementary attributes of 2 purebreds	**2-Breed terminal cross:** Mate sires of 1 breed to cows of another	Easy if all crossbred progeny are sold	Required unless only some of the cows are mated to a second breed	This system is often geared to supply particular market requirements	Cows 100 Calves 50:50	Cows 0 Calves 100
Use hybrid vigor	**2-Breed rotation:** Produce first-cross animals and then backcross females to bulls of the alternative breed to that of the dam's sire	Herd needs to be separated into 2 groups for mating but otherwise all cattle can be run together. A simple ear-marking system is required to denote breed of the calf's sire	Inbuilt but not feasible in small herds unless using AI	Minimal for similar breeds, but more if diverse breeds are involved	67:33 or 33:67	67

(continued on next page)

Table 6
(continued)

Primary Objective for Crossbreeding	Crossing System	Ease of Management	Female Replacements	Marketing Problems	Breed Composition (When Herd is Stable)	Expression of Heterosis (When Herd is Stable) (%)
To combine the attributes of 2 breeds	**2-Breed composites:** Produce first-cross females and then a. Mate to first-cross bulls and so on, or b. Backcross and then interbreed the backcross progeny and so on, depending on the composition required	Two (a) or maybe 3 (b) types of bulls are involved initially but later, the latest generation of bulls is used. Several generations are on hand in the female herd, which is more difficult in early years	Inbuilt	Depends on the divergence between the breeds chosen	a. 50:50 b. 75:25 or 25:75	50 38
Use hybrid vigor and combine the attributes of several breeds. Need to maintain a population size large enough that the increased heterozygosity is not dissipated by early inbreeding of composite populations	**(a) 3-Breed terminal cross or 2-breed backcross** Use first-cross females mated to bulls of a third breed or backcrossed to 1 of the parent breeds	Difficult if a supply of first-cross females is not available, because a 2-herd system is required	Need to be bought or bred	Depends on the breeds chosen and whether first-crosses need to be bred	First-cross cows 50:50 Calves a. Outcross 50:25:25 b. Backcross 75:25	First-cross cows 100 Calves a. Outcross 100 b. Backcross 50
	(b) 4-Breed composite Produce the first-crosses (in at least 2 and preferably 4 combinations) and then mate those together to give the desired composition	If attempted properly this is complex in the early years but becomes easier when the composite develops	Inbuilt	Could be large depending on the breeds chosen	25:25:25:25	75[a]

[a] Assumes large herds with no inbreeding (ie, many sires of each breed) and that hybrid vigor is related to the degree of heterozygosity.
Adapted from Barlow R. Crossbreeding - where and how it can be used to increase beef production. Proceedings: Refresher Course for Veterinarians, Beef Cattle Production. University of Sydney 1984;68;491–504.

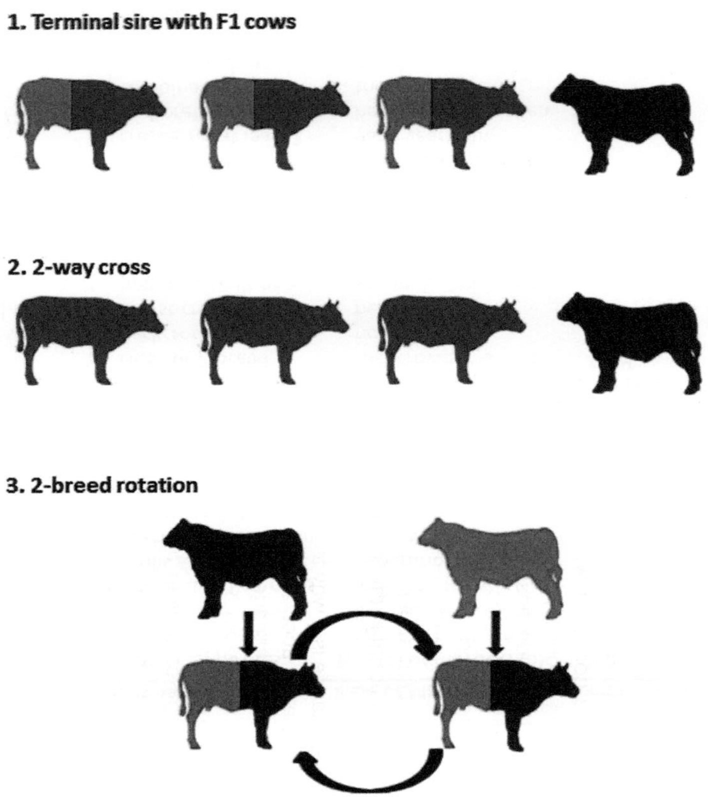

Pros	Cons
1. Terminal sire with F1 cows	
- Most productive - + 20-40% weaning weight turnoff - Maximum hybrid vigor - Maximum heterosis in cow and calf - Optimize cow/bull traits - All calves marketed have same breed composition	- Replacement heifers needed - Heifers may have to be mated to different breeds
2. 2-way cross (topcross)	
- Simple system - + 5-10% weaning weight turnoff - Easy replacements - Increased value of heifers as F1 breeders, 'steer' value	- Replacement heifers have to be purchased or bred in separate herd - No benefits of maternal heterosis
3. 2-breed rotation (criss-cross)	
- Simple system - +10-20% weaning weight turnoff - Generates replacements - Retains calf heterosis - Capitalizes on dam heterosis	- Need maternal breeds - Variability of sale progeny - Identification of progeny sire breed essential for management

1. Terminal sire with F1 cows

2. 2-way cross

3. 2-breed rotation

Fig. 1. Three simple crossbreeding systems.

and remain pregnant, and others to the prompt resumption of estrus after calving. In addition, cows need to be able to successfully deliver viable calves, preferably unassisted. In those segments of the industry that try to calve heifers at 2 years of age, much of the success of the cow-calf enterprise depends on breeding and calving heifers by the age of 2 years. Therefore, it is important to select heifers with higher genetic potential for fertility that breed early in their first season to calve as 2-year-olds and then continue to rebreed and calve each year as mature females.

Effective selection tools for genetic improvement of reproduction are limited.[14] Several traits have been used as possible indicators of fertility in cattle. These traits include pregnancy rate, first-service conception rate, scrotal circumference (SC), age at puberty, postpartum interval, length of the estrous cycle immediately before breeding, days to first breeding, HP rate, size of the ovulatory follicle, the total number of follicles in the ovary, days to calving, calving interval, longevity, and stayability (STAY). Several US breed associations have implemented total-herd reporting systems, in which data are recorded from all of the cows in a herd each year, with the objective of being able to develop better genetic evaluations of reproductive traits.

EPD, Accuracy, and Possible Change

EPD are predictions of an animal's genetic merit for a given trait. They predict the difference in performance expected from the offspring of 1 individual compared with the offspring of another individual, within the same breed. They are calculated by breed associations using pedigree and performance information on an individual and its relatives. A listing of the EPD available for different US breed associations is shown in **Table 7**. Although EPD are the best estimate of an animal's genetic worth, they are still an expectation, and as more information on an animal becomes available, the more confident we are in the estimate. Each EPD is associated with an accompanying accuracy ranging between 0 and 1. In the United States, this value is based on the guidelines of the Beef Improvement Federation (BIF). Young animals tend to have low BIF accuracy (eg, 0.05) EPD, whereas well-proven artificial insemination (AI) sires tend to have high BIF accuracy (eg, 0.95) EPD, because of the large number of progeny performance records that are available on proven sires. The EPD of an AI sire having a high accuracy is close to his true genetic merit, which means that we are confident in the estimate based on the observed performance of progeny he has sired.

Possible change is a way to express the uncertainty associated with an EPD based on its associated accuracy. In the case of a low-accuracy EPD, more change is possible. Possible change can move in either a positive or a negative direction, and moving in an undesired direction can have serious consequences depending on the trait. For example, an important consideration when selecting a bull to breed heifers is the accuracy of calving ease direct (CED) EPD, which measures the ability of offspring of an individual to be born unassisted. CED EPD are calculated using information from birth weight information of the bull's progeny and problems experienced in calvings of 2-year-old females only (no older calvings are included). A higher value of this EPD indicates a higher percentage of unassisted calving heifers. If a yearling Angus bull and a proven AI sire both have the same EPD value for CED, the possible change value associated with a low 0.05 BIF accuracy CED EPD is ±7.8% of unassisted births, whereas it is ±0.8% for a 0.9 BIF accuracy CED EPD (http://www.angus.org/Nce/Accuracy.aspx). Although unlikely, the consequence of the yearling bull having an EPD that increases the percentage of unassisted birth by 7.8% could be dramatic come calving time. Using high-accuracy sires minimizes the risk of a large adverse EPD change, which is associated with low-accuracy bulls.

Table 7
Current EPD available from breeds in the United States

Breed	Growth								Maternal							Carcass									Other		
	Birth Weight	Weaning Weight	Milk	Yearling Weight	Total Maternal	Yearling Height	Mature Height	Mature Weight	SC	CED	Calving Ease	Maternal HP	Gestation Length	Maternal Birth Weight	Maternal Weaning Weight	Carcass Weight	Ribeye Area	Fat Thickness	Marbling	Retail Product	Yield Grade	Tenderness	Intramuscular Fat (%)	Warner-Bratzler Shear Force	STAY	Maintenance Energy	Docility
Angus	X	X	X	X	X	X	X	X	X	X	X	X				X	X	X	X								X
Beefmaster	X	X	X	X	X				X							X	X	X	X				X				
Brahman	X	X	X	X										X								X					
Brangus/Red Brangus	X	X	X	X	X					X	X					X	X	X	X				X				
Braford	X	X	X	X	X									X		X		X	X								
Braunvieh	X	X	X	X	X					X	X					X	X	X	X	X							
Charolais	X	X	X	X	X				X	X	X					X	X	X	X	X							
Chianina	X	X	X	X												X	X	X	X	X							
Gelbvieh	X	X	X	X	X					X	X		X	X		X	X	X	X		X				X		
Hereford	X	X	X	X	X				X	X	X					X	X	X	X								
Limousin	X	X	X	X	X					X	X					X	X	X	X	X	X				X		X
Maine-Anjou	X	X	X	X	X										X	X	X	X	X	X							
Red Poll	X	X	X	X	X																						
Red Angus	X	X	X	X	X					X	X	X				X	X	X	X	X	X	X			X	X	
Salers	X	X	X	X	X				X	X	X				X	X	X	X	X	X					X		X
Santa Gertrudis	X	X	X	X	X				X							X	X	X	X	X							
Senepol	X	X	X	X																							
Shorthorn	X	X	X	X	X					X	X					X	X	X	X								
Simmental[a]	X	X	X	X	X					X	X				X	X	X	X	X	X	X		X		X		
South Devon	X	X	X	X	X				X	X	X				X	X	X	X	X	X							
Tarentaise	X	X	X	X	X					X	X																

[a] Simmental EPD include Simangus and Simbrah breed associations.

EPD that are directly associated with fertility include yearling bull SC, which has been shown to be genetically correlated with age at puberty in heifers.[15] Researchers have also shown a favorable relationship between SC and age at first breeding and subsequent rebreeding in females as reviewed.[16] HP measures the ability to become pregnant and calve as a 2-year-old. A higher EPD is the more favorable direction and the EPD is reported in percentage units. STAY is defined as the probability (in percent) of a cow surviving or staying in a herd to a given age provided it has the opportunity. The higher the EPD value, the higher the probability that the bull's daughters will remain in the herd until 6 years of age. Heritability of STAY has been estimated to range from 0.02 to 0.23, depending on the end point chosen.[17] A recent study of a large population of Nellore cattle[18] reported the genetic correlation between HP and STAY to be high 0.64 (±0.07). The investigators went on to suggest that EPD for HP could be used "to select bulls for the production of precocious, fertile, and long-lived daughters."

Other EPD associated indirectly with fertility include CED and calving ease total maternal (CEM), which measures the ability of an individual's daughters to give birth unassisted. Depending on the breed association, this EPD is sometimes referred to as the calving ease daughters or CEM. Several other EPD, such as mature size, mature weight, docility, and birth weight may also influence reproduction either directly or indirectly.

Commercial producers often place selection emphasis on CED EPD when purchasing heifer herd bulls to avoid dystocia. As these heifer bulls mature and get too heavy to breed the heifers, they are often moved across to breed the cows, despite the fact that cows have little calving difficulty and selection for bulls to breed cows ideally emphasizes a different suite of traits. A preferable approach might be to artificially inseminate heifers using semen from a high-accuracy calving ease bull, and focus herd bull selection on maternal traits of importance to breeding cows. Using an AI bull with a favorable CED EPD and a high BIF accuracy reduces the possible change associated with his CED EPD, providing some assurance that his calves are unlikely to cause calving problems in heifers. Using semen from high-accuracy, genetically superior AI bulls on heifers also helps to accelerate the rate of genetic progress, because of a decrease in the generation interval, and concomitantly reduces the selection emphasis on CED when considering herd bulls to breed cows.

There are few beef EPD that are directly correlated with reproductive traits, and even fewer multitrait beef cattle economic selection indexes that appropriately weight the relative importance of reproductive traits in selection decisions. Multitrait selection indexes combine EPDs for several traits into a single economic value. The index values are interpreted like an EPD; the difference in index value between 2 bulls is the expected difference in average dollar value of their progeny when the bulls are bred to similar cows. Indexes are expressed in dollars per head, and higher indexes mean a higher dollar value per head. An index value has meaning only when it is compared with the index value of another animal of the same breed. Currently, indexes are calculated for Angus, Charolais, Gelbvieh, Hereford, Limousin, Simmental, and Simangus bulls (**Table 8**).

In most cases, these indexes encompass only postweaning and carcass performance. Other factors drive profitability, especially fertility. Improvements in reproductive performance can be up to 4-fold more important than improvements in end-product traits in a conventional cow-calf operation selling market calves at weaning.[19] The relative importance of fertility in cow-calf production selection has been observed consistently across many different production systems and countries. The ratio of relative weightings in phenotypic standard deviation units for

Table 8
US beef cattle breed association indexes. Those that are designed for a self-replacing herd are in bold type

Angus	http://www.angus.org/Nce/ValueIndexes.aspx

$W, weaned calf value. This is the expected average of future progeny for preweaning performance, within a typical beef cowherd. It accounts for the economic impact of birth weight, weaning weight, maternal milk, and mature cow size.

Cow energy value ($EN). This is a component of $W and is measured in dollars of savings per cow per year, accounting for energy requirements because of mature size and milking ability.

$F, feedlot value. This is the expected average of future progeny for postweaning feedlot performance, and includes EPD for weaning and yearling weight.

$QG, quality grade. This is the quality grade segment of $G. The carcass marbling and ultrasound % intramuscular fat EPDs contribute to $QG.

$YG, yield grade. This is the yield grade segment of $G. It combines ribeye, fat thickness, and weight into an economic value for red meat yield.

$G, grid value. This is the expected average of future progeny for carcass grid merit. It combines $QG and $YG, so it focuses on quality and red meat yield simultaneously.

$B, beef value. This is the expected average of future progeny for postweaning performance and carcass value. The $B value combines information from $F and $G. This index includes EPD for yearling weight, carcass weight, and carcass or ultrasound traits.

$W, weaned calf value. This is the expected average of future progeny for preweaning performance, within a typical beef cowherd. It accounts for the economic impact of birth weight, weaning weight, maternal milk, and mature cow size.

Charolais	http://www.charolaisusa.com/terminalprofitindex.html

Terminal sire profitability index. This index is intended for use by commercial producers to address profitability and selection of sires depending on the cow base they would be bred to. The index allows producers to input data for their own cow herd profiled against the Charolais database to identify the most profitable sires (weighed economic values).

Gelbvieh	http://www.gelbvieh.org/education/library/epdinformation.html

CV, carcass value. This is the expected average carcass value of future progeny when sold on a grid. It incorporates carcass weight, yield grade, and quality grade information.

FM, feedlot merit. This is the expected average of future progeny for postweaning feedlot performance.

Hereford	http://www.hereford.org/node/310

BMI$, baldy maternal index. This is the expected average performance of progeny of Hereford bulls used in rotational crossbreeding programs on Angus-based cows and heifers, with the progeny marketed on a Certified Hereford Beef, LLC pricing grid.

CEZ$, calving ease index. This is similar to BMI$, except that the bulls are mated only to yearling heifers. It has increased emphasis on calving ease.

BII$, Brahman influence index. This is similar to BMI$, except that the bulls are mated to Brahman-based cows. It puts more emphasis on fertility and age at puberty, and less on growth and calving ease.

CHB$, certified Hereford beef index. This is the expected average performance of progeny of Hereford bulls mated to British-cross cows, with all progeny sold as fed cattle on a certified Hereford beef LLC pricing grid. It is a terminal sire index, including growth and carcass information only, because all progeny are marketed and no females are retained in the herd.

Limousin	http://www.nalf.org/pdf/2012/06.04/Reading-the-Whole-Herd-Report-June-2012.pdf

(continued on next page)

Table 8
(*continued*)

$MTI, mainstream terminal index. The mainstream terminal index takes both genetics and economics into account to rank animals in terms of expected profit per carcass produced from weaning to mainstream market end points of yield grade 1s and 2s and select to low-choice quality grades. It is based on the assumption that Angus-Hereford cows in a 2-breed rotation are mated to Limousin-influenced terminal sires and is determined primarily by genetics and economics associated with postweaning growth and yield and quality grade. The mainstream terminal index does not have an associated accuracy value.

Shorthorn	http://www.shorthorn.org/images/shperformance/helpfultools/ValueDefinitions.pdf

$ CEZ ($ calving ease) This index assumes a bull is mated only to heifers, not cows. The potential profitability of the sire is measured by the incidence of live calves at birth. Moderate mature size is also emphasized in the index, but performance is not a priority. This index is also a good measure of Shorthorn females' ability to produce calving ease sires. Overemphasis of $CEZ may cause unwanted depression of weaning and yearling performance.

$F ($ feedlot) Similar to a terminal sire scenario, $feedlot places strong emphasis on growth and carcass traits. This multitrait index assumes that the sire is mated to a mix of heifers and cows and attempts to measure profitability when progeny are sold on the fed market. On the female side, mature size should be monitored closely when selecting for $F. Overselection may cause detrimental harm to longevity, reproductive efficiency, and fleshing ability.

$BMI ($ British maternal index) As the name implies, this multitrait selection index attempts to measure a bull's potential profitability when complementing the British cow base (eg, Angus, Red Angus, Hereford). Shorthorn females can likewise be gauged at adding value to British or British-composite bulls of other breeds. A balance of growth and carcass traits is desired with a strong maternal component aimed at optimum reproductive efficiency and cow longevity.

Simmental/Simangus	http://simmental.org/site/pdf/other/quick_reference_epds_indexes.pdf

API, all-purpose index. This is the expected average performance of progeny of Simmental bulls used on the entire Angus cowherd, with a portion of the daughters being retained for breeding and the remaining progeny being put on feed and sold grade and yield.

TI, terminal index. This is the expected average performance of progeny of Simmental bulls mated to mature Angus cows, with all offspring placed in the feedlot and sold grade and yield. It includes growth and carcass information only, because all progeny are marketed.

reproductive/growth/carcass traits across several studies in different countries were as follows when based on phenotypic scale[20]:

Country	Reproductive/Growth/Carcass
Australia	6:2:1 and 3:2:1
Canada	4:1:1
New Zealand	2:1
Ireland	9:3:1, 8:3:1, and 9:4:6

Reproductive traits have a high relative importance in almost all systems in which the goal is to produce herd replacements, but in certain marketing situations growth and carcass traits can make an approximately equal contribution to the objective.[20] The relative emphasis depends on how much the value derived from genetic gain in feedlot and carcass traits is shared with the cow-calf producer in the integrated system.

Breeding for increased production in dairy cattle resulted in negative side effects on fertility traits. **Table 9** shows the 10 dairy traits that are included in the US dairy selection index, with the year when each trait was introduced. The US dairy cattle selection net merit index (NM$) is defined as expected lifetime profit compared with the breed base cows born in 2005. Over the years, emphasis on yield traits has declined as genetic evaluation for other fitness traits has been introduced. As protein yield became more important, milk volume became less important. Fertility evaluations were included in NM$ a decade ago. Approximately 33% of the selection emphasis in the current NM$ is focused on direct (daughter pregnancy rate/fertility) and indirect (productive life/longevity) fertility traits. No selection emphasis is placed on milk yield, and production traits receive only a 35% emphasis.[21] Developing a fertility genetic evaluation has enabled the dairy industry to reverse the genetic trend for fertility since inclusion of this trait in NM$ in 2003 (**Fig. 2**).

COMMERCIAL REPLACEMENT HEIFER SELECTION

In practice, not all replacement heifers are registered, and so EPDs are frequently not available to inform replacement heifer selection decisions. Selection is frequently driven by size, because heifers that are born late(r) in the calving season are often too immature to be cycling in time for the first potential breeding season. Commercial producers typically select on at least a visual estimate of a heifer's 400-day weight, in addition to visual evaluations of structural and udder soundness. This size criterion tends to put indirect selection on fertility traits of the dam (eg, early calving); however, it can lead to inadvertent selection for increased mature weight.

One promising phenotype that can be used to assess the maturity of the reproductive tract is an evaluation of the uterus and ovary by rectal palpation.[22] Reproductive tract scoring (RTS) is a method of assigning a numerical score from 1 to 5 based on the maturity of the ovaries and uterine horns in developing heifers. Heifers that lack palpable structures on the ovaries and have immature uterine horns are assigned an RTS of 1. As the uterine horns develop and follicles become prominent on the ovary, the RTS increases. An RTS of 5 is assigned to a heifer that has been in heat, and has a palpable corpus luteum. Heifers with higher, more mature reproductive scores have higher pregnancy rates and calve earlier in the breeding season.[1] This score was found to be repeatable,[23] heritable 0.24[1] to 0.32 ($\pm$0.17),[22] and offers a

Table 9		
Year that genetic rankings began and emphasis placed on dairy traits in 2010 US national dairy selection indexes		
Trait	**Year Begun**	**Emphasis (%)**
1. Milk	1935	0
2. Milk fat	1935	16
3. Milk protein	1977	19
4. Calving ease/stillbirth	1978/2006	5
5. Udder shape and support	1983	7
6. Feet and leg conformation	1983	4
7. Body size/weight	1983	−6
8. Productive life/longevity	1994	22
9. Mastitis resistance	1994	10
10. Daughter pregnancy rate/fertility	2003	11

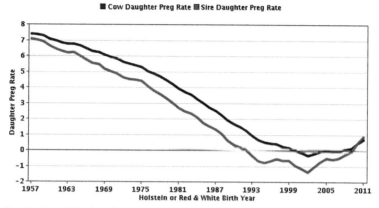

Fig. 2. Genetic trend in daughter pregnancy rate for US Holstein or Red and White dairy cattle since the inclusion of this fertility trait in the dairy selection index in 2003. (*From* Agricultural Research Service. Trend in daughter preg rate for Holstein or red & white. Available at: http://aipl.arsusda.gov/eval/summary/trend.cfm?R_Menu=HO.d#StartBody. Accessed August 8, 2013.)

phenotypic approach to identify sexual maturity independent of age or size considerations.

Recently, some DNA tests have become available to help commercial producers make heifer selection decisions. These tests do not predict fertility traits, and accuracy estimates for these tests have not been published, making it difficult to assess their worth. Unless DNA tests have high accuracy for reproductive traits, they should be used judiciously for heifer selection and in conjunction with selection on the available phenotypic data for reproductive traits (eg, date of birth, structural soundness, RTS). Technologies to improve the accuracy of heifer selection need to be evaluated objectively to determine if they are cost-effective. The break-even cost of improving HP rate by 1% was estimated to be $4.30/cow.[24] At $3 to $5/heifer, the cost of RTS provides a useful phenotypic selection criterion for reproductive maturity that generates a value that is approximately matched to the cost of the test.[24]

THE FUTURE AND DEVELOPING TECHNOLOGIES

The combination of AI and gender-selected or sexed semen offers the opportunity to rethink the logistics and economics associated with different breeding systems. Semen can be sorted as to gender because the X (female) chromosome has slightly more DNA than the Y (male) chromosome. If semen is stained with a fluorescent dye, the female-producing sperm with the larger X chromosome absorb more dye and hence shine brighter. Sorting machines can read this difference and sort the sperm as they go through the machine in single file. This process takes time, results in a lot of discarded sperm, and is not 100% efficient (meaning that some X and Y sperm are sorted into the wrong group), and so sexed-semen is more expensive than conventional semen.[25] Hall and Glaze[26] provided a review of the pregnancy rates obtained using sexed semen in beef heifers and cows. These investigators reported that there were 70 beef bulls with gender-sorted semen available from the major US AI studs in 2011.[26] Sexed semen tends to give pregnancy rates that are 10% to 20% lower than conventional semen. In some cases, inseminating only females detected in estrus results in pregnancy rates approaching conventional semen.

Gender-selected semen provides the opportunity to develop novel breeding scenarios, and avoid some of the logistical problems associated with the various cross-breeding systems. Some of these opportunities have been reviewed elsewhere.[27,28] One use is the heifer-heifer system, which uses bred replacement heifers to produce only enough heifer calves to produce the next generation of replacements, thereby allowing the mature cows to be bred to terminal-type sires. From a geneticist's perspective, this is an attractive proposition because such a system enables faster genetic progress by decreasing the generation interval (average age of the parents when the next generation is born) of females. In addition, heifers should always be genetically superior to cows in any herd that is undergoing continuous genetic improvement to ensure faster genetic progress. Heifer calves are associated with less dystocia than bull calves.

The advent of reliable fixed-time AI protocols opens up the opportunity to develop a crossbreeding strategy that obtains the benefit of hybrid vigor from the semen tank. A hypothetical example of a 100-cow herd that uses a combination of sexed semen on heifers, heterosis, and breed complementarity to sell products into different markets (purebred females and steers for premium markets, terminal-sired calves with maximum heterosis raised on ranch-bred F1 crossbred females) while still using natural service bulls (one terminal, 2 straightbred bulls selected on a maternal index) on the cow herd is shown in **Fig. 3**. The reader is cautioned not to interpret this schema literally in the absence of an economic and feasibility analysis, but rather to use it to contemplate various scenarios of how gender-selected semen might be strategically used to achieve desired outcomes.

Genomics and Selection for Heifers

Genomic selection (GS) refers to the use of genome-wide DNA markers to predict the genetic merit of selection candidates. GS relies on using many individuals in a genotyped and phenotyped training population to derive a genomic prediction equation that can then be used to estimate the genetic merit of unphenotyped individuals from a selection candidate population based solely on their genotype. It was shown early on that 50,000 single nucleotide polymorphism (SNP) (50K) DNA marker-based prediction equations trained in 1 breed have low predictive ability in other breeds. This finding is believed to be because much of the accuracy of genomic breeding values results from the effect of large chromosome segments that segregate within closely related animals in 1 breed, but not across breeds. Practically, this observation means that each breed has had to develop its own training population. There are several breeds (Angus, Hereford, Simmental, Red Angus, Brangus, Gelbvieh, and Limousin) that have achieved this population by genotyping approximately 1000 or more animals with EPDs to develop prediction equations. This genomic information is starting to be incorporated into national cattle evaluations, and the resulting genomic-enhanced EPD have improved accuracies, especially on young animals, thus decreasing the possible change associated with their EPD. There are also many composite cattle represented in the Red Angus, Simmental, and Gelbvieh breed databases, and it is hoped that prediction equations can be developed that will improve the accuracy of composite bull EPD.

It has long been recognized that the advantage of GS over traditional selection based on phenotype and pedigree was the ability to accurately predict the genetic merit of young animals for traits that are difficult to measure, like fertility. However, the collection of 1000 or more genotyped animals with comprehensive fertility data to comprise the training population will be both time consuming and expensive,[29] especially if each breed needs to assemble a separate population to obtain accurate within-breed genomic predictions for fertility.

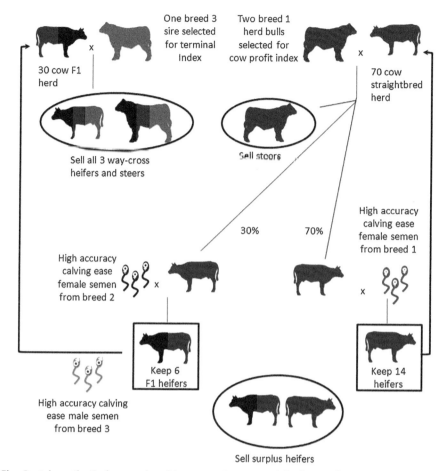

One breed 3 sire selected for terminal Index

Two breed 1 herd bulls selected for cow profit index

30 cow F1 herd

70 cow straightbred herd

Sell all 3 way-cross heifers and steers

Sell steers

High accuracy calving ease female semen from breed 1

High accuracy calving ease female semen from breed 2

30%   70%

High accuracy calving ease male semen from breed 3

Keep 6 F1 heifers

Keep 14 heifers

Sell surplus heifers

Fig. 3. A hypothetical example of how sexed semen might be used in combination with crossbreeding to create a self-replacing 70% straightbred: 30% F1 100 cow herd assuming a 20% replacement rate.

Whole-Genome Resequencing

There are efforts to obtain the full genome sequence of key sires from a variety of breeds to identify SNPs that are predicted to have a disruptive effect on protein structure (also called causative DNA sequence variants) and impair fertility.[30,31] In the most extreme case, an SNP that causes harmful fertility effects (ie, embryonic lethality) would never be found in the homozygous condition in the population and would be detected as a marker with a significant departure from the expected number of homozygotes in the population based on Hardy-Weinberg equilibrium. This approach has already been used to identify missing homozygotes using 50K data in dairy cattle.[32] It is hoped that identifying these causative mutations or fertility-reducing markers will enable the development of inexpensive DNA tests that can accurately identify animals carrying these fertility-reducing markers, perhaps across breeds, and suggest optimum mate selection strategies that maximize the rate of genetic gain and minimize the frequency of carrier matings, with resultant improvements in fertility.

SUMMARY

The choice of breed(s) and breeding system plays an important role in overall ranch profitability. The reproductive fitness of females is a major economic driver and fertility considerations should be given high priority when selecting both the most appropriate breeding system and the best replacement heifers for a given set of environmental, resource, management, and market constraints. Some breed associations calculate EPD (HP, STAY, SC) that have been directly associated with measures of female fertility. These EPD can be used to incorporate fertility in selection decisions, although the amount of fertility data entering national cattle genetic evaluations is limited. By necessity, female selection tends to focus on heifers derived from early calving, fertile cows, which inherently favors the inclusion of fertility in heifer selection. There are some extant and emerging reproductive and genomic technologies, including RTS, timed AI, sexed semen, GS, and the resequencing of prominent bulls to identify causative fertility-reducing markers, that offer innovative opportunities to redesign breeding programs, improve fertility genetic merit evaluations, and optimize mate selection. As with all new technologies, enthusiasm needs to be tempered with a realistic and objective evaluation of the costs and expected benefits of implementation before widespread industry adoption.

REFERENCES

1. Martin LC, Brinks JS, Bourdon RM, et al. Genetic effects on beef heifer puberty and subsequent reproduction. J Anim Sci 1992;70:4006–17.
2. Cundiff LV, Szabo F, Gregory KE, et al. Breed comparisons in the Germplasm evaluation program at MARC. Presented at: Beef Improvement Federation 25th Anniversary Conference. Asheville (SC), May 26–29, 1993.
3. Laster DB, Glimp HA, Gregory KE. Age and weight at puberty and conception in different breeds and breed-crosses of beef heifers. J Anim Sci 1972;34:1031–6.
4. Cundiff LV, Gregory KE, Koch RM. Effects of heterosis on reproduction in Hereford, Angus and shorthorn cattle. J Anim Sci 1974;38:711–27.
5. Cundiff LV, Núñez-Dominguez R, Dickerson GE, et al. Heterosis for lifetime production in Hereford, Angus, shorthorn, and crossbred cows. J Anim Sci 1992; 70:2397–410.
6. Heins BJ, Hansen LB, Seykora AJ. Fertility and survival of pure Holsteins versus crossbreds of Holstein with Normande, Montbeliarde, and Scandinavian red. J Dairy Sci 2006;89:4944–51.
7. Olson TA, Peacock FM, Koger M. Reproductive and maternal performance of rotational three-breed, and inter se crossbred cows in Florida. J Anim Sci 1993;71:2322–9.
8. Winder JA, Rankin BJ, Bailey CC. Maternal performance of Hereford, Brangus, and reciprocal crossbred cows under semidesert conditions. J Anim Sci 1992; 70:1032–8.
9. Wall E, Brotherstone S, Kearney JF, et al. Impact of nonadditive genetic effects in the estimation of breeding values for fertility and correlated traits. J Dairy Sci 2005;88:376–85.
10. Williams JL, Aguilar I, Rekaya R, et al. Estimation of breed and heterosis effects for growth and carcass traits in cattle using published crossbreeding studies. J Anim Sci 2010;88:460–6.
11. Cundiff LV, Gregory KE. What is systematic crossbreeding? Presented at: Cattlemen's College, Cattle Industry Annual Meeting and Trade Show. Charlotte (NC), February 11, 1999.

12. Daley DA, Earley SP. Impacts of crossbreeding in a vertically coordinated beef industry marketing systems. In: Harris Heterosis Report. Available at: http://www.hereford.org/static/files/HarrisHeterosisReport.pdf. Accessed August 8, 2013.

13. Pierce V. Comparison of the economic value of Hereford sired herds vs. Angus sired herds on long run economics. A simulation based on performance data provided by the Hereford Association. 2009. Available at: http://hereford.org/static/files/pierce_circleareprt.pdf. Accessed August 8, 2013.

14. Gutiérrez JP, Alvarez I, Fernández I, et al. Genetic relationships between calving date, calving interval, age at first calving and type traits in beef cattle. Livestock Production Science 2002;78:215–22.

15. Evans JL, Golden BL, Bourdon RM, et al. Additive genetic relationships between heifer pregnancy and scrotal circumference in Hereford cattle. J Anim Sci 1999;77:2621–8.

16. Burns BM, Gazzola C, Holroyd RG, et al. Male reproductive traits and their relationship to reproductive traits in their female progeny: a systematic review. Reprod Domest Anim 2011;46:534–53.

17. Capper JL, Cady RA, Bauman DE. The environmental impact of dairy production: 1944 compared with 2007. J Anim Sci 2009;87:2160–7.

18. Van Melis MH, Eler JP, Rosa GJ, et al. Additive genetic relationships between scrotal circumference, heifer pregnancy, and stayability in Nellore cattle. J Anim Sci 2010;88:3809–13.

19. Melton BF. Conception to consumption: the economics of genetic improvement. In: The Proceedings of the Beef Improvement Federation 27th Research Symposium and Annual Meeting. Sheridan (WY): 1995. p. 40–7.

20. Roughsedge T, Amer PR, Thompson R, et al. Development of a maternal breeding goal and tools to select for this goal in UK beef production. Animal Science 2005;81:221–32.

21. Cole JP, VanRaden PM, Multi-State Project S-10402. Net merit as a measure of lifetime profit: 2010 revision. Available at: http://aipl.arsusda.gov/reference/nmcalc.htm. Accessed August 8, 2013.

22. Anderson KJ, LeFever FG, Brinks JS, et al. The use of reproductive tract scoring in beef heifers. AgriPractice 1991;12:19–26.

23. Rosenkrans KS, Hardin DK. Repeatability and accuracy of reproductive tract scoring to determine pubertal status in beef heifers. Theriogenology 2003;59:1087–92.

24. Snelling WM, Cushman RA, Fortes MR, et al. Physiology and Endocrinology Symposium: how single nucleotide polymorphism chips will advance our knowledge of factors controlling puberty and aid in selecting replacement beef females. J Anim Sci 2012;90:1152–65.

25. Seidel GE. Sexing mammalian sperm–where do we go from here? J Reprod Dev 2012;58:505–9.

26. Hall JB, Glaze JB. Can sexed semen work in your herd? In: Proceedings, Applied Reproductive Strategies in Beef Cattle. Sioux Falls (SD): 2012. p. 363–74.

27. Hohenboken WD. Applications of sexed semen in cattle production. Theriogenology 1999;52:1421–33.

28. Seidel GE Jr. Sexing mammalian sperm–intertwining of commerce, technology, and biology. Anim Reprod Sci 2003;79:145–56.

29. Cammack KM, Thomas MG, Enns RM. Review: reproductive traits and their heritabilities in beef cattle. Professional Animal Scientist 2009;25:517–28.

30. Hayes BJ, Lewin HA, Goddard ME. The future of livestock breeding: genomic selection for efficiency, reduced emissions intensity, and adaptation. Trends Genet 2013;29(4):206–14.

31. Georges M. Impact of high-throughput genotyping and sequencing on the identification of genes and variants underlying phenotypic variation in domestic cattle. In: Womack JE, editor. Bovine genomics. Oxford (United Kingdom): John Wiley; 2012. p. 211–58.

32. VanRaden PM, Olson KM, Null DJ, et al. Harmful recessive effects on fertility detected by absence of homozygous haplotypes. J Dairy Sci 2011;94:6153–61.

33. Corah LR, Hixon DL. Replacement heifer development. In: Beef cattle handbook. Extension Beef Cattle Resource Committee; 1999. p. 1–4 BCH-2100.

34. Ferrell CL. Effects of postweaning rate of gain on onset of puberty and productive performance of heifers of different breeds. J Anim Sci 1982;55:1272–83.

35. Freetly HC, Cundiff LV. Postweaning growth and reproduction characteristics of heifers sired by bulls of seven breeds raised on different levels of nutrition. J Anim Sci 1997;75:2841–51.

36. Fanning M, Selph J, Eubanks S. Florida cow-calf management, 2nd edition - managing reproduction (#AN119). Gainesville (FL): University of Florida Institute of Food and Agricultural Sciences; 2007. Available at: http://edis.ifas.ufl.edu/an119. Accessed February 27, 2013.

37. Laster DB, Smith GM, Gregory KE. Characterization of biological types of cattle IV. Postweaning growth and puberty of heifers. J Anim Sci 1976;43:63–70.

38. Koch RM, Cundiff LV, Gregory KE. Heterosis and breed effects on reproduction. In: Fields MJ, Sand RS, editors. Factors affecting calf crop. Boca Raton (FL): CRC Press; 1994. p. 223–42.

39. Hruska RL. Beef Research Program Progress Report No. 2. Ames (IA): US Meat Animal Research Center; 1985. p. 1–90.

40. Reynolds WL. Breeds and reproduction. In: Cunha TJ, Warnick AC, Koger M, editors. Factors affecting calf crop. Gainesville (FL): University of Florida Press; 1967. p. 244–59.

41. McCartor MM, Randel RD, Carroll LH. Dietary alteration of ruminal fermentation of efficiency of growth and onset of puberty in Brangus heifers. J Anim Sci 1979;48: 488–94.

42. Cundiff LV, Gregory KE, Koch RM, et al. Genetic diversity among cattle breeds and its use to increase beef production efficiency in a temperate environment. In: Proceedings of the 3rd World Congress on Genetics Applied to Livestock Production. Lincoln (NE): 1986. p. 271–82.

43. Cundiff LV, Gregory K, Koch RM, et al. Characteristics of diverse breeds in cycle IV of the Cattle Germ Plasm Evaluation Program at the US Meat Animal Research Center. In: Range Beef Cow Symposium XII Proceedings. Fort Collins (CO): 1991.

44. Thallman RM, Cundiff LV, Gregory KE, et al. Germplasm evaluation in beef cattle–cycle IV: postweaning growth and puberty of heifers. J Anim Sci 1999;77:2651–9.

45. Greiner SP. Beef cattle breeds and biological types (#400–803). Virginia Cooperative Extension. 2009. Available at: http://pubs.ext.vt.edu/400/400-803/400-803.html. Accessed February 27, 2013.

46. Romano MA, Barnabe VH, Kastelic JP, et al. Follicular dynamics in heifers during pre-pubertal and pubertal period kept under two levels of dietary energy intake. Reprod Domest Anim 2007;42:616–22.

47. Hopper HW, Williams SE, Byerley DJ, et al. Effect of prepubertal body weight gain and breed on carcass composition at puberty in beef heifers. J Anim Sci 1993;71: 1104–11.

48. Freking B. Heifer management. In: 2000 beef progress report–1. 2000. Available at: http://www.kerrcenter.com/publications/HeiferManagement.pdf. Accessed February 27, 2013.

Effect of Prenatal Programming on Heifer Development

Richard N. Funston, PhD[a],*, Adam F. Summers, PhD[b]

KEYWORDS

- Fetal programming • Maternal nutrition • Epigenetic modification • Beef cow

KEY POINTS

- Two main mechanisms responsible for fetal programming include DNA methylation and histone modifications.
- Alterations in the genome can be passed through multiple generations.
- Gestational nutrition can affect placental efficiency, fetal organ development, and progeny weaning body weight.
- Late-gestation protein supplementation can decrease heifer progeny age at puberty and increase reproductive efficiency.
- Maternal environment (nutrition, age, physiologic status) can program progeny heifer growth and reproductive performance.

INTRODUCTION

There are several characteristics suggesting the "ideal" beef cow. First, she calves at 2 years of age, does not require human intervention to calve or assistance in nursing her calf, maintains a 365-day calving interval, and weans a marketable calf each year. Furthermore, this animal must remain structurally sound, be able to graze the forages provided in her area, and be tolerant of environmental stressors and disease.[1] Profitability of beef cattle producers is tied directly to the productive life span of mature cows. Heifer development costs are recovered through subsequent calf crops. Reproductive failure represents a major reason females leave the herd, affecting producers' ability to recoup heifer development costs. Nutrition plays a major role in all aspects of beef cattle productivity. Furthermore, it is suggested the fetus is rarely able to

Disclosure: Portions of this review were previously published by the authors in *Annual Reviews: Animal Bioscience* 1:14.1–25. "Epigenetics: setting up lifetime production of cows by managing nutrition."

[a] Department of Animal Science, West Central Research and Extension Center, University of Nebraska – Lincoln, 402 West State Farm Road, North Platte, NE 69101, USA; [b] Department of Animal Science, University of Nebraska – Lincoln, A224b Animal Science, Lincoln, NE 68583, USA

* Corresponding author.

E-mail address: Rick.funston@unl.edu

http://dx.doi.org/10.1016/j.cvfa.2013.07.001
0749-0720/13/$ – see front matter © 2013 Elsevier Inc. All rights reserved.
vetfood.theclinics.com

completely express its full genetic potential for growth, owing to insults caused by the maternal environment.[2]

The main factors influencing nutrient partitioning between the dam and fetus include age of the dam, number of fetuses, production demand, and environmental stress.[3] These factors play a critical role in programming the fetus for its future environment and available resources. Moreover, fetal programming reportedly affects neonatal mortality and morbidity, postnatal growth rate, body composition, health, and reproduction.[4]

EPIGENETIC MODIFICATIONS

Epigenetics is defined as heritable changes in gene expression resulting from alterations in chromatin structure but not DNA sequence. Two mechanisms known to be involved in causing epigenetic changes to the genome include DNA methylation and histone modification.[5] These processes regulate both the intensity and timing of gene expression during cell differentiation.[6,7] Current understanding of these genomic modifications has led to the hypothesis that epigenetics is a key mechanism allowing for phenotypic plasticity with regard to a fixed genotype.[7]

Human epidemiologic studies report associations between low birth body weight (BW) and adult disease. Researchers propose that a fetal programming mechanism occurs whereby environmental stimuli in utero affect fetal growth and health not only during gestation but also later in life.[8,9] Animal models that report intrauterine growth retardation caused by maternal undernutrition indicate altered organ and tissue development in utero.[10,11] These studies suggest modification of the growing fetus to allow environmental adaptation. Epigenetic modifications can result from internal, as well as external, stimuli,[12] thus allowing gene expression in the fetus to best fit with environmental stimulation.

To help explain the main events and processes linking dietary exposures to epigenetic marks and, later, health outcomes, Mathers and McKay[12] developed the 4 Rs of nutritional epigenomics. From this model, one learns that nutrition stimuli and other exposures are (1) received and (2) recorded by the genome. Exposures are also (3) remembered across successive cell generations, and finally, (4) revealed in altered gene expression, cell function, and overall health.[12]

DNA Methylation

Most mammalian DNA, including exons, intergenic DNA, and transposons, is methylated. Methylation sites are located at cytosine bases, followed by a guanosine (CpG).[13] Although most CpG sites are methylated, specific CpG-rich areas of the genome, known as CpG islands, are not methylated. These regions span the 5' end of the regulatory region of a gene.[6] The pattern of CpG-island DNA methylation varies based on tissue type, and this variation likely results in the differing expression of genes in diverse tissues.[14]

The DNA methyltransferase (Dnmt) family of enzymes plays an important role in DNA methylation and, ultimately, embryonic development and survival. Dnmt1, Dnmt3a, and Dnmt3b catalyze cytosine methylation. Furthermore, Dnmt3a and Dnmt3b can establish methylation patterns on unmodified DNA, whereas Dnmt1 maintains these patterns[15] when DNA is duplicated before cell division. Dnmt-null mice die in early gestation,[16] and methyltransferase mutations can cause not only abnormal fetal growth but also immunodeficiency and brain abnormalities in humans.[17]

Methyltransferases use S-adenosylmethionine (SAM) as a methyl donor, and SAM can be directly influenced by diet. Methyl donors for SAM include choline, methionine, and methyltetrahydrofolate, which are related metabolically at the point homocysteine is converted to methionine.[6] Owing to the close relation and interaction among pathways, if the metabolism of any of these methyl donors is altered, compensatory changes will occur in the other methyl donors. A metabolite of 1-carbon metabolism, SAM acts as a methyl donor for methylation reactions, whereas S-adenosylhomocysteine (SAH) acts as a product inhibitor for methyltransferases in DNA and histone methylation. Thus, alterations of folate, vitamin B_{12}, methionine, choline, and betaine through nutrition can alter 1-carbon metabolism and disrupt the availability of methyl donor groups.[18] Restriction of folate, vitamin B_{12}, and methionine from the periconceptional diet of ewes resulted in offspring that were obese as adults and had impaired immune function.[19] Furthermore, studies in rats indicate that DNA methylation of the liver increased 14% for individuals provided a low-folate diet from weaning to puberty.[20] These reports indicate that reducing dietary methyl nutrients may alter methylation patterns and potentially increase disease susceptibility later in life.

Histone Modifications

Extensive wrapping of the DNA during packaging occurs in the nucleus, forming chromatin. The fundamental unit of chromatin is the nucleosome, which consists of an octamer of the 4 core histones (H3, H4, H2A, H2B), wrapped with 147 base pairs of DNA.[21] Histone tails protrude from the globular core and allow for further epigenetic modification via posttranslational modifications of specific amino acid residues.[7,21] Histones can undergo more than 100 distinct posttranslational modifications.[21] For example, similar to DNA, histones can be modified by methylation. However, unlike DNA, histones can also be modified through several types of N-terminal tail modifications, including acetylation, phosphorylation, biotinylation, ubiquitination, and adenosine diphosphate ribosylation,[5] and these modifications can lead to further compaction of DNA and alter the access of transcription factors.[22] Dnmt1 and Dnmt3a reportedly can also act with histone deacetylases to repress transcription.[23]

Protein restriction in maternal diets has resulted in reduced DNA methylation and histone modification in rat offspring as both juveniles and adults.[24,25] However, high-protein maternal diets during gestation and lactation result in sex-specific differences in progeny. Male rat pups from mothers fed a high-protein diet had higher blood pressure compared with male pups from control-fed rats. Female pups born to high-protein intake rats had greater fat pad and body mass compared with females from control-fed rats.[26]

Intergenerational Effects of Fetal Programming

Genome programming can have lasting effects on future generations through intergenerational influences described as factors, conditions, exposures, and environments in one generation that affect the health, growth, and development of subsequent generations.[27] Drake and Walker[28] suggested 3 possible explanations for the occurrence of intergenerational effects: (1) genetic attributes may manifest themselves similarly in mother and offspring; (2) adverse extrinsic environmental conditions may persist across generations; and (3) adverse in utero experiences may permanently affect maternal growth and development, altering the mother's metabolism in a way that provides an adverse fetal environment.[28] In a recent review, Ford and Long[29] report data from human, rat, and sheep studies indicating an intergenerational effect of maternal nutrition on offspring. Zamenhof and colleagues[30] reported reduced birth BW in rats born 2 generations after protein restriction. In addition, Susser and Stein[31] reported that women undernourished during late pregnancy had babies with reduced birth BW, who subsequently had lower birth BW babies in the next generation.

Stewart and colleagues[32] reported that rats maintained on a control diet for 12 generations had greater first-generation birth BW compared with individuals born to rats fed a diet marginally deficient in protein. Epigenetic adaptations also occurred approximately halfway through the experiment when a more unpalatable diet was supplied accidentally to rats on both diets. The subsequent generation of rats had more reduced birth BW for the protein-deficient colony as well as a slight reduction in birth BW for pups born in the control colony. Following readministration of a more palatable diet, birth BW in the control-born pups increased, but colony birth BW did not return to the baseline level for approximately 3 generations despite adequate maternal nutrition.[32]

IMPACT OF EARLY GESTATIONAL NUTRITION

Robinson and colleagues[33] reported that 75% of ruminant fetal growth occurs during the last 2 months of gestation. Owing to the minimal nutrient requirement during early gestation, inadequate nutrition during this time was thought to have little significance. However, Rhind and colleagues[34] indicated that maternal undernutrition affected the conceptus as early as gestation day 11 in sheep, before implantation; the conceptus from ewes fed 50% maintenance requirement was nearly one-third the size of the conceptus from ewes fed 1.5 times their nutrient requirements. During the early phase of fetal development, critical events for normal conceptus development occur, including differentiation, vascularization, fetal organogenesis, and placental development.[35]

Maternal Nutrition and Placental Development

The ability to alter placental development in domesticated livestock through maternal nutrition has been reviewed.[36–38] Establishment of functional uteroplacental and fetal circulation is one of the earliest events of embryonic and placental development.[39,40] This process allows for transportation of all respiratory gas, nutrient, and waste exchanges between the maternal and fetal systems.[41,42] In the ruminant this involves the development of the placentome, the physiologic exchange site between the mother and fetus. The placentome comprises 2 components, cotyledons (fetal portion) and caruncles (maternal portion), which are located on the uterine wall and bind together to allow nutrient exchange. Nutrient transport efficiency through the placentome is related to uteroplacental blood flow.[41] Under normal conditions, placental weights and fetal weights are highly correlated, and reports indicating reduced fetal growth rates also suggest reduced placental blood flow and nutrient uptake.[43,44] Placental growth occurs throughout gestation, although the greatest amount of growth occurs during the first two-thirds of gestation.[44] Although placental growth slows during late gestation, blood flow to the placenta increases 4.5-fold during the last half of gestation to support the exponential rate of fetal growth occurring at the same time.[37,42,45]

Restricting beef cow nutrient intake for 90 days during early to mid-gestation results in altered placental vascularity and function.[46,47] Zhu and colleagues[48] reported that nutrient restriction (NR) of beef cows from days 30 to 125 of gestation resulted in reduced caruncular and cotyledonary weights in comparison with control cows. Fetal weights from NR cows also tended to be reduced when compared with control cows. Following realimentation during days 125 to 250 of gestation, caruncular and cotyledonary weights in NR cows were still reduced; however, fetal weight was not different. Vonnahme and colleagues,[49] using the same cows, reported increased placental angiogenesis as well as angiogenic factor mRNA abundance in the caruncular and cotyledonary tissues at the end of the NR period. Capillary vascularity from days 30 to 125 of gestation was not different; however, from days 125 to 250, significant differences existed when comparing control (CON) and NR cows, which suggests that capillary areas, numbers, and surface densities had been hindered on realimentation.[49]

In a recent review, Vonnahme and Lemley[38] reported that providing protein supplementation to cows beginning on day 190 of gestation resulted in a doubling of uterine blood flow when compared with nonsupplemented cows. It is hypothesized that increased uterine blood flow may increase progeny performance (see later discussion) owing to increased nutrient transfer to the fetus. Sullivan and colleagues[50] fed composite beef heifers in a 2×2 factorial design in which heifers were assigned a high- or low-protein and dietary energy diet during the first trimester of gestation. During the second trimester of gestation, half of each treatment group was offered the oppo site diet, leading to 4 treatment groups: high/high (HH), high/low (HL), low/high (LH), and low/low (LL). Cotyledonary weight was dependent on both first-trimester and second-trimester diets; pregnant heifers fed the HH diet had the most cotyledons present, and heifers fed the LL diet had the fewest cotyledons in the expelled placenta. Caruncles are present in the bovine uterus as early as month 4 of gestation, and thus the number of caruncles may be determined before birth.[51] Of note, altering maternal dietary protein level during the first or second trimester did not influence the number of caruncles present in nonpregnant adult progeny uterus.[50] This finding would suggest that maternal NR affects the number of cotyledons developed on the placenta and available to bind to the maternal caruncle.

Maternal Nutrition and Fetal Organ Development

Fetal organ formation occurs simultaneously with placental development, and by gestation days 50 to 60 ovarian development begins in female calves. Maternal nutrient status can affect fetal organ development. Long and colleagues[52] reported enlarged hearts and brains in fetuses from NR cows from days 30 to 125 of gestation, in comparison with fetuses from control cows. However, after realimentation of NR cows to achieve weight and body condition score (BCS) similar to those of control cows by day 220 of gestation, brain or heart weights did not differ among groups by day 245 of gestation. Meyer and colleagues[53] reported no differences in fetal visceral organ weights at day 125 of gestation, using the same fetuses reported by Long and colleagues.[52] However, at day 245 of gestation, fetuses from NR cows had greater reticular mass and total intestinal vascularity compared with fetuses from control cows.[53] Other organs affected by maternal nutrition include liver,[54] lung,[55] pancreas,[56] kidney,[57] perirenal fat,[58,59] and small intestine.[60]

Primordial Follicle Assembly

Cow longevity is related to the ability to annually produce a live calf. Subsequently, reproductive failure (inability to maintain pregnancy) is one of the main reasons cows leave the production herd.[61,62] Furthermore, fertility is closely related to ovarian characteristics.[63] Follicle assembly is the developmental process by which individual oocytes develop from oocyte nests and assemble into primordial follicles. Initiation of primordial follicle assembly is species specific[64–68] and is reported to occur around day 80 of gestation in cattle, with most primordial follicles formed by day 143.[69] Primordial follicle numbers are highly variable at birth in cattle, ranging from an estimated 14,000 to 250,000.[70,71] Over the course of the cow's lifetime nearly 99% of all follicles within the ovarian reserve will become atretic.[72]

Primordial follicles remain arrested at the diplotene stage of the first meiotic division until hormonal regulation stimulates the transition from primordial to primary follicle.[69] Transition of follicles to the primary stage is an important process allowing follicle growth and ovulation; however, it is also irreversible. Follicles stimulated to the primary stage will either proliferate and ovulate, or undergo atresia.[73]

Follicle-stimulating hormone (FSH) is important for folliculogenesis, allowing for growth and differentiation of antral follicles during follicular waves.[74] However, concentration of FSH has a negative relationship with the number of healthy follicles and oocytes reported during follicular waves.[75] Ovaries are the primary source of androgen production in the female. High variability in the number of growing follicles within individuals is hypothesized to be related to androgen production by individual follicles, and the total follicle pool, which is highly variable.[76] Conversely, anti-Müllerian hormone (AMH) concentrations have a positive relationship with the number of healthy follicles.[74,77]

Antral Follicle Counts

One method of predicting ovarian reserve is to measure antral follicle counts (AFC) in the ovary via ultrasonography. Classifications are made based on number of antral follicles identified by ultrasonography, with animals having 15 or fewer being classified as low, 16 to 24 as moderate, and 25 or more as high follicle count.[77] These follicles, at least 3 mm in size, represent a subpopulation of total ovarian reserve. Typically AFC are conducted in heifers before their first breeding season (13–15 months old), and approximately 15% to 20% of the herd are classified as low or high AFC while the remaining 80% to 85% are classified as moderate AFC.[78] Previous reports state that although variation in follicle number is present among individuals, the peak number of antral follicles growing during a follicular wave is highly repeatable within individuals when ovarian ultrasonography is used.[79,80] Low-AFC heifers had lower pregnancy rates and reduced numbers of morphologically healthy oocytes and follicles[62,77,81] when compared with high-AFC heifers. Furthermore, Mossa and colleagues[81] reported that high-AFC dairy cows had a 3.34 times greater odds ratio of being pregnant at the end of the breeding season and a reduced duration from calving to conception compared with low-AFC heifers. The decreased timing from calving to conception could be due to an increase in the number of estrous cycles experienced by high-AFC cows earlier in the breeding season. Byerley and colleagues[82] observed increased pregnancy rates for heifers bred on third estrus compared with those bred on pubertal estrus, and perhaps similar improvements in fertility can be associated with first estrous after calving and later estrous cycles. Cow reproductive longevity has been associated with AFC. Mossa and colleagues[81] reported that dairy cows with high-AFC had an average of 2.6 lactations compared with 1.9 lactations for low-AFC, also suggesting increased longevity of cows with greater AFC. Furthermore, Mossa and colleagues[81] reported a trend for decreased median calving to conception period for high-AFC cows (100 days) compared with low-AFC cows (114 days).

Reports of differences in hormone profiles between high-AFC and low-AFC heifers can also be found in the literature. Ireland and colleagues[74] reported a 2-fold increase in follicular fluid estrogen concentration, as well as increased FSH concentration, when comparing low-AFC with high-AFC animals. Furthermore, heifers classified as low AFC have increased gonadotropin secretion and reduced progesterone levels in comparison with high-AFC heifers.[78] Decreased progesterone levels have been reported to increase embryonic mortality in cattle,[78,83] and could possibly play a role in the decreased pregnancy rates reported in low-AFC heifers.[62,77,81]

Impact of Maternal Nutrition on Progeny Follicle Development

Rae and colleagues[84] reported that maternal undernutrition in sheep during the first 110 days of gestation results in reduced ovulation rates, most likely through a direct effect on folliculogenesis. Furthermore, limiting the duration of undernutrition to 1 to 2 months during the first 110 days of gestation also reduces the number of follicles that develop beyond the primordial stage.[84] Maternal nutrient restriction can also have long-term influences on plasma progesterone levels in progeny.[85,86] In a small group of heifers, NR and NR with protein supplementation resulted in reduced wet ovarian weight and decreased luteal tissue mass in a comparison with heifers born to control-fed cows.[87]

Mossa and colleagues[88] reported a 60% reduction in AFC for heifers born to dams fed 60% of their energy requirements compared with heifers from control-fed dams. However, Da Silva and colleagues[54] reported reduced ovarian follicles from progeny of ewe lambs fed to achieve rapid maternal growth rates throughout pregnancy when compared with progeny from ewe lambs fed to gain 50 to 75 g/d through the first 100 days of gestation. Sullivan and colleagues[63] also reported a negative influence of high protein and dietary energy fed to heifers during the second trimester on primordial and primary follicle density (n per 100 mm^2). Progeny born to heifers fed the HH or LH diets had lower primordial and primary follicle densities compared with progeny from heifers fed the LL or HL diets; however, total AFC density was not different.[63] Reduced follicle densities in the LH and HH groups coincided with high maternal plasma urea nitrogen (PUN) concentration.[63] The effect of PUN on fetal ovarian follicle development is unknown; however, it has been well established high PUN affects reproductive characteristics and fertility, with reports indicating an increased interval from calving to first ovulation, altered uterine pH, and decreasing pregnancy rates.[89–93]

Impact of Maternal Undernutrition on Female Progeny Performance

The majority of studies evaluating the effect of maternal nutrition on heifer progeny performance are limited to first-calf heifer data. However, Roberts and colleagues[94] conducted a study over a 7-year period monitoring the production of composite (one-half Red Angus, one-quarter Charolais, one-quarter Tarentaise) cows from dams fed either marginal or adequate levels of harvested feeds from December to March (**Table 1**). Groups of cows were placed in separate pastures, and a supplement of alfalfa cake or hay, depending on year, was provided either daily or every other day at an average of 1.8 kg/d for adequate cows or 1 kg/d for marginal cows. During the winter supplementation period, pasture forage was generally accessible for grazing. On days when snow limited pasture availability, cows were fed at a rate of 10.9 and 9.1 kg/d for adequate and marginal cows, respectively. Each year at weaning, heifer calves were assigned to a pen for a 140-day feeding period and either offered a control diet, fed to appetite, or given a restricted diet, offered at 80% of the amount consumed by heifers on the control diet adjusted to a common BW. Heifers were managed similarly after the feeding period through the breeding season and fall. Control heifers were then provided the adequate level of feed during each subsequent winter, and restricted heifers were provided marginal levels. Heifers born to marginal dams had greater BW later in life compared with heifers of adequate dams.[95] This difference may be caused in part by the increased BCS of the cows from marginal dams. Furthermore, calves born to restricted dams and marginal grand dams were lighter at both birth and weaning compared with calves born to control dams and adequate grand dams; however, pregnancy rates for bred heifers did not differ.[94] Corah and colleagues[96] reported increased morbidity and mortality rates in calves born to primiparous heifers receiving 65% of their dietary energy requirement over the last 90 days of gestation, in comparison with calves from primiparous heifers receiving 100% of their energy requirement. Furthermore, these investigators reported that heifers born to primiparous heifers fed 100% of their dietary energy requirement during the last 90 days

Table 1
Effects of level of feed input provided to dam and progeny on progeny performance

| Heifer Development and Treatment[b] | Level of Winter Supplement to Dam[a] | | | |
| | Marginal | | Adequate | |
	Restricted	Control	Restricted	Control
Five-year BW[c], kg	515	530	490	505
BCS at 5 y[d]	4.9	5.1	4.7[e]	5.0
Retention at 5 y, %	48	46	39	49
Calf birth weight, kg	33.6[e]	35	35	35
Calf weaning weight[d], kg	196[e]	201	202	204

[a] Level of supplementation provided to cows from December to March. Marginal = equivalent of 1.1 kg/d; Adequate = equivalent of 1.8 kg/d.
[b] Dietary level offered to heifers during 140-day postweaning development period. Restricted = 80% of feed provided to control and 1.1 kg/d supplement each subsequent winter. Control = fed ad libitum during postweaning and 1.8 kg/d supplement each winter.
[c] $P<.01$ for effect of dam treatment and heifer development treatment.
[d] $P<.001$ for interaction of dam treatment and heifer development treatment.
[e] Differs from others in same row.
Data from Roberts AJ, Grings EE, MacNeil MD, et al. Implications of going against the dogma of feed them to breed them. Wes Sect Anim Sci Proc 2009;60:87–8; and Roberts AJ, Funston R, Mulliniks T, et al. Feed efficiency—how should it be used for the cow herd? Presented at Range Beef Cow Symposium XXII. Mitchell, November 30, 2011.

of gestation were pubertal 19 days earlier than heifers born to primiparous heifers fed 65% of their dietary energy requirement, although this difference was not significant.

Effect of Late-Gestation Protein Supplementation on Heifer Progeny Performance

Rolfe and colleagues[97] reported that birth BW was affected by previous maternal weaning date and grazing treatment. Progeny of October (OCT)-weaned dams receiving 0.91 kg/d protein supplement while grazing winter range (WR2) had greater birth BW than calves from nonsupplemented dams grazing winter range (WR0). Calves from December (DEC)-weaned WR0 dams had reduced birth BW compared with all other groups except DEC-weaned calves from dams grazing winter range and receiving 0.45 kg/d protein supplement (WR1). OCT BW was reduced 15 to 23 ± 3 kg in calves born to WR0 dams compared with all other groups. Dam winter treatment also affected DEC and prebreeding BW; WR0-born calves had reduced BW compared with other winter treatment groups.[97]

Martin and colleagues[98] conducted a study with cows grazing winter range (WR) during late gestation. One group received a 42% crude protein (CP, dry-matter [DM] basis) cube offered 3 times weekly at the equivalent of 0.45 kg/d, and another group received no supplement. After calving, pairs were offered cool-season grass hay or placed on subirrigated meadows during early lactation. Calf birth BW was not different between heifer progeny from supplemented and nonsupplemented dams; however, heifer progeny from supplemented cows had increased adjusted 205-day weaning BW (226 vs 218 ± 7 kg), prebreeding BW (276 vs 266 ± 9 kg), BW at pregnancy diagnosis (400 vs 386 ± 31 kg), and improved pregnancy rates (93% vs 80%) compared with heifers from nonsupplemented dams (**Table 2**). Martin and colleagues[98] also reported that after a subset of these heifers was placed in a Calan gate individual feeding system, DMI, ADG, and residual feed intake (RFI) did not differ between heifer progeny from supplemented and nonsupplemented dams (see **Table 2**).

Table 2
Effect of maternal protein supplementation on heifer progeny performance

| Item | Dietary Treatment | | | |
| | Martin et al,[98] 2007[a] | | Funston et al,[99] 2010[b] | |
	NS	SUP	NS	SUP
Birth weight, kg	35	36	35	35
Weaning weight, kg	207	212	225[c]	232[d]
Adjusted 205-day weight, kg	218[c]	226[d]	213	217
Dry matter intake, kg/d	6.50	6.75	9.48	9.30
Average daily gain, kg/d	0.41	0.40	0.85	0.79
Residual feed intake	−0.12	0.07	0.08	−0.04
Final BW,[e] kg	290[f]	304[g]	—	—
Age at puberty, d	334	339	366[f]	352[g]
Prebreeding weight, kg	266[c]	276[d]	317	323
Pregnancy diagnosis weight, kg	386[c]	400[d]	364	368
Pregnant, %	80[c]	93[d]	80	90
Calved in first 21 d, %	49[c]	77[d]	85	77

[a] NS = dams did not receive protein supplement while grazing dormant Sandhills range during the last third of gestation; SUP = dams were supplemented 3 times per week with the equivalent of 0.45 kg/d of 42% CP cube (dry-matter basis) while grazing dormant Sandhills range during the last third of gestation.

[b] NS = dams did not receive protein supplement while grazing dormant Sandhills range or corn residue during the last third of gestation; SUP = dams were supplemented 3 times per week with the equivalent of 0.45 kg/d of a 31% CP cube (dry-matter basis) while grazing dormant Sandhills range or corn residue during the last third of gestation.

[c,d] Means within a study with different superscripts differ ($P \leq 05$).

[e] Final weight of heifers after 84-day individual feeding period.

[f,g] Means within a study with different superscripts differ ($P \leq .10$).

Data from Martin JL, Vonnahme KA, Adams DC, et al. Effects of dam nutrition on growth and reproductive performance of heifer calves. J Anim Sci 2007;85:844–6; and Funston RN, Martin JL, Adams DC, et al. Winter grazing system and supplementation of beef cows during late gestation influence heifer progeny. J Anim Sci 2010;88:4098–99.

Using the same cow herd (see **Table 2**), Funston and colleagues[99] offered a distillers-based supplement (31% CP; DM basis) 3 times weekly at the equivalent of 0.45 kg/d or no supplement during late gestation to cows grazing either WR or corn residue (CR). Calf weaning BW was greater for heifers from protein-supplemented dams (232 vs 225 ± 6 kg).[99] Martin and colleagues[98] also reported increased weaning BW, though not significant, for heifers from protein-supplemented dams. Using distillers' grains as an energy source during late gestation and early lactation, Gunn and colleagues[100] reported greater birth BW and increased calving difficulty in progeny compared with progeny from corn silage and haylage-fed dams. However, weaning BW were also greater in progeny from distillers' grains–fed dams.

Funston and colleagues[99] also reported that heifers from protein-supplemented cows attained puberty 14 days earlier than heifers from nonsupplemented dams. Furthermore, there was a trend for higher pregnancy rates when comparing heifers from protein-supplemented dams with heifers from nonsupplemented dams, possibly related to decreased age at puberty. The studies conducted by Martin and colleagues[98] and Funston and colleagues[99] both used experiments of 2 × 2 factorial design. The slight differences reported between these investigators may be explained by differences in study design and animal allotment to treatment. Both treatment factors studied by Funston and colleagues[99] were applied to the cow prepartum, and cows in this study remained on the same treatment all 3 years. By contrast, Martin and colleagues[98] studied the effect of protein supplementation or no supplementation during late gestation but also the effect of grazing cow/calf pairs on subirrigated meadow or meadow hay provided during early lactation. In this experiment the researchers used a crossover design in the first 2 years of the study and randomly assigned cows to a treatment group during the third year of the experiment. Moreover, Martin and colleagues[98] used a 42% CP supplement consisting of 50% sunflower meal and 47% cottonseed meal, whereas Funston and colleagues[99] provided a 31% crude protein supplement consisting of mostly dried distillers' grains with solubles. Using NRC[101] feed values, the protein in the supplement fed by Martin and colleagues[98] contained approximately 33% rumen undegradable protein (RUP), whereas the supplement administered by Funston and colleagues[99] provided approximately 48% of the protein as RUP. Increased levels of RUP would provide increased levels of diet-supplied amino acids to the intestine for use by the animal, compared with protein degraded in the rumen and utilized by rumen microbes.

Warner and colleagues[102] reported no differences in pregnancy rates for heifers from dams grazing CR and receiving protein supplement when compared with dams grazing CR and receiving no supplement during late gestation. These results coincide with data presented by Funston and colleagues[99] showing that pregnancy rates for heifers from protein-supplemented cows were affected by dam wintergrazing treatment, with pregnancy rates being similar for heifers born to cows grazing CR regardless of protein-supplementation treatment.[99] Rolfe and colleagues[97] reported a similar proportion of heifers cycling, and overall pregnancy rates did not differ based on maternal weaning treatment or winter treatment when analyzing the first year of data. However, the investigators did report a numeric increase in pregnancy rates in all groups compared with WR0, similar to data reported by Funston and colleagues[99] whereby heifers born to supplemented dams had greater pregnancy rates than heifers of nonsupplemented dams.

Compared with heifer progeny from supplemented and nonsupplemented cows, Funston and colleagues[99] reported no differences in heifer BW at prebreeding, calf birth BW, calf production, or second-calf rebreeding. Gunn and colleagues[103] reported a decrease in the proportion of singleton births and an increase in the proportion of multiple births over 3 parities in progeny born to ewes offered a protein supplement while grazing native pastures during the last 100 days of gestation, compared with progeny from nonsupplemented ewes. Late-gestation supplementation did not alter the proportion of barren ewe progeny; however, supplementation during lactation did.[103] Martin and colleagues[98] reported a 28% increase in the proportion of heifers that calved in the first 21 days of the calving season from protein-supplemented dams compared with heifers from nonsupplemented dams.

Impact of Maternal Body Reserves on Progeny Performance

BCS is an estimate of energy reserves available to help the animal with maintenance and production requirements. Pryce and colleagues[104] reported no difference in progeny heifer reproductive performance considering dairy cow maternal nutritional status, determined by BCS, DMI, and milk yield of fat and protein. Rolfe and colleagues[97] reported similar cow BCS and BW at the October weaning; however, by December, BCS and BW for DEC cows was reduced in comparison with OCT-weaned cows. Cow BCS precalving remained greater for OCT-weaned cows than for DEC-weaned cows, but BCS did not differ for weaning treatment by prebreeding.[97] The difference in BCS and BW can be attributed to the added requirements of lactation during the 2-month difference in weaning treatment. In October, calves from OCT-weaned dams had greater BW compared with calves from DEC-weaned dams. BW was greater for heifers born to OCT-weaned calves at the December weaning, and greater BW continued to the breeding season.[97] Although BW in OCT-weaned heifers differed from that of DEC-weaned heifers, steer progeny BW, feedlot performance, and carcass characteristics were similar among weaning treatments.

Impact of Maternal Overnutrition on Progeny Performance

Although producers typically manage animals in such a way that there is no overabundance of nutrients, researchers have studied the effects of overnutrition on progeny performance. Overnutrition in cattle has been reported to increase BW and skeletal size, decrease milk production, and decrease reproductive life and longevity.[105–108] Of note, maternal overnutrition has been reported to decrease birth BW of lambs.[54,109,110] Furthermore, reproductive phenotypes were altered in sheep born to overnourished dams, with female progeny having reduced ovarian size and male progeny increased age at puberty.[54,110]

In many reports in human and livestock species, it appears that maternal overnutrition results in progeny phenotypes similar to progeny from undernourished females.[29] The investigators hypothesize that the mechanism involving the similarities in phenotypes is due in part to the reduction of placental vascularity and nutrient transporter in animals fed 150% maintenance requirements from 60 days before conception through gestation.[111] Ewes fed 50% maintenance requirements from early to mid-gestation and then 100% requirement until lambing had fetal BW approximately 60% below fetal BW from overnourished ewes at mid-gestation day 110. However, after nutrient realignment in nutrient restricted ewes (late gestation), placental vascularity and nutrient transporter activity increased, unlike in the overnourished model, giving rise to lambs born from each treatment with similar birth BW.[111]

Effect of Maternal Age, Milk Production, and Birth Date on Progeny Performance

Cows becoming pregnant at a young age must not only provide energy for developing fetal growth but also supply energy for their own growth requirements. In fact, Caton and colleagues[112] reported that primiparous heifers require an additional 1.46 Mcal/d of net energy during the last trimester of gestation compared with mature cows. This increase in daily energy requirements is associated directly with the heifer's growth requirement. Increasing cow longevity is advantageous to producers because it allows them to spread heifer development costs across more units of output (calves) or a greater number of lactations in dairy cattle.

One potential side effect of the developing fetuses of older dams is a possible increase in chromosome abnormalities owing to reduced oocyte competence.[113] Extremes in age, both old and young, resulted in mice pups with reduced BW and delayed puberty.[114] Old cows (13–16 years old) recovered fewer embryos and had a greater proportion of unfertilized oocytes compared with their younger daughters (3–6 years old).[113] Fuerst-Waltl and colleagues[115] analyzed records of approximately 217,000 Austrian dual-purpose Simmental cows and reported that energy-corrected milk yield, milk fat, and protein yield decrease as maternal age increases through the first 3 lactations.

Although lactation coincides with fetal growth and development, thus competing for energy, it appears that maternal milk production has no effect on progeny milking performance.[116,117] Banos and colleagues[116] reported that heifers born to young cows (18–23 months old) had greater daily milk yield and BCS, and calved 3 days earlier than heifers born to older cows (30–36 months old). However, heifers born to younger dams had reduced fertility, requiring 7% more inseminations per conception compared with heifers from older cows.[116] Cows born to young, second-calving dams (36–41 months old) had improved productivity with increased fertility and daily milk yield during first lactation compared with cows from dams who were older (47–55 months old) at second calving.[116]

Thirteen years of spring calving records at the University of Nebraska Gudmundsen Sandhills Laboratory (GSL) were reviewed to examine the impact of heifer birth date on productivity.[118] Heifers were classified as being born in the first, second, or third 21-day periods of the calving season based on birth date. Heifers born in the first 21 days had reduced birth BW (36 ± 0.70 kg) compared with the other groups. Heifers born in the third 21 days had the greatest birth BW (38 ± 0.70 kg). One possible cause for increased birth BW in calves born later in the calving season is improved quality of forage. Records were reported from spring calving cows, with the average Julian birth date of calves from the first 21 days being 72 (March 13). The third group categorized was born on Julian date 113 (April 23). Previous research conducted at the GSL suggests a 2% improvement in range crude protein and nutrient value from February, coinciding with late gestation for calves born in the first 21-day period, to March/April, corresponding with late gestation for calves born in the third 21-day period of the calving season.[119] As previously mentioned, nutrient demand for fetal growth is greatest during late gestation because of the increased growth rate of the fetus before birth. Increased quality of forage before birth for calves born later in the calving season could cause improved nutritional status of the cow, and thus increase nutrient supply to the growing fetus to increase birth BW.

Weaning BW, prebreeding BW, proportion of heifers cycling at the beginning of the breeding season, and percentage of pregnant animals were greatest for heifers born in the first 21 days of the calving season.[118] Because more heifers born in the first 21 days of the calving season were cycling at the beginning of the breeding season, heifers from that group likely had more estrous cycles before breeding compared with heifers born later in the calving season. Byerley and colleagues[82] observed increased pregnancy rates for heifers bred on third estrus compared with those bred on pubertal estrus. A greater proportion of heifers born in the first 21 days also calved in the first 21 days as first-calf heifers, and weaned heavier calves.[117] In addition, heifers calving earlier in their first calving season have greater lifetime productivity than those calving later.[120]

SUMMARY

Several factors influence cow productivity and performance, including maternal age, maternal milking ability, weaning weight, and maternal nutrition during gestation. Maternal nutrient status can alter the epigenome via posttranslational modifications. The timing of maternal nutrient alteration also plays an important role in determining the effect nutrition will have on the developing placenta, fetus, and progeny performance (**Fig. 1**). Fetal programming can occur before implantation, and placental development can be compromised through reduced nutrient intake (see **Fig. 1**). At present, the amount of literature reporting maternal nutrition effects on heifer progeny longevity is limited; however, in most of these studies performance through the first production cycle has been documented. Providing adequate nutrition has resulted in improved progeny health and increased BW. Furthermore, studies have reported reduced age at puberty, increased fertility, and earlier calving dates for heifers born to dams supplemented with protein while grazing winter range (see **Fig. 1**). Early

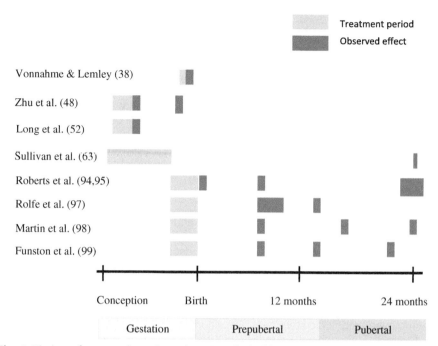

Fig. 1. Timing of maternal nutrient alteration (*light blue*) affects fetal development and progeny performance (*dark blue*) in beef cattle. (*Adapted from* Rhind SM, Rae MT, Brooks AN. Effects of nutrition and environmental factors on the fetal programming of the reproductive axis. Reproduction 2001;122:206; with permission.)

neonatal life is also crucial for future calf performance. Milk production and puberty attainment can be altered based on nutrient intake as well as time of weaning. Studies have also reported that by limiting feed during the developmental period, heifer development costs can be reduced without compromising reproductive efficiency. Exposing heifers to the environment where they will be managed as cows early in development may potentially improve productivity and longevity.

REFERENCES

1. Hohenboken WD. Bovine nirvana—from the perspective of an experimentalist. J Anim Sci 1988;66:1885–91.
2. Gluckman PD, Liggins GC. Regulation of fetal growth. In: Beard RW, Nathanielsz PW, editors. Fetal physiology and medicine. 2nd edition. London: Butterworths; 1984. p. 511–57.
3. Reynolds LP, Borowicz PP, Caton JS, et al. Developmental programming: the concept, large animal models, and the key role of uteroplacental vascular development. J Anim Sci 2010;88(Suppl E):E61–72.
4. Wu G, Bazer FW, Wallace JM, et al. Board-invited review: intrauterine growth retardation: implications for the animal sciences. J Anim Sci 2006;84:2316–37.
5. Canani RB, Costanzo MD, Leone L, et al. Epigenetic mechanisms elicited by nutrition in early life. Nutr Res Rev 2011;24:198–205.
6. Zeisel SH. Epigenetic mechanisms for nutrition determinants of later health outcomes. Am J Clin Nutr 2009;89:S1488–93.

7. McKay JA, Mathers JC. Diet induced epigenetic changes and their implications for health. Acta Physiol (Oxf) 2011;202:103–18.

8. Barker DJ. Fetal origins of coronary heart disease. BMJ 1995;331:171–4.

9. Barker DJ. Fetal programming and public health. In: O'Brien PM, Wheeler T, Barker DJ, editors. Fetal programming: influences on development and disease in later life. London: TCOG Press; 1999. p. 3–11.

10. Vonnahme KA, Hess BW, Hansen TR, et al. Maternal undernutrition from early to midgestation leads to growth retardation, cardiac ventricular hypertrophy, and increased liver weight in the fetal sheep. Biol Reprod 2003;69:133–40.

11. Ford SP, Zhang L, Zhu M, et al. Maternal obesity accelerates fetal pancreatic β-cell but not α-cell development in sheep: prenatal consequences. Am J Physiol Regul Integr Comp Physiol 2009;297:R835–43.

12. Mathers JC, McKay JA. Epigenetics—potential contribution to fetal programming. Adv Exp Med Biol 2009;646:119–23.

13. Holliday R, Grigg GW. DNA methylation and mutation. Mutat Res 1993;285:61–7.

14. Suzuki MM, Bird A. DNA methylation landscapes: provocative insights from epigenomics. Nat Rev Genet 2008;9:465–76.

15. Cheng X, Blumenthal RM. Mammalian DNA methyltransferases: a structural perspective. Structure 2008;16:341–50.

16. Lei H, Oh SP, Okano M, et al. De novo DNA cytosine methyltransferase activities in mouse embryonic stem cells. Development 1996;122:3195–205.

17. Clouaire T, Stancheva I. Methyl-CpG binding proteins: specialized transcriptional repressors or structural components of chromatin? Cell Mol Life Sci 2008;65:1509–22.

18. Choi SW, Friso S. Epigenetics: a new bridge between nutrition and health. Adv Nutr 2010;1:1–16.

19. Sinclair KD, Allegrucci C, Singh R, et al. DNA methylation, insulin resistance, and blood pressure in offspring determined by maternal periconceptional B vitamin and methionine status. Proc Natl Acad Sci U S A 2007;104:19351–6.

20. Kotsopoulos J, Sohn KJ, Kim YI. Postweaning dietary folate deficiency provided through childhood to puberty permanently increases genomic DNA methylation in adult rat liver. J Nutr 2008;138:703–9.

21. Kouzarides T. Chromatin modifications and their function. Cell 2007;128:693–705.

22. Faulk C, Dolinoy DC. Timing is everything the when and how of environmentally induced changes in the epigenome of animals. Epigenetics 2011;6(7):791–7.

23. Burgers WA, Fuks F, Kouzarides T. DNA methyltransferases get connected to chromatin. Trends Genet 2002;18:275–7.

24. Lillycrop KA, Slater-Jefferies JL, Hanson MA, et al. Induction of altered epigenetic regulation of the hepatic glucocorticoid receptor in the offspring of rats fed a protein- restricted diet during pregnancy suggests that reduced DNA methyltransferase-1 expression is involved in impaired DNA methylation and changes in histone modifications. Br J Nutr 2007;97:1064–73.

25. Lillycrop KA, Phillips ES, Torrens C, et al. Feeding pregnant rats a protein-restricted diet persistently alters the methylation of specific cytosines in the hepatic PPARα promoter of the offspring. Br J Nutr 2008;100:278–82.

26. Thone-Reineke C, Kalk P, Dorn M, et al. High-protein nutrition during pregnancy and lactation programs blood pressure, food efficiency, and body weight of the offspring in a sex-dependent manner. Am J Physiol Regul Integr Comp Physiol 2006;291:R1025–30.

27. Emanuel I. Maternal health during childhood and later reproductive performance. Ann N Y Acad Sci 1986;477:27–39.
28. Drake AJ, Walker BR. The intergenerational effects of fetal programming: nongenomic mechanisms for the inheritance of low birth weight and cardiovascular risk. J Endocrinol 2004;180:1–16.
29. Ford SP, Long NM. Evidence for similar changes in offspring phenotype following either maternal undernutrition or overnutrition: potential impact on fetal epigenetic mechanisms. Reprod Fertil Dev 2012;24:105–11.
30. Zamenhof S, van Marthens E, Grauel L. DNA (cell number) in neonatal brain: second generation (F2) alteration by maternal (F0) dietary protein restriction. Science 1971;172:850–1.
31. Susser M, Stein Z. Timing in postnatal nutrition: a reprise of the Dutch Famine Study. Nutr Rev 1994;52:84–94.
32. Stewart RJ, Sheppard H, Preece R, et al. The effect of rehabilitation at different stages of development of rats marginally malnourished for ten to twelve generations. Br J Nutr 1980;43:403–12.
33. Robinson JJ, McDonald I, Fraser C, et al. Studies on reproduction in prolific ewes. I. Growth of the products of conception. J Agric Sci 1977;88:539–52.
34. Rhind SM, McKelvey WA, McMillen SR, et al. Effect of restricted food intake, before and/or after mating, on the reproductive performance of Greyface ewes. Anim Prod 1989;48:149–55.
35. Funston RN, Larson DM, Vonnahme KA. Effects of maternal nutrition on conceptus growth and offspring performance: implications for beef cattle production. J Anim Sci 2010;88(Suppl E):E205–15.
36. Redmer DA, Wallace JM, Reynolds LP. Effect of nutrient intake during pregnancy on fetal and placental growth and vascular development. Domest Anim Endocrinol 2004;27:199–217.
37. Reynolds LP, Caton JS, Redmer DA, et al. Evidence for altered placental blood flow and vascularity in compromised pregnancies. J Physiol 2006;572:51–8.
38. Vonnahme KA, Lemley CO. Programming the offspring through altered uteroplacental hemodynamics: how maternal environment impacts uterine and umbilical blood flow in cattle, sheep, and pigs. Reprod Fertil Dev 2012;24:97–104.
39. Patten BM. Foundations of embryology. 2nd edition. New York: McGraw-Hill; 1964.
40. Ramsey EM. The placenta, human and animal. New York: Praeger; 1984.
41. Reynolds LP, Redmer DA. Utero-placental vascular development and placental function. J Anim Sci 1995;73:1839–51.
42. Reynolds LP, Redmer DA. Angiogenesis in the placenta. Biol Reprod 2001;64: 1033–40.
43. Wootton R, McFayden IR, Cooper JE. Measurement of placental blood flow in the pig and its relation to placental and fetal weight. Biol Neonate 1977;31: 333–9.
44. Reynolds LP, Millaway DS, Kirsch JD, et al. Growth and in-vitro metabolism of placental tissues of cows from day 100 to day 250 of gestation. J Reprod Fertil 1990;89:213–22.
45. Reynolds LP, Ferrell CL, Robertson DA, et al. Metabolism of the gravid uterus, foetus and uteroplacenta at several stages of gestation in cows. J Agric Sci 1986;106:437–44.
46. Vonnahme KA, Ford SP, Nijland MJ, et al. Alteration in cotyledonary (COT) vascular responsiveness to angiotensin II (ANF II) in beef cows undernourished during early pregnancy [abstract]. Biol Reprod 2004;70(Suppl 1):110.

47. Vonnahme KA, Reynolds LP, Nijland MJ, et al. Impacts of undernutrition during early to mid gestation on basal vascular tone of the cotyledonary and caruncular arterial beds in bovine placentomes. J Soc Gynecol Investig 2004;11(Suppl):222A.

48. Zhu MJ, Du M, Hess BW, et al. Maternal nutrient restriction upregulates growth signaling pathway in the cotyledonary artery of cow placentomes. Placenta 2007;28:361–8.

49. Vonnahme KA, Zhu MJ, Borowicz PP, et al. Effect of early gestational undernutrition on angiogenic factor expression and vascularity in the bovine placentome. J Anim Sci 2007;85:2464–72.

50. Sullivan TM, Micke GC, Magalhaes RS, et al. Dietary protein during gestation affects placental development in heifers. Theriogenology 2009;72:427–38.

51. Atkinson BA, King GJ, Amoroso EC. Development of caruncular and intercaruncular regions in the bovine endometrium. Biol Reprod 1984;30:763–74.

52. Long NM, Vonnahme KA, Hess BW, et al. Effects of early gestational undernutrition on fetal growth, organ development, and placentomal composition in the bovine. J Anim Sci 2009;87:1950–9.

53. Meyer AM, Reed JJ, Vonnahme KA, et al. Effects of stage of gestation and nutrient restriction during early to mid-gestation on maternal and fetal visceral organ mass and indices of jejunal growth and vascularity in beef cows. J Anim Sci 2010;88:2410–24.

54. Da Silva P, Aitken RP, Rhind SM, et al. Impact of maternal nutrition during pregnancy on pituitary gonadotrophin gene expression and ovarian development in growth-restricted and normally grown late gestation sheep fetuses. Reproduction 2002;123:769–77.

55. Gnanalingham MG, Mostyn A, Dandrea J, et al. Ontogeny and nutritional programming of uncoupling protein-2 and glucocorticoid receptor mRNA in the ovine lung. J Physiol 2005;565:159–69.

56. Limesand SW, Rozance PJ, Zerbe GO, et al. Attenuated insulin release and storage in fetal sheep pancreatic islets with intrauterine growth restriction. Endocrinology 2006;147:1488–97.

57. Gilbert JS, Ford SP, Lang AL, et al. Nutrient restriction impairs nephrogenesis in a gender specific manner in the ovine fetus. Pediatr Res 2007;61:42–7.

58. McMillin IC, Muhlhausler BS, Duffield JA, et al. Prenatal programming of postnatal obesity: fetal nutrition and the regulation of leptin synthesis and secretion before birth. Proc Nutr Soc 2004;63:405–12.

59. Matsuzaki M, Milne JL, Aitken RP, et al. Overnourishing pregnant adolescent ewes preserves perirenal fat deposition in their growth-restricted fetuses. Reprod Fertil Dev 2006;18:357–64.

60. Greenwood PL, Bell AW. Consequences of intra-uterine growth retardation for postnatal growth, metabolism and pathophysiology. Reprod Suppl 2003;61:195–206.

61. Renquist BJ, Oltjen JW, Sainz RD, et al. Effects of age on body condition and production parameters of multiparous beef cows. J Anim Sci 2006;84:1890–5.

62. Cushman RA, Allen MF, Kuehn LA, et al. Evaluation of antral follicle count and ovarian morphology in crossbred beef cows: investigation of influence of stage of the estrous cycle, age, and birth weight. J Anim Sci 2009;87:1971–80.

63. Sullivan TM, Micke GC, Greer RM, et al. Dietary manipulation of Bos indicus × heifers during gestation affects the reproductive development of their heifer calves. Reprod Fertil Dev 2009;21:773–84.

64. Sakai T. Studies on the development of the embryonic ovary in swine, cattle and horse. Jap J Vet Res 1955;3:183–94.
65. Tanaka Y, Nakada K, Moriyoshi M, et al. Appearance and number of follicles and change in the concentration of serum FSH in female bovine fetuses. Reproduction 2001;121:777–82.
66. Mauleon P. The establishment of the primordial follicle reserve in the sheep embryo studied by labeling of oocytes with tritiated thymidine. Eur J Obstet Gynecol Reprod Biol 1974;4:S133–9.
67. Sawyer HR, Smith P, Heath DA, et al. Formation of ovarian follicles during fetal development in sheep. Biol Reprod 2002;66:1134–50.
68. Hirshfield AN. Relationship between the supply of primordial follicles and the onset of follicular growth in rats. Biol Reprod 1994;50:421–8.
69. Nilsson EE, Skinner MK. Progesterone regulation of primordial follicle assembly in bovine fetal ovaries. Mol Cell Endocrinol 2009;313:9–16.
70. Erickson BH. Development and senescence of the postnatal bovine ovary. J Anim Sci 1966;25:800–5.
71. Erickson BH. Development and radio-response of the prenatal bovine ovary. J Reprod Fertil 1966;10:97–105.
72. Ireland JJ. Control of follicular growth and development. J Reprod Fertil Suppl 1987;34:39–54.
73. Kezele P, Skinner MK. Regulation of ovarian primordial follicle assembly and development by estrogen and progesterone: endocrine model of follicle assembly. Endocrinology 2003;144:3329–37.
74. Ireland JJ, Zielak-Steciwko A, Jimenez-Krassel F, et al. Variation in the ovarian reserve is linked to alterations in intrafollicular estradiol production and ovarian biomarkers of follicular differentiation and oocyte quality in cattle. Biol Reprod 2009;80:954–64.
75. Singh J, Dominguez M, Jaiswal R, et al. A simple ultrasound test to predict the superstimulatory response in cattle. Theriogenology 2004;62:227–43.
76. Jimenez-Krassel F, Folger JK, Ireland JL, et al. Evidence that high variation in ovarian reserves of healthy young adults has a negative impact on the corpus luteum and endometrium during estrous cycles in cattle. Biol Reprod 2009;80:1272–81.
77. Ireland JL, Scheetz HD, Jimenez-Krassel F, et al. Antral follicle count reliably predicts number of morphologically healthy oocytes and follicles in ovaries of young adult cattle. Biol Reprod 2008;79:1219–25.
78. Ireland JJ, Smith GW, Scheetz D, et al. Does size matter in females? An overview of the impact of the high variation in the ovarian reserve on ovarian function and fertility, utility of anti-Müllerian hormone as a diagnostic marker for fertility and cases of variation in the ovarian reserve in cattle. Reprod Fertil Dev 2011;23:1–14.
79. Burns DS, Jimenez-Krassel F, Ireland JL, et al. Numbers of antral follicles during follicular waves in cattle: evidence for high variation among animals, very high repeatability in individuals, and an inverse association with serum follicle-stimulating hormone concentrations. Biol Reprod 2005;73:54–62.
80. Ireland JJ, Ward F, Jimenez-Krassel F, et al. Follicle numbers are highly repeatable within individual animals but are inversely correlated with FSH concentrations and the proportion of good-quality embryos after ovarian stimulation in cattle. Hum Reprod 2007;22:1687–95.
81. Mossa F, Walsh SW, Butler ST, et al. Low numbers of ovarian follicles ≥3 mm in diameter are associated with low fertility in dairy cows. J Dairy Sci 2012;95:2355–61.

82. Byerley DJ, Staigmiller RB, Berardinelli JG, et al. Pregnancy rates of beef heifers bred either on pubertal or third estrus. J Anim Sci 1987;65:645–50.

83. Inskeep EK. Preovulatory, postovulatory and postmaternal recognition effects of concentrations of progesterone on embryonic survival in the cow. J Anim Sci 2004;82(Suppl 13):E24–9.

84. Rae MT, Palassio S, Kyle CE, et al. Maternal undernutrition during pregnancy retards early ovarian development and subsequent follicular development in fetal sheep. Reproduction 2001;122:915–22.

85. Long NM, Nijland MJ, Nathananielsz PW, et al. The impact of early to mid-gestational nutrient restriction on female offspring fertility and hypothalamic-pituitary-adrenal axis response to stress. J Anim Sci 2010;88:2029–37.

86. Nurmamat T, Long NM, Nathanielsz PW, et al. Early to mid-gestational nutrient restriction reduced steroidogenic enzyme expression in luteal tissue of mature offspring [abstract]. Biol Reprod 2011;85(Suppl 1):216.

87. Long NM, Tousely CB, Underwood KR, et al. Effects of early to mid gestational undernutrition with or without protein supplementation on offspring growth, carcass characteristics, and adipocyte size in beef cattle. J Anim Sci 2012; 90:197–206.

88. Mossa F, Carter F, Walsh SW. Maternal undernutrition in cows impairs ovarian and cardiovascular systems in their offspring. Biol Reprod 2013. http://dx.doi.org/10.1095/biolreprod.112.107235.

89. Jordan ER, Swanson LV. Effect of crude protein on reproductive efficiency, serum total protein, and albumin in the high producing dairy cow. J Dairy Sci 1979;62:58–63.

90. Canfield RW, Sniffen CJ, Butler WR. Effects of excess degradable protein on postpartum reproduction and energy balance in dairy cattle. J Dairy Sci 1990; 73:2342–9.

91. Elrod CC, Van Amburgh M, Butler WR. Alterations of pH in response to increased dietary protein in cattle are unique to the uterus. J Anim Sci 1993;71:702–6.

92. Sinclair KD, Kuran M, Gebbie FE, et al. Nitrogen metabolism and fertility in cattle: II. Development of oocytes recovered from heifers offered diets differing in their rate of nitrogen release in the rumen. J Anim Sci 2000;78:2670–80.

93. Moellam U, Blanck R, Lehrer H, et al. Effects of high dietary crude protein on the characteristics of preovulatory follicles in dairy heifers. J Dairy Sci 2001;94: 785–92.

94. Roberts AJ, Grings EE, MacNeil MD, et al. Implications of going against the dogma of feed them to breed them. West Sect Anim Sci Proc 2009;60:85–8.

95. Roberts AJ, Funston R, Mulliniks T, et al. Feed efficiency—how should it be used for the cow herd? Presented at Range Beef Cow Symposium. XXII. Mitchell, November 30, 2011.

96. Corah LR, Dunn TG, Kaltenbach CC. Influence of prepartum nutrition on the reproductive performance of beef females and the performance of their progeny. J Anim Sci 1975;41:819–24.

97. Rolfe KM, Stalker LA, Klopfenstein TJ, et al. Influence of weaning date and prepartum plane of nutrition on cow-calf productivity. West Sect Anim Sci Proc 2011;62:375–8.

98. Martin JL, Vonnahme KA, Adams DC, et al. Effects of dam nutrition on growth and reproductive performance of heifer calves. J Anim Sci 2007;85:841–7.

99. Funston RN, Martin JL, Adams DC, et al. Winter grazing system and supplementation of beef cows during late gestation influence heifer progeny. J Anim Sci 2010;88:4094–101.

100. Gunn PJ, Schoonmaker JP, Lemenager RP, et al. Feeding distiller's grains as an energy source to gestating and lactating heifers: impact on calving and pre-weaning progeny performance [abstract]. J Anim Sci 2011;88(E-Suppl 2):627.

101. NRC. Nutrient requirements of beef cattle. 7th edition. Washington, DC: National Academy Press; 1996.

102. Warner JM, Martin JL, Hall ZC, et al. The effects of supplementing beef cows grazing cornstalk residue with dried distillers grains based cube on cow and calf performance. Prof Anim Sci 2011;27:540–6.

103. Gunn RG, Sim DA, Hunter EA. Effects of nutrition in utero and in early life on the subsequent lifetime reproductive performance of Scottish Blackface ewes in two management systems. Anim Sci 1995;60:223–30.

104. Pryce JE, Simm G, Robinson JJ. Effects of selection for production and maternal diet on maiden dairy heifer fertility. Anim Sci 2002;74:415–21.

105. Hansen K, Steensberg V. Forskelligt opdraettede Koers hildbarked og ydelse. 246. Bertn Forsoglab. (Kbh) 1950. Cited by Hansson A. Influence of rearing intensity on body development and milk production. Proc Brit Soc Anim Prod 1956; p. 51–66.

106. Hansson A. Influence of rearing intensity on body development and milk production. Proc Brit Soc Anim Prod 1956;51–66.

107. Pinney DO. Performance of range beef cows as affected by supplemental winter feed and age at first calving [master's thesis]. Stillwater (OK): Oklahoma State University; 1962.

108. Arnett DW, Holland GL, Totusek R. Some effects of obesity in beef females. J Anim Sci 1971;33:1129–36.

109. Wallace JM, Aitken RP, Cheyne MA. Nutrient partitioning and fetal growth in rapidly growing adolescent ewes. J Reprod Fertil 1996;107:183–90.

110. Da Silva P, Aitken RP, Rhind SM, et al. Influence of placentally mediated fetal growth restriction on the onset of puberty in male and female lambs. Reproduction 2001;122:375–85.

111. Ma Y, Zhu MJ, Zhang L, et al. Maternal obesity and overnutrition alter fetal growth fate and cotyledonary vascularity and angiogenic factor expression in the ewe. Am J Physiol Regul Integr Comp Physiol 2010;299:R249–58.

112. Caton JS, Grazul-Bilska AT, Vonnahme KA, et al. Nutritional management during gestation: impacts on lifelong performance. Proceedings of the 18th Annual Florida Ruminant Nutrition Symposium. Gainesville (FL): 2010. p. 1–20.

113. Malhi PS, Adams GP, Mapletoft RJ, et al. Oocyte development competence in a bovine model of reproductive aging. Reproduction 2007;134:233–9.

114. Wang MH, von Saal FS. Maternal age and traits in offspring. Nature 2000;407: 469–70.

115. Fuerst-Waltl B, Reichl A, Fuerst C, et al. Effect of maternal age on milk production traits, fertility, and longevity in cattle. J Dairy Sci 2004;87:2293–8.

116. Banos G, Brotherstone S, Coffey MP. Prenatal maternal effects on body condition score, female fertility, and milk yield of dairy cows. J Dairy Sci 2007;90: 3490–9.

117. Berry DP, Lonergan P, Butler ST, et al. Negative influence of high maternal milk production before and after conception on offspring survival and milk production in dairy cattle. J Dairy Sci 2008;91:329–37.

118. Funston RN, Musgrave JA, Meyer TL, et al. Effect of calving distribution on beef cattle progeny performance. J Anim Sci 2012;90:5118–21.

119. Geisert BG. Development of a set of forage standards to estimate in vivo digestibility of forages and prediction of forage quality of diets consumed by cattle

grazing Nebraska Sandhills range and pasture [PhD thesis]. Lincoln (NE): University of Nebraska; 2007. p. 108–10.

120. Lesmeister JL, Burfening PJ, Blackwell RL. Date of first calving in beef cows and subsequent calf production. J Anim Sci 1973;36:1–6.

Nutritional Development and the Target Weight Debate

John B. Hall, PhD, PAS[a,b],*

KEYWORDS

- Beef heifer • Nutrition • Development • Puberty • Target weight • Management

KEY POINTS

- Postnatal nutrition has a profound effect on reproductive efficiency and lifetime productivity of beef heifers.
- Preweaning and postweaning nutrition influence age at puberty. Preweaning nutrition may have a greater effect on onset of puberty, but the impact of management is limited preweaning.
- Postweaning gain can overcome nutrient deficiencies preweaning.
- Energy is the primary limiting nutrient in heifer diets; however, protein must be adequate and heifers may benefit from rumen undegradable protein.
- A planned nutritional program based on the Beef NRC should be used to develop heifers in an efficient and economic manner.
- Source of nutrients and pattern of growth do not have a significant effect on heifer reproductive success as long as the planned target weight is achieved.
- Achieving a target weight of 65% of mature weight by the beginning of the breeding season ensures nutrition does not limit reproductive success of heifers; however, it seems a target weight of 55% has application for some operations and may have positive effects on heifer longevity.

INTRODUCTION

Beef heifers that attain puberty at an early age and conceive early in the breeding season have greater lifetime productivity and longevity.[1] To conceive early in the breeding season, heifers should have several estrous cycles before insemination.[2] Therefore,

Funding: Idaho Agricultural Experiment Station, VPI & SU Agricultural Experiment Station, Pfizer, Select Sires, ABS, Powell River Project.
Conflict of Interest: Previously Consultant for World Wide Sires, Inc.
[a] Department of Animal and Veterinary Science, University of Idaho, 875 Perimeter Drive MS 2330, Moscow, ID 83844-2330, USA; [b] Idaho Agricultural Experiment Station, Nancy M. Cummings Research, Extension, and Education Center, University of Idaho, 16 Hot Springs Ranch Road, Carmen, ID 83462, USA
* Nancy M. Cummings Research, Extension, and Education Center, University of Idaho, 16 Hot Springs Ranch Road, Carmen, ID.
E-mail address: jbhall@uidaho.edu

management strategies that allow heifers to reach puberty 45 days before the initiation of breeding could be economically and biologically beneficial.

Nutrition is the management tool that can have the greatest impact on the age at which heifers reach puberty. Heifers of a similar breed composition can reach puberty several months apart when fed different diets.[3,4] In addition, feed costs account for 60% to 70% of the costs of raising replacement heifers. Therefore, the financial impact of puberty onset is dictated by the age at puberty, and the feed costs associated with achieving a younger age at puberty. The cost of feeding heifers to reach puberty early should be weighed against the income gained by increased conception rates and heavier weaning weights.

The reproductive development of heifers can be affected by nutrition at any phase of prepubertal growth. Effects of postweaning nutrition are well characterized followed by preweaning growth rates.[5,6] More recently, prenatal nutrition was recognized as a significant factor in reproductive performance in heifers.[7] In some cases, nutritional deprivation at one stage of development may be overcome in the following stages of development. In contrast, effects at certain stages (ie, prenatal phase) seem to be permanent and may be independent of subsequent growth rate or age at puberty.

The mechanisms by which nutrition alters reproductive development are not completely understood. However, current research indicates that there are direct effects of individual nutrients on various portions of the hypothalamic-pituitary-ovarian-uterine axis.[6] Unfortunately, monitoring of individual nutrients or metabolic status by clinicians or beef producers at the ranch level is neither practical nor efficacious.

Diagnostic and management strategies that can be used at the ranch level include body condition, average daily gain, and target weight. There is considerable, and sometimes conflicting, information on the effects of different nutritional management, patterns of growth, and the use of target weights for proper heifer development. This article reviews current concepts of postnatal beef heifer nutritional development and suggests management strategies for use by clinicians and producers to help ensure heifer reproductive success. In addition, the current debate on the ideal target weight is examined.

INFLUENCE OF BIRTH WEIGHT ON HEIFER DEVELOPMENT

Birth weight in cattle is a function of genetics of the parents, dam uterine environment, and prenatal nutrition.[7,8] The effects of prenatal nutrition and specific nutrients or deficiencies are discussed elsewhere in this issue. However, actual birth weight regardless of cause may have an impact on heifer development. Heifer birth weight has a weak negative correlation with age at puberty[9] and a positive correlation with weight at puberty. However, others did not find a relationship between birth weight and heifer fertility.[10] Therefore, heifers that are heavier at birth tend to be younger and heavier at puberty, but pregnancy rates may not necessarily be influenced by heifer birth weight.

The decision to retain heifers that have high birth weights as replacement heifers may have other impacts beyond age and weight at puberty. Heifers with high birth weights may have a genetic potential to increase birth weights of their calves. In purebred operations, more emphasis should be placed on expected progeny difference for birth weight and calving ease than actual heifer birth weight. In commercial cow-calf operations, retention of heifers with extremely high birth weights should be avoided.

PREWEANING NUTRITION
Preweaning Growth and Dam Milking Ability

Well-controlled studies on preweaning nutrition are limited. Most studies estimate preweaning nutrition from preweaning growth rate and weaning weight. Both of these observations are a function of dam milking ability, calf genetics for growth, and forage/nutrients consumed by the calf.

- Increased weaning weights or adjusted weaning weights were associated with younger age and heavier weight at puberty.[11]
- Greater average daily gain from birth to weaning was negatively correlated with age at puberty.[12]
- Rapid growth preweaning results in a higher incidence of precocious puberty (puberty before 9 months of age).[13]
- Heifers from breeds selected for increased milking ability are younger at puberty.[14]

It is difficult to separate the genetic component from the nutrition of the developing heifer.

Increased growth rate caused by enhanced preweaning nutrition can reduce age at puberty (**Table 1**) and may increase weight at puberty. Body weight gain during the preweaning period may have a greater influence on puberty onset than postweaning gain.[15] In addition, rapid growth during the preweaning phase may reduce the impact of nutritional manipulations later in development.[12] However, under standard management conditions of a cow-calf operation where calves are not weaned until 6 or 7 months of age there are limited management options to alter heifer development. Among the few options are creep grazing and creep feeding.

Creep Feeding

Creep feeding provides calves with increased energy and protein usually in the form of grains and other concentrates by access to a self-feeder that excludes their dams. Creep feeding increases growth rate and may hasten the onset of puberty.[16] Most studies reported limited effects on heifer reproductive development beyond earlier age at puberty and a greater percentage of heifers cycling at the beginning of the breeding season.[16-18] However, creep-fed heifers may have impaired milking ability and produce less kilograms of calf during their lifetime.[16,17] In contrast, several researchers observed no impact on weaning weights of calves born to creep-fed heifers despite decreased milk production as long as high-quality forage is available to the calves.[16,18]

Creep Grazing

Creep grazing allows calves access to portions of pasture or range than have not been grazed recently and from which their dams are excluded. This allows for selective grazing by the offspring, which results in ingestion of a diet higher in protein and energy than the diet they can graze with their dams.[19] Creep-grazed calves are 10 to 30 kg heavier at weaning than their non–creep grazed counterparts.[20] Although heifers

Table 1
Effect of periweaning growth rate on percentage of heifers expressing precocious puberty and age at precocious puberty

Year	Average Daily Gain (kg/d)	Precocious Puberty (%)	Age at Precocious Puberty (d)
1990	0.75 ± 0.03^a	25^a	206 ± 14.8
1991	0.57 ± 0.02^a	16.6^a	158 ± 14.2

[a] Effect of year ($P<.02$).

Data from Wehrman ME, Kojima FN, Sanchez T, et al. Incidence of precocious puberty in developing beef heifers. J Anim Sci 1996;74(10):2462–7.

that were creep grazed as calves seem to reach puberty at a slightly earlier age than their non–creep grazed counterparts, creep-grazed heifers exhibit a similar decrease in milk production and calf performance as heifers that are creep fed on concentrates.[21]

EARLY WEANING NUTRITION

In cow-calf operations, early weaning refers to permanent separation of calves from their dams at less than or equal to 5 months of age. Early weaning is usually conducted for the following reasons:

1. Improve rebreeding rates of 2-year-old (primiparous) and 3-year-old (diparous) cows. Calves are usually weaned at 30 to 60 days of age.
2. Increase cyclicity in thin (body condition score <4) or late calving (<40 days postpartum) cows. Calves are generally weaned at 45 to 90 days of age.
3. Reduce cow nutrient requirements during times of drought. Weaning age is 60 days to 5 months.

Multiple studies investigated the impact of early weaning on cow and calf performance including carcass performance of calves.[22–24] Reproductive performance of cows whose calves are early weaned is greatly improved as evidenced by greater pregnancy rate and increased percentage of cows calving early in the subsequent calving season. Depending on the nutritional management of early weaned calves, these calves weigh more, less, or the same as their normal-weaned cohorts. When calves are early weaned onto high-energy diets carcass quality is improved, whereas carcass weight is similar or decreased compared with normal-weaned calves.[25] However, only a few studies have examined the long-term effects of early weaning on the developing female.

Early weaned heifers were reported to be lighter or heavier than their normal-weaned cohort by the time both cohorts were 7 to 9 months old.[18,26] The body weight differences were dependent on the type of diet received by early weaned heifers, and environment in which they were placed. Early weaned heifers placed in drylot tended to be heavier than normal-weaned heifers. In contrast, normal-weaned heifers were heavier than early weaned heifers that remained on similar pastures but were creep fed a high-energy diet. The percent crude protein (CP) in early weaned heifer diets needs to be 17% CP, and most of that protein should be in a rumen undegradable form.[18,26]

Several studies indicate that early weaned heifers supplied with high-energy (concentrate) diets exhibit high rates of precocious puberty or a high percentage of heifers are cyclic by 8 to 9 months of age (**Fig. 1**).[18,26,27] However, the percentage of heifers puberal by the beginning of the breeding season was nearly similar regardless of weaning treatment.[18,26]

Pregnancy rates in early weaned heifers were reported as greater[18] or similar[26] to heifers weaned at a normal age. Certainly, the effects of early weaning had no detrimental effects on reproduction (**Fig. 2**).

Precocious puberty whether a result of early weaning or preweaning nutrition is not always a positive occurrence. Heifers exhibiting precocious puberty do not necessarily maintain cycles until normal breeding age. In addition, the potential for young heifers to become pregnant before weaning exists.

POSTWEANING NUTRITION

One of the most critical factors affecting the success of reproduction in replacement heifers is postweaning nutrition. This phase is subject to the most control by

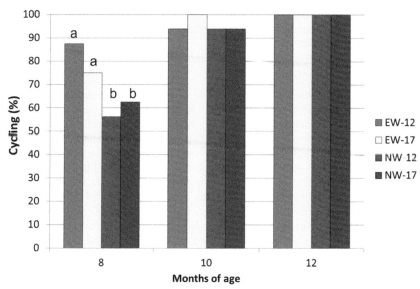

Fig. 1. Percentage of heifers cycling by 8, 10, or 12 months of age as affected by early (EW) or normal (NW) age at weaning and percentage of CP (12% vs 17%) in supplement provided. Blue, EW + 12% CP; Yellow, EW + 17% CP; Red, NW + 12% CP; Purple, NW + 17% CP. [a,b] Within month, percentage of heifers cycling affected by treatment (P<.05). (*Data from* Sexten WJ, Faulkner DB, Dahlquist JM. Supplemental feed protein concentration and weaning age affects replacement beef heifer performance. Prof Anim Sci 2005;21:278–85.)

management. Therefore, this phase may have considerable impact on heifer development and costs or profitability.

Considerable research has investigated the role of nutrition and specific nutrients on puberty onset and reproduction in heifers.[6,28] From a management perspective, the

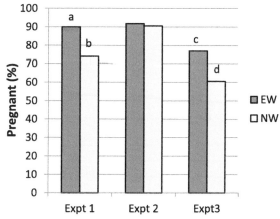

Fig. 2. Effect of early (EW) or normal (NW) age at weaning on percentage of heifers becoming pregnant. [a,b] Effect of weaning age (P<.09). [c,d] Effect of weaning age (P<.05). (*Data from* Refs.[18,26,27])

most important consideration is that heifers reach a critical or "target" body weight before the breeding season.[29] The target weight concept and determination of a target weight are discussed later.

Impacts of Average Daily Gain

Several experiments investigated the effect of growth rate as measured by average daily gain on heifer development. Heifers raised on low-energy diets are delayed in reaching puberty and have lower pregnancy rates their first breeding season than heifers raised on a high-energy diet.[4,30] Results from the experiment shown in **Table 2** exemplify the effect of postweaning nutrition on replacement heifer reproductive efficiency. The high-gain heifers reached puberty earlier than the other two groups. In addition, 60% of the heifers in the medium- and high-gain groups conceived in the first 20 days of the breeding season, and overall conception rates were greater for the medium- and high-gain heifers compared with low-gain heifers.

Nutrient needs are affected by growth rate (average daily gain) and body weight of the heifer (**Table 3**). This table provides a limited example. Heifer nutritional needs should be calculated from the Nutrient Requirements of Beef Cattle (Beef NRC) or commercial programs that use the Beef NRC to calculate requirements.

Does Pattern of Gain Affect Heifer Development?

After a target weight is determined, managers can focus on the mechanics of heifer development. The route (pattern of gain) toward the target weight may not be as important as attaining the target weight by the breeding season (**Table 4**). Heifers achieved their target weight by three different methods: (1) rapid gain followed by slow gain, (2) steady gain, or (3) slow gain then rapid gain had similar pregnancy rates.[31] Similarly, spring-born heifers that were roughed through the winter then pushed to gain most of their target weight during the last 60 days before the breeding season had pregnancy rates equal to[32] or less than[33] heifers on a steady rate of gain. Heifers developed on stair step gain (fast-slow-fast) had enhanced or equal pregnancy rates to heifers on a steady gain system.[34,35] Therefore, managers can design feeding programs to maximize gain during times of abundant forage, low-cost feed supplies, or favorable environmental conditions.

Sorting heifers into feeding groups by body weight at weaning decreases feed costs and improves reproductive performance (**Fig. 3**).[36,37] Light-weight heifers at weaning benefited from separate feeding as indicated by increased body weights at breeding and enhanced pregnancy rates. Feed costs are reduced because heavier heifers can be grown at a slower rate on less expensive feedstuffs.

Table 2
Effect of feed level on reproductive performance in beef heifers

	Low	Medium	High
Gain (kg/d)	0.23	0.45	0.68
Age at first estrus (d)	434	412	388
Weight at first estrus (kg)	237	247	255
Conception rate first 20 d of breeding season (%)	30	62	60
Overall conception rate (%)	50	86	87

Data from Short RE, Bellows RA. Relationships among weight gains, age at puberty and reproductive performance in heifers. J Anim Sci 1971;32:127.

Table 3								
Examples of nutrient requirements of heifers postweaning								
				Daily Nutrients per Animal				
Body Weight (kg)	ADG (kg)	DMI (kg/d)	TDN (kg)	NEm (Mcal)	NEg (Mcal)	CP (kg)	Ca (g)	P (g)
227 (500 lb)	0.45	5.5	3.3	4.5	1.32	0.54	18.6	10
	0.68	5.7	3.7	4.5	2.06	0.64	24.5	12.2
272 (600 lb)	0.45	6.3	3.8	5.16	1.51	0.59	19.5	10.9
	0.68	6.5	4.2	5.16	2.36	0.69	24.4	12.7
317 (700 lb)	0.45	7.2	4.2	5.79	1.70	0.64	20	11.8
	0.68	7.4	4.7	5.79	2.65	0.74	24.5	13.6

Abbreviations: ADG, average daily gain; CP, crude protein; DMI, dry matter intake; NEg, net energy - gain; NEm, net energy - maintenance; TDN, total digestible nutrients.

ENERGY INTAKE

Energy is the primary nutrient regulating reproduction in female beef cattle. Under-nourished heifers are delayed in the resumption or initiation of estrous cycles. Energy availability seems to control reproduction primarily through pathways that permit or inhibit the release of gonadotropin-releasing hormone from the hypothalamus and luteinizing hormone and follicle-stimulating hormone from the pituitary.[6] Energy substrates or metabolic responses to energy availability may also act on the ovary to influence follicular growth, estrogen production, and circulating progesterone levels.[38] In addition to overall energy availability, the timing of energy increase or deprivation seems to be important in determining pregnancy rates.

SOURCE OF CALORIES

Most of the studies discussed to this point have investigated varying levels of dietary energy with little regard to the source of calories. Starch, fiber, and fats all supply energy to ruminants, but each of these sources of energy produces different physiologic effects in cattle. Isoenergetic diets in which calories come from different energy sources may have different effects on reproduction.

A few studies in developing heifers have examined all three sources of energy in a single experiment. Heifers grazing stockpiled fescue were fed isonitrogenous-isoenergetic supplements constructed with corn-soy (high starch), whole cotton-seed (high fat), or soy hulls (high fiber). There was no effect of type of supplement on heifers cycling at the beginning of the breeding season or percentage pregnant

Table 4					
Impact of pattern of gain on pregnancy rates in replacement beef heifers[a]					
		Pattern of Gain			
Study	No. of Heifers	Even Gain (%)	Slow-Fast (%)	Fast-Slow (%)	Fast-Slow-Fast (%)
Clanton et al,[31] 1983	180	82	75	73	—
Lynch et al,[32] 1997	160	87.4	87.2	—	—
Poland et al,[34] 1998	96	75	—	—	89.6
Grings et al,[35] 1999	210	81.8	—	—	86.6

[a] Within row no effect of pattern of gain (*P*>.05).
Data from Refs.[31,32,34,35]

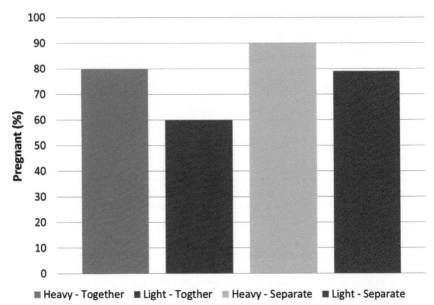

Fig. 3. Effect of sorting heifers into heavyweight and lightweight feeding groups on percentage of heifers cycling by the beginning of the breeding season. Orthogonal contrasts indicated there was no effect of feeding method for heavy heifers; however, in light heifers feeding separately improved (*P*<.05) pregnancy rate. (*Data from* Varner LW, Bellows RA, Christensen DS. A management system for wintering replacement heifers. J Anim Sci 1977;44:165–71.)

to artificial insemination (AI) or clean-up natural service (**Table 5**). Extremely high temperatures and drought may have reduced overall percentage pregnant; however, supplement did not influence heifer performance. Similarly, Howlett and co-workers[39] found no advantage to whole soybeans or whole cottonseed compared with soyhulls or a corn-soy supplement. Both experiments had only small numbers of heifers so only drastic changes in reproductive performance would have been detected.

Dried distillers grains plus soluble is a product that contains energy in the form of fat and by-pass protein. Supplementing pregnant heifers with dried distillers grains plus soluble increased pregnancy rates as first calf heifers compared with heifers supplemented with other grain coproducts.[40,41] Other studies did not see a significant advantage to distillers grains over other supplements.[42]

Table 5
Impact of source of energy in supplements for developing heifers on pregnancy rate[a]

Supplement	Percentage Pregnant to AI	Overall Percentage Pregnant
Soyhulls	45.8 (11/24)	79.2 (19/24)
Whole cottonseed	45.8 (11/24)	75 (18/24)
Corn-soybean meal	54.1 (13/24)	83.3 (20/24)

[a] No effect of supplement (*P*>.05).
Data from Wuenschel JC, Cuddy DL, Greiner SP, et al. Effect of source of energy on growth and reproduction of replacement beef heifers. J Anim Sci 2005;83(Suppl 2):23.

FATS

The impact of fats on reproduction in cattle is a focus of considerable research.[43,44] Because fatty acids and cholesterol are substrates for hormone synthesis, increasing fat in the diet may increase levels of reproductive hormones (progesterone, prostaglandins) or fats may act directly on the reproductive axis. Therefore, the effects of fat may be independent of or additive to those of increased energy availability.

Cattle diets usually contain less than 2% or 3% fat. Supplementing fat to improve reproduction was initially attempted to increase the energy density in the diet. High-fat diets for cattle contain 5% to 8% fat. Exceeding these dietary fat levels impairs rumen function.

Early studies[45,46] indicated that feeding high-fat diets to cycling heifers and postpartum cows increased progesterone production and the lifespan of the corpus luteum. Higher progesterone levels during the luteal phase generally result in improved fertility.

Increasing dietary fat also results in increased follicular growth. More small and medium follicles are present in cows and heifers fed high-fat diets.[47–49] In addition, this increased follicular growth is often accompanied by increased estrogen or progesterone production. These changes in follicular growth and hormone production may enhance reproduction.

Developing Heifers: Is There an Advantage to Fat?

The research on reproductive effects of fat supplementation in developing heifers indicates varied results. Lammoglia and coworkers[50] reported a high-fat diet increased pregnancy rates and cyclicity in heifers of a double muscled breed, but it had little effect or a negative effect in other breeds. In contrast, pregnancy rates to AI were increased in developing heifers that received whole cottonseed (5% fat diet) compared with heifers receiving the same amount of energy from starch sources (**Fig. 4**).[51] The effectiveness of fat to increase fertility in heifers may be related to duration of feeding with shorter feeding periods (45–75 days) having the most impact. In summaries of multiple studies, Hess and colleagues[44] concluded that fat

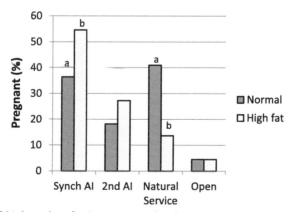

Fig. 4. Effect of high- or low-fat isoenergetic development diets on pregnancy rates to AI and subsequent natural service in replacement beef heifers. [a,b] Within insemination type, effect of dietary fat ($P<.07$). (*Data from* Cuddy DL, Hall JB, Beal WE, et al. Effect of high fat diet on reproduction in replacement beef heifers. J Anim Sci 2002;80(Suppl 1):410.)

supplementation increased heifer pregnancy rates by approximately 10%, whereas Funston[43] found fat supplementation was of little value to well-developed heifers.

Does Source of Fat Matter?

In general, unsaturated fat sources should give better results for all production phases. Linoleic acid serves as a precursor for prostaglandin $F_{2\alpha}$, whereas linolenic, eicosapentanoic, and docosahexanoic acids may inhibit prostaglandin $F_{2\alpha}$ production.[43] Oil seeds, such as safflower, sunflower, soybeans, and cottonseed, contain high concentrations of polyunsaturated fatty acids, and all of these oilseeds have given positive results. Rumen-protected saturated fatty acids seem not to be as effective as oil seeds.

Replacement heifers supplemented with whole soybeans may have impaired reproduction.[52] It is hypothesized that high levels of phytoestrogens may be detrimental to development of the replacement beef heifer. The phytoestrogen content of specific oil seeds should be considered.

Fish oil or fish meal may also be of benefit, but little beef cattle reproductive research has been completed with this product. Fish meal reduced the oxytocin-induced increase in prostaglandin $F_{2\alpha}$ in heifers with low progesterone production.[53] However, feeding 0.45 kg of a supplement that was high in eicosapentanoic and docosahexanoic did not influence AI or overall pregnancy rates in heifers (**Table 6**).[54]

PROTEIN INTAKE

Protein effects on reproduction are often confounded with energy deficiency or general poor nutrition. Developing replacement heifers grazing protein-deficient forages respond to combined protein and energy supplementation with decreased age at puberty and enhanced pregnancy rates.[55] Increasing the amount of digestible intake protein (DIP) enhances digestibility of and energy intake from medium- to low-quality forages. There needs to be at least 7% CP in the diet for proper rumen function. Below 7% CP the digestibility of the forage is increased by supplementing protein. Therefore, whether protein-induced improvements in reproductive efficiency are a direct effect of protein or amino acids or a result of improved energy availability is unclear.

The measurement of protein content in the diet used to balance diets for cows and heifers seems to be important. The commonly used measure of protein in the diet for cattle is CP, which is based on the nitrogen content of the feedstuff. Metabolizable protein (MP) is a measure (or estimate) of the protein reaching and absorbed by the small intestine. Using MP-designed supplements for pregnant heifers did not alter body weights or body condition of heifers compared with heifers fed supplements

Table 6
Effect of normal or eicosapentanoic-docosahexanoic containing supplements on AI and overall pregnancy percentages in replacement beef heifers

Pregnancy Status	Supplement		P Value
	EnerGII[a]	Corn-Soy	
% Pregnant AI	51.4 (54/105)	49.1 (53/108)	.73
% Pregnant overall	87.6 (92/105)	93.5 (101/108)	.14

[a] EnerGII, Vitus Nutrition, LLC, Corcoran, CA.

Data from Wuenschel JC. Effects of feeding supplemental eicosapentanoic acid and decosahexanoic acid to beef females on reproductive responses and free fatty acids [master's thesis]. Blacksburg (VA): Virginia Polytechnic Institute & State University; 2006.

based on CP.[56] However, heifers consuming supplements based on MP had 5% greater pregnancy rates as 2 year olds, which increased the value of each bred heifer by $13.64.

Although a more refined estimate of protein content of the diet, MP cannot be measured directly by chemical analysis and must be estimated from in situ digestion trials of similar feedstuffs. For grains and oilseeds, estimates of MP are fairly accurate; however, estimating MP values of forage is more challenging because of wide variations caused by species, soil fertility, and plant maturity.

BY-PASS OR UNDEGRADABLE INTAKE PROTEIN

Because forages, especially pasture, contain mostly DIP, there has been interest in the use of undegradable intake protein (UIP) or rumen by-pass protein to enhance beef production. Supplying part of the protein requirement by UIP enhances growth in most trials with stocker and finishing cattle. Impacts of UIP supplementation on reproduction are equivocal.

The value of UIP in replacement heifer diets is unclear. In one study, feeding 250 g of UIP to heifers delayed puberty compared with heifers fed monensin, but did not hurt overall conception rates.[57] In contrast, feeding 100 g of UIP decreased age at puberty and increased pelvic area (**Table 7**).[58] Developing heifers grazing dormant forage that receive increased amounts of UIP in supplements had increased pregnancy rates and greater longevity.[59] The effects of UIP on replacement heifers seem to depend on UIP supplied and UIP in the base diet.

At present, there are many unanswered questions about the impacts of UIP on reproduction. Producers and clinicians should continue to watch for new developments in UIP feeding. More research is needed to correctly match the level of UIP to the forage and to stage of production of the cow. In addition, the cost/benefit ratios of UIP supplementation must be considered.

EXCESSIVE PROTEIN

Overfeeding of DIP either as protein or urea is associated with decreased pregnancy rates in female dairy and beef cattle.[60,61] Exposure to high levels of ammonia or urea may impair maturation of oocytes and subsequent fertilization or maturation of developing embryos. However, supplying adequate energy for excretion of excess ammonia or urea may prevent decreases in fertility in dry cows or heifers.[62] In addition, not all studies have observed negative effects of elevated blood-urea-nitrogen concentrations on embryo quality or pregnancy rates.[63]

Table 7
Effect of undegradable intake protein on developing replacement heifers

	Undegradable Intake Protein (g/d)	
	0[a]	100[a]
Average daily gain	1.86	2.1
Pelvic area (cm^2)	150.6	162.8
Cycling %	54	77

[a] Effect of level of undegradable intake protein ($P<.05$).

Data from Kerley M and Patterson DJ. The reproductive effects associated with fat and rumen undegradable protein supplementation in heifers and cows. Proceedings of Reproductive Management Tools & Techniques II. February 1–2, 2000. Columbia, MO: University of Missouri; 2000. p. 5–5.

MINERALS

Mineral supplementation that supports normal growth seems to be sufficient for reproductive development in heifers. Concentrations of calcium and phosphorus adequate for the expected growth rate of developing heifers (see **Table 3**) support pubertal development in heifers. Various studies indicated only relatively small alterations in reproductive efficiency in response to trace mineral supplementation unless there are severe deficiencies or antagonisms.[64,65] Mineral supplementation should be based on analysis of feed supplied to developing heifers.

Growth Promotants: Ionophores and Implants

Because age at puberty can be reduced by increased growth rates as a result of improved nutrition, producers are often interested in the effects of growth-promoting implants and feed additives. Although the results may be similar (increased growth rate), ionophores (monensin, lasalocid) and growth implants work differently in the animal. Therefore, their effects on reproduction can be different.

Ionophores act by altering the types of microbes in the rumen, thereby enhancing digestion and growth rate. Addition of ionophores to replacement heifer diets can reduce age at puberty by 15 to 30 days while increasing growth rate.[66] Although some of the effect may be caused by ionophores action in the rumen, there may be direct actions on the reproductive axis. Response to ionophores seems to be less dramatic in light-weight or poorly fed heifers.

Most growth implants are steroids (estrogens or androgens) or have steroid-like activity. Steroids increase the release of growth hormones or growth factors to improve muscle and bone growth, but they also act on the reproductive system. Therefore, if given at the wrong time or in improper doses, growth implants have a detrimental effect on reproduction. Many different studies have investigated implants and reproduction and the results are varied.[67,68] The effects on replacement heifers can be summarized as follows:

- Implanting heifers at birth dramatically impairs reproduction.
- One Zeranol or estrogen-progesterone implant between 1 and 3 months resulted in highly variable effects on pregnancy rate ranging from 10% less to 19% greater. Thirteen studies reported negative effects of implants on pregnancy rate; nine experiments had positive or no effects.
- One implant at or near weaning had similar variable effects on pregnancy rate as implanting at 1 to 3 months of age.
- Multiple implants during a heifer's life reduces pregnancy rate.

THE TARGET WEIGHT DEBATE

Many theories have been proposed on the mechanisms by which nutrition affects onset of puberty. The critical body weight theory[69] and critical body fat hypothesis[70] are not applicable to heifers.[5,30] Current theories hypothesize that availability of nutrients to the central nervous system may be altered as somatic growth slows[71] or that signals, such as leptin from adipose tissue, may create a permissive environment for sexual maturation to occur.[72]

Although achievement of a specific body weight or fatness may not trigger onset of puberty,[33,44] it is well established that heifers do not attain puberty below a "threshold weight."[73,74] Lamond[29] suggested that managers could use a "target weight" (percentage of mature cow weight) by breeding to ensure heifers were sufficiently developed to have a high probability of conception. Achieving the target weight before breeding ensures that breeding success is not limited by nutrition. Currently, there is considerable debate as to the ideal target weight for beef heifers.

The Argument for the 65% Target Weight

For many years, the target weight for heifers suggested by research and experience has been set at 65% of mature weight (MW).[28]

- The 65% level seems to be effective across a wide range of cattle biologic types and nutritional environments.
- Heifers developed to 65% of MW by breeding had less calving difficulty than heifers developed to 55% of MW.[28]
- If the 65% weight can be achieved economically or if heifer value or pasture costs are high, raising heifers to 60% to 65% of MW is advantageous.

The Argument Against the 65% Target Weight

- Current high feed prices make supplementation of heifers to achieve the 65% target too costly.
- The 65% target may reduce selection pressure on early puberty because age at puberty is decreased by heavy feeding.
- Some heifers may become overconditioned and the decrease in nutrient intake when heifers go to pasture may decrease pregnancy rates.[75]

The Argument for the 55% Target Weight

Several articles reported advantages to developing heifers to a 53% to 55% of MW target weight compared with 60% to 65% target weight.[76–78]

- Developing spring calving heifers to 53% of MW compared with a 58% to 60% target weight reduced heifer development costs without any impacts on initial pregnancy rates.
- Dystocia, rebreeding rates, or calf production traits were not compromised by the lower target weight.[76]
- Heifers bred at a restricted target weight had greater or similar longevity compared with heifers developed to "normal" target weight when weights were equal by calving.[79]

The Argument Against the 55% Target Weight

- The studies supporting the 55% target weight were conducted with crossbred/composite heifers, which tended to reach puberty early as evidenced by 74% of the 53% MW heifers and 85% of 58% MW heifers cycling by the start of the breeding season.
- A follow-up study[80] indicated that developing heifers to 50% MW compared with 55% MW resulted in similar overall pregnancy rates, but decreased calf weaning weight from 2-year-old cows and delayed calving in 3-year-old cows.
- The decrease in calf value offset any gain by reducing heifer development costs.
- Although overall pregnancy rates were not compromised by the 55% target weight, several studies indicated decreased conception early in the breeding season or to AI.[81]
- Heifers that continued to be restricted postbreeding have compromised rebreeding rates and longevity.[79]

Box 1
Factors for consideration when selecting a target weight (percentage of mature weight) for replacement heifers to attain by the beginning of the breeding season

65% of Mature Weight	55% Mature Weight
Purebred or straightbred heifers	Crossbred heifers
Later-maturing breeds	Earlier-maturing breeds
Large-frame cows	Moderate-framed cows
Limited cow numbers	Large herd (>200 cows)
Good forage resources	Limited forage resources
High replacement heifer value	Average replacement heifer value
Limited marketing options for open heifers	Ability to retain ownership on heifers in feedlot

---

Which is the "Right" Target Weight?

Consideration must be given to heifer biologic type, breeding (purebred vs crossbred), development costs, and marketing options before selecting or recommending a target weight (percentage of MW) goal (**Box 1**). Reducing development costs for replacement heifers by lowering target weights is not without risks.

For the reduced development program to work effectively for producers, they must (1) effectively market open heifers, (2) provide sufficient nutritional resources postbreeding for proper heifer growth to mature size, and (3) incorporate a progestin-based synchronization system to induce puberty in a maximum number of heifers.

REFERENCES

1. Lesmeister JL, Burfening PJ, Blackwell RL. Date of first calving in beef cows and subsequent calf production. J Anim Sci 1973;36:1.
2. Byerley DJ, Staigmiller RB, Berardinelli JG, et al. Pregnancy rates of beef heifers bred either on puberal or third estrus. J Anim Sci 1987;65:1571–5.
3. Wiltbank JN, Kasson CW, Ingalls JE. Puberty in crossbred and straightbred beef heifers on two levels of feed. J Anim Sci 1969;29:602–5.
4. Short RE, Bellows RA. Relationships among weight gains, age at puberty and reproductive performance in heifers. J Anim Sci 1971;32:127.
5. Hall JB. Interfaces between metabolism and onset of puberty in ruminants [PhD dissertation]. Lexington (KY): University of Kentucky; 1991.
6. Schillo KK, Hall JB, Hileman SM. Effects of nutrition and season on puberty onset in the beef heifer. J Anim Sci 1992;70:3994–4005.
7. Funston RM, Larson DM, Vonnahme KA. Effects of maternal nutrition on conceptus growth and offspring performance: Implications for beef cattle production. J Anim Sci 2010;88(E Suppl):E205–15.
8. Ferrell CL. Maternal and fetal influences on uterine and conceptus development in the cow: I. Growth of tissues of the gravid uterus. J Anim Sci 1991;69: 1945–53.
9. Martin LC, Brinks JS, Bourdon RM, et al. Genetic effects on beef heifer puberty and subsequent reproduction. J Anim Sci 1992;70:4006–17.
10. Bergmann JA, Hohenboken WD. Prediction of fertility from calfhood traits of Angus and Simmental heifers. J Anim Sci 1992;70:2611–21.
11. Wolfe MW, Stumpf TT, Wolfe PL, et al. Effect of selection for growth traits on age and weight at puberty in bovine females. J Anim Sci 1990;68:1595–602.

12. Arije GF, Wiltbank JN. Age and weight at puberty in Hereford heifers. J Anim Sci 1971;33:401–6.
13. Weherman ME, Kojima FN, Sanchez T, et al. Incidence of precocious puberty in developing beef heifers. J Anim Sci 1996;74:2462–7.
14. Gregory KE, Lunstra DD, Cundiff LV, et al. Breed effects and heterosis in advanced generations of composite populations for puberty and scrotal traits of beef cattle. J Anim Sci 1991;69:2795–807.
15. Witbank JN, Gregory KE, Swiger LA, et al. Effects of heterosis on age and weight at puberty in beef heifers. J Anim Sci 1966;25:744–51.
16. Buskirk DD, Faulkner DB, Ireland FA. Subsequent productivity of beef heifers that received creep feed for 0, 28, 56, or 84 d before weaning. Prof Anim Sci 1996;12:37–43.
17. Hixon DL, Fahey GC, Kesler DJ, et al. Effects of creep feeding and monensin on reproductive performance and lactation of beef heifers. J Anim Sci 1982;55: 467–74.
18. Sexten WJ, Faulkner DB, Dahlquist JM. Supplemental feed protein concentration and weaning age affects replacement beef heifer performance. Prof Anim Sci 2005;21:278–85.
19. Jordan RM, Marten GC. Forward-creep grazing vs conventional grazing for production of suckling lambs. J Anim Sci 1970;31:598–600.
20. Bagley CP. Nutritional management of replacement beef heifers: a review. J Anim Sci 1993;71:3155–63.
21. Morrison DG, Feazel JI, Carpenter JC Jr, et al. The effect of creep grazing on the subsequent production of beef replacement heifers [abstract]. J Anim Sci 1984; 59(Suppl 1):44.
22. Lusby KS, Wettemann RP, Turman EJ. Effects of early weaning calves from first-calf heifers on calf and heifer performance. J Anim Sci 1981;53:1193–7.
23. Arthington JD, Kalmbacher RS. Effect of early weaning on the performance of three-year-old, first-calf beef heifers and calves reared in the subtropics. J Anim Sci 2003;81:1136–41.
24. Myers SE, Faulkner DB, Ireland FA, et al. Comparison of three weaning ages on cow-calf performance and steer carcass traits. J Anim Sci 1999;77:323–9.
25. Myers SE, Faulkner DB, Ireland FA, et al. Production systems comparing early weaning to normal weaning with or without creep feeding for beef steers. J Anim Sci 1999;77:300–31.
26. Waterman RC, Geary TW, Paterson JA, et al. Early weaning in Northern Great Plains beef cattle production system: II. Development of replacement heifers weaned at 80 or 215 d of age. Livest Sci 2012;148:36–45.
27. Day ML, Huston JE, Grum DE. Early weaning, puberty and cow reproduction [abstract]. J Anim Sci 2001;79(Suppl 2):44.
28. Patterson DJ, Perry RC, Kiracofe GH, et al. Management considerations in heifer development and puberty. J Anim Sci 1992;70:4018–35.
29. Lamond DR. The influence of undernutrition on reproduction in the cow. Anim Breeding Abstr 1970;38:359–71.
30. Hall JB, Staigmiller RB, Bellows RA, et al. Body composition and metabolic profiles associated with puberty in beef heifers. J Anim Sci 1995;73:3409–20.
31. Clanton DC, Jones LE, England ME. Effect of rate and time of gain after weaning on the development of replacement beef heifers. J Anim Sci 1983;56:280–5.
32. Lynch JM, Lamb GC, Miller BL, et al. Influence of timing of gain on growth and reproductive performance of beef replacement heifers. J Anim Sci 1997;75: 1715–22.

33. Hall JB, Staigmiller RB, Short RE, et al. Effect of age and pattern of gain on induction of puberty with a progestin in beef heifers. J Anim Sci 1997;75:1606–11.

34. Poland WW, Ringwall KA, Schroeder JW, et al. Nutritionally-directed, compensatory growth regimen in beef heifer development. Research report. Dickinson Research Extension Center, Fargo (ND): North Dakota State University; 1998. Available at: http://www.ag.ndsu.edu/archive/dickinso/research/1998/beef98h.htm. Accessed January 12, 2013.

35. Grings EE, Grings RB, Staigmiller RB, et al. Effects of stair-step nutrition and trace mineral supplementation on attainment of puberty in beef heifers of three sire breeds. J Anim Sci 1999;77:810–5.

36. Varner LW, Bellows RA, Christensen DS. A management system for wintering replacement heifers. J Anim Sci 1977;44:165–71.

37. Bellows RA, Hall JB. Physiology and management of the replacement beef heifer [review]. In: Proceedings of the Canadian Society of Animal Science Annual Meeting. Quebec: 1996. p. 217–34.

38. Webb R, Garnsworthy PC, Gong JG. Control of follicular growth: local interactions and nutritional influences. J Anim Sci 2004;82:E63–74.

39. Howlett CM, Vanzant ES, Anderson LH, et al. Effects of supplemental nutrient source on heifer growth and reproductive performance, and on utilization of corn silage based diets by beef steers. J Anim Sci 2003;81:2367.

40. Engle CL, Patterson HH, Perry GA. Effect of dried corn distillers grains plus solubles compared with soybean hulls, in late gestation heifer diets, on animal and reproductive performance. J Anim Sci 2008;86:1697–708.

41. Martin JL, Cupp AS, Rasby RJ, et al. Utilization of dried distillers grains for developing beef heifers. J Anim Sci 2007;85(9):2298–303.

42. Jaeger JR, Waggoner JW, Olson KC, et al. Growth and reproductive performance of beef replacement heifers fed development diets containing soybean meal or wet distillers grains. Prof Anim Sci 2012;28:300–5.

43. Funston RN. Fat supplementation and reproduction in beef females. J Anim Sci 2004;82(E Suppl):E154–61.

44. Hess BW, Moss GE, Rule DC. A decade of developments in the area of fat supplementation research with beef cattle and sheep. J Anim Sci 2008;86: E188–204.

45. Talavera E, Park CS, Williams GL. Relationships among dietary lipid intake, serum cholesterol and ovarian function in Holstein heifers. J Anim Sci 1985; 60:1045.

46. Williams GL. Modulation of luteal activity in postpartum beef cows through changes in dietary lipid. J Anim Sci 1989;67:785–93.

47. Thomas MG, Bao B, Williams GL. Dietary fats varying in their fatty acid composition differentially influence follicular growth in cows fed isoenergetic diets. J Anim Sci 1997;75:2512–9.

48. Ryan DP, Spoon RA, Williams GL. Ovarian follicular characteristics, embryo recovery, and embryo viability in heifers fed high-fat diets and treated with follicle-stimulating hormone. J Anim Sci 1992;70:3505–13.

49. Lammoglia MA, Willard ST, Hallford DM, et al. Effects of dietary fat on follicular development and circulating concentrations of lipids, insulin, progesterone, estradiol-17b,13,14-dihydro-15-keto-prostaglandin F2a, and growth hormone in estrous cyclic Brahman cows. J Anim Sci 1997;75:1591–600.

50. Lammoglia MA, Bellows RA, Grings EE, et al. Effects of dietary fat and sire breed on puberty, weight, and reproductive traits of F1 beef heifers. J Anim Sci 2000;78:2244–52.

51. Cuddy DL, Hall JB, Beal WE, et al. Effect of high fat diet on reproduction in replacement beef heifers. J Anim Sci 2002;80(Suppl 1):410.

52. Harris HL, Cupp AS, Creighton KW, et al. Reproductive response in heifers fed soybeans during post weaning development. 2005. Nebraska beef cattle report. Lincoln (NE): University of Nebraska; 15–7.

53. Wamsley NE, Burns PD, Engle TE, et al. Fish meal supplementation alters uterine prostaglandin F2α synthesis in beef heifers with low luteal-phase progesterone. J Anim Sci 2005;83:1832–8.

54. Wuenschel JC. Effects of feeding supplemental eicosapentanoic acid and decosahexanoic acid to beef females on reproductive responses and free fatty acids [master's thesis]. Blacksburg (VA): Virginia Polytechnic Institute & State University; 2006.

55. Oyedipe EO, Osori DIK, Akerejola O, et al. Effect of level of nutrition on onset of puberty and conception rate in Zebu heifers. Theriogenology 1982;18:525–39.

56. Patterson HH, Adams DC, Klopfenstein TJ, et al. Supplementation to meet metabolizable protein requirements of primiparous beef heifers: II. Pregnancy and economics. J Anim Sci 2003;81:563–70.

57. Lalman DL, Petersen MK, Ansotegui RP, et al. The effects of ruminally undegradable protein, propionic acid, and monensin on puberty and pregnancy in beef heifers. J Anim Sci 1993;71:2843–52.

58. Kerley MS, Patterson DJ. The reproductive effects associated with fat and rumen undegradable protein supplementation in heifers and cows. Proceedings of Reproductive management tools & techniques II. Columbia, MO: University of Missouri; 2000. p 5–5.

59. Mulliniks JT, Hawkins DE, Kane KK, et al. Metabolizable protein supply while grazing dormant winter forage during heifer development alters pregnancy and subsequent in-herd retention rate. J Anim Sci 2013;91(3):1409–16. Available at: http://www.journalofanimalscience.org/content/early/2013/01/07/jas.2012-5394. Accessed February 14, 2013.

60. Blanchard T, Ferguson J, Love L, et al. Effect of dietary crude-protein type on fertilization and embryo quality in dairy cattle. Am J Vet Res 1990;51(6):905–8.

61. Sinclair KD, Kuram M, Gebbie FE, et al. Nitrogen metabolism and fertility in cattle: II. Development of oocytes recovered from heifers offered diets differing in their rate of nitrogen release in the rumen. J Anim Sci 2000;78:2670–80.

62. Garcia-Bojalil CM, Staples JC, Thatcher WW, et al. Protein intake and development of ovarian follicles and embryos of superovulated nonlactating dairy cows. J Dairy Sci 1994;77:2537–48.

63. Jousan FD, Utt MD, Beal WE. Effects of differences in dietary protein on the production and quality of bovine embryos collected from superovulated donors. J Anim Sci 2002;80(Suppl 1):99.

64. Grings EE, Hall JB, Bellows RA, et al. Effect of nutritional management, trace mineral supplementation, and norgestomet implant on attainment of puberty in beef heifers. J Anim Sci 1998;76:2177–81.

65. Ahola JK, Baker DS, Burns PD, et al. Effects of copper, zinc, and manganese source on mineral status, reproduction, immunity, and calf performance in young beef females over a two-year period. Prof Anim Sci 2005;21:297–304.

66. Moseley WM, Dunn TG, Kaltenbach CC, et al. Relationship of growth and puberty in beef heifers fed monensin. J Anim Sci 1982;55:357.

67. Deutscher GH, Zerfoss LL, Clanton DC. Time of zeranol implantation on growth, reproduction and calving of beef heifers. J Anim Sci 1986;62:875–86.

68. Selk G. Implants for suckling steer and heifer calves and potential replacement heifers. OSU Implant Symposium. November 21–23, 1996.
69. Frisch RE, Revelle R. Height and weight at menarche and a hypothesis of critical body weights and adolescent events. Science 1970;169:397–9.
70. Frisch RE, McAuthur J. Menstrual cycles: fatness as a determinant of minimum weight for height necessary for their maintenance or onset. Science 1974;185: 949–51.
71. Schillo KK. Effects of dietary energy on control of luteinizing hormone secretion in cattle and sheep. J Anim Sci 1992;70:1271–82.
72. Zieba DA, Amstalden M, Williams GL. Regulatory roles of leptin in reproduction and metabolism: a comparative review. Domest Anim Endocrinol 2005;29(1): 166–85.
73. Kiser TE, Krealing RR, Rampacek GB, et al. Luteinizing hormone secretion before and after ovariectomy in prepubertal and pubertal beef heifers. J Anim Sci 1998;53:1545–50.
74. Day ML, Imakawa I, Zalesky DD, et al. Effect of restriction of dietary energy intake during the prepuberal period on secretion of luteinizing hormone and responsiveness of the pituitary to luteinizing hormone-releasing hormone in heifers. J Anim Sci 1986;82:1641–8.
75. Perry GA. Physiology and Endocrinology Symposium: Harnessing basic knowledge of factors controlling puberty to improve synchronization of estrus and fertility in heifers. J Anim Sci 2012;90:1172–82.
76. Funston RN, Deutscher GH. Comparison of target breeding weight and breeding date for replacement beef heifers and effects on subsequent reproduction and calf performance. J Anim Sci 2004;82:3094–9.
77. Martin JL, Creighton KW, Musgrave JA, et al. Effect of prebreeding body weight or progestin exposure before breeding on beef heifer performance through the second breeding season. J Anim Sci 2008;86:451–9.
78. Larson DM, Cupp AS, Funston RN. Extending grazing in heifer development systems decreases costs without compromising production. J Anim Sci 2009; 87(E-Suppl 3):140.
79. Endecott RL, Funston RN, Mulliniks JT, et al. Joint Alpharma-Beef Species Symposium: implications of beef heifer development systems and lifetime productivity. J Anim Sci 2012;91:1329–35. http://dx.doi.org/10.2527/jas2012-5704.
80. Creighton KW, Musgrave JA, Klopfenstein, et al. Comparison of two development systems for March-born replacement beef heifers. 2005. Nebraska beef cattle report. Lincoln (NE): University of Nebraska; p. 3–6.
81. Roberts AJ, Geary TW, Grings EE, et al. Reproductive performance of heifers offered ad libitum or restricted access to feed for a one hundred forty-day period after weaning. J Anim Sci 2009;87:3043–52.

Setting the Stage for Long-term Reproductive Health

Craig A. Payne, DVM, MS[a],*, Brian Vander Ley, DVM, PhD[b],
Scott E. Poock, DVM[a]

KEYWORDS

- Reproductive health • Heifer development • Disease prevention • Parasite control
- Body condition score

KEY POINTS

- Replacement heifers are the future of the breeding herd and mismanagement can have long-term consequences.
- Veterinarians are key to long-term reproductive health in the breeding herd.
- Health events and parasitism can have negative impacts on heifer development programs.
- Body condition scoring at strategic times can increase the rebreeding success of first-calf heifers.

INTRODUCTION

Profitability of cow-calf production depends largely on reproductive performance. Successful cow-calf operations tend to have a large percentage of cows that wean a calf every year, whereas less successful operations struggle with reproductive performance.

Achieving reproductive success requires that producers manage all aspects of the breeding herd; however, heifer development may be the most important given that heifers are the future of the herd. Mistakes and setbacks in heifer development compound over time and have negative long-term consequences on productivity and profitability of cow-calf operations. Because of their expertise in animal health management, veterinarians are well positioned to help producers manage heifer development sucessfully.[1] This article addresses some of the areas veterinarians should be involved in to ensure the long-term health and productivity of replacements heifers.

Disclosures: The authors have nothing to disclose.
[a] Department of Veterinary Extension and Continuing Education, University of Missouri College of Veterinary Medicine, 900 East Campus Drive, Columbia, MO 65211, USA;
[b] Department of Food Animal Medicine & Surgery, University of Missouri College of Veterinary Medicine, 900 East Campus Drive, Columbia, MO 65211, USA
* Corresponding author.
E-mail address: payneca@missouri.edu

Vet Clin Food Anim 29 (2013) 555–565
http://dx.doi.org/10.1016/j.cvfa.2013.07.006
0749-0720/13/$ – see front matter © 2013 Elsevier Inc. All rights reserved.

DISEASE PREVENTION

In order for a heifer to calve at approximately 24 months of age she needs to reach 60% to 65% of her mature body weight to become pubertal and she must do this before 15 months of age. In addition, the heifer must continue to grow while gestating and lactating, and then rebreed the following year in a timely manner. The veterinarian should be involved in every step of the way to ensure that heifers remain healthy so they can meet these challenges.

A logical place for the veterinarian to be involved in a heifer development program is in disease prevention, which is one of the most important aspects of heifer development because infectious diseases can have a major impact on growth and development as well as the reproductive efficiency of a herd.[2]

Efforts to control disease in replacement heifers should begin early in life. A disease event such as bovine respiratory disease in a young heifer can have long-term consequences and negatively affect growth, reproductive performance, and longevity.[3]

Biosecurity and biocontainment are integral parts of any disease control program[4] and no disease program can be effective without them. Biosecurity involves the precautionary measures taken by each operation to prevent the introduction of new diseases onto a farm, whereas biocontainment is the control of the spread of infectious agents that are already present on the farm.[5]

Designing effective biosecurity and biocontainment plans is a team effort and individuals playing a significant role in the operation, such as the veterinarian, owner, farm hands, and feed suppliers, should be asked to provide input. It is the responsibility of managers and veterinarians not only to develop the plan, but to ensure its implementation and to monitor its effectiveness.

Biosecurity plans should be developed within the framework of Hazard Analysis and Critical Control Points.[4,6] With this method there are 4 steps to apply[4]:

1. Hazard identification: identify potential infectious agents that can pose a threat
2. Exposure assessment: identify possible routes by which animals can be exposed to the infectious agents
3. Risk characterization: determine the level of exposure risk for each agent
4. Risk management: design, implement, and monitor biosecurity and biocontainment plans

A primary consideration in replacement heifer biosecurity is the source of the heifers. Some operations purchase heifers. Other operations ship their heifers elsewhere to have them developed and then bring them back to the farm to calve them out. In either case, the biosecurity plan needs to specifically address the disease risk associated with heifers not raised on the farm and how they will be handled once brought onto the operation. Because reproductive diseases most commonly enter a herd through importation of infected animals,[2] quarantine and possibly testing for certain diseases are warranted. It is just as important to know the health history of the location where the heifers originated.[2]

VACCINATION PROGRAM

The vaccination program is part of the biosecurity/biocontainment plan but is not a substitute for it. The replacement heifer vaccination program should begin early in life and the vaccines to be administered depend on the operation and its needs.

As a general rule, the vaccine program should be designed to prevent diseases early in life that can be life threatening or affect growth and performance. Some examples are clostridials and bovine respiratory disease. The program also needs to include vaccines that prevent reproductive losses. With that in mind, the following discussion provides the suggested minimum requirements for reproductive vaccines that should be included in the vaccination program.

Bovine Virus Diarrhea Virus

Bovine virus diarrhea virus (BVDV) infections in cow-calf operations usually manifest as reproductive losses or as an immunosuppressive event before a respiratory or diarrhea outbreak.[7] The greatest economic impact of BVDV on a cow-calf operation is through reproductive losses.[8] BVDV infection can cause early embryonic death, abortion, and fetal malformations.[9] Fetal infection with BVDV during the first trimester of infection often results in development of calves born persistently infected (PI) with BVDV.[10] PI calves go on to become the principal source of new infections within a herd.[11] Herds that experience reproductive loss caused by BVDV often harbor PI cattle, thereby maintaining a cycle of reproductive loss and generation of new PI cattle.

At a minimum, producers should test replacement heifers before breeding. Producers ideally should test all calves, cows without calves, bulls, and all purchased cattle before the beginning of each breeding season to break the cycle of reproductive loss and PI generation. Cattle that test negative remain negative for life and do not need to be retested in subsequent years. Contact between breeding females and cattle of unknown status (eg, neighboring cattle, purchased cattle) should be avoided from the onset of breeding until all cows have reached the second trimester of gestation.

BVDV vaccination is another important tool to prevent losses associated with infections. Vaccination does not replace detection and removal of PI cattle. Vaccination serves as defense against brief exposure. Developing heifers should be vaccinated at least twice before breeding.

Infectious Bovine Rhinotracheitis

Infectious bovine rhinotracheitis (IBR), like BVDV, can affect several different physiologic systems, including reproductive and respiratory systems. From a reproductive standpoint, IBR has been diagnosed as a significant cause of abortion in the past with one article reporting that herds with abortion epidemics saw greater than 50% abortion rates because of the virus.[12] Although IBR abortion storms of that magnitude are infrequent, especially in the United States, it is still one of the most common viral abortifacients.[12,13]

IBR is a herpesvirus. The significance of this is that, once an animal is infected, the infection may become indefinite. The virus can remain dormant in sensory ganglia of the trigeminal nerve, sacral spinal ganglia, tonsillar lymphoid cells, and peripheral blood lymphocytes.[14] During times of stress the virus can recrudesce, leading to viral shedding and thus exposure of other cattle. For this reason, vaccination is important for preventing outbreaks of clinical disease; however, vaccination may not prevent infection or prevent the establishment of latency.[15] Biosecurity and biocontainment processes therefore are an important part of IBR control programs.

Leptospirosis

Leptospirosis has long been recognized as a cause of reproductive loss. It is most often thought of as causing late-term abortions but may also be a cause of stillbirths, weak born calves, and occasionally infertility and early embryonic death.[16]

In studies compiled by Anderson[13] from veterinary diagnostic laboratory surveys in the United States, leptospirosis accounted for up to 10.6% of the abortion cases in which a causal agent was found. Estimates of prevalence of leptospira infection in US dairies and cow-calf operations indicate that overall herd infection prevalence was approximately 35% to 50%, with most of the infections being caused by serovar hardjo.[15]

Leptospira strains colonize the kidney and reproductive tracts of cattle and the organism is shed in the urine. The persistence of the infection and shedding depends on the serovar. With serovar hardjo, cattle seem to be the primary maintenance host, so infections may last for longer than 12 months.[16] Other serovars persist for shorter periods of time.[17] Susceptible animals that come into contact with infected urine are at risk of becoming infected themselves. When conditions are right, this organism may survive in the environment for up to 6 months.

In the United States, the primary means of controlling leptospirosis is through the use of a whole-cell inactivated vaccine containing Leptospira interrogans serovars hardjo, canicola, pomona, grippotyphosa, and icterohaemorrhagiae.[18] It has recently been suggested that these 5-way vaccines may not provide adequate protection because these vaccines do not contain Leptospira borgpetersenii serovar hardjo type hardjo-bovis, which is the most common cause of leptospirosis in cattle and the only type of serovar hardjo isolated from cattle in the United States.[19] To address this, some animal health companies are providing vaccines that contain hardjo-bovis, whereas other companies have conducted studies to show the protection their current 5-way Leptospira vaccine provides against hardjo-bovis.

Regardless of the choice of vaccine, it is recommended that 2 doses be given initially within the time frame indicated on the vaccine label, and this should be done before breeding occurs. Even with vaccination, protection is not guaranteed, so biosecurity and biocontainment processes are also an important part of leptospirosis control.

CHOOSING A VACCINE

The choice of whether to use a modified live (MLV) or inactivated viral vaccine is not easy. The literature contains many studies comparing their effectiveness and each has shown the ability to prevent respiratory disease or reproductive losses.[20–23]

This article therefore does not attempt to establish that one type of vaccine is more effective than another. That decision and recommendation is up to the veterinarian and is based on personal experience. Instead, this article discusses precautions for when MLVs are used in a heifer development program. This advice is not intended to discourage the use of MLVs but instead to create awareness of some of the unintended reproductive losses that may arise when using MLVs in breeding-age heifers.

Although MLVs are commonly used in breeding-age animals, certain problems with their use have been described. The problem that pertains specifically to breeding-age heifers is the effect that MLV IBR viruses can have if administered to naive heifers close to breeding time. In one study, heifers were synchronized using 2 doses of a commercially available prostaglandin $F_{2\alpha}$ 10 days apart and were vaccinated intramuscularly with a modified live viral IBR when the last dose of prostaglandin $F_{2\alpha}$ was administered.[24] The heifers were then placed with a proven sire for 35 days. The conception rate in the vaccinated group was estimated to be 35% based on their calving dates, whereas the conception rate was 78% in the control group.

More recently, a study was conducted comparing the effects of vaccinating naive beef heifers with an MLV or inactivated vaccine at the time of first induced ovulation of a fixed-time artificial insemination (AI) synchronization protocol.[25] Outcomes measured were plasma hormone concentration, estrous cycle length, and pregnancy success. Heifers in this study were either given an MLV vaccine (8 days before AI), 1 dose of killed vaccine (8 days before AI), 2 doses of killed vaccine (36 days and 8 days before AI), or a placebo (inactivated sterile water 36 and 8 days before AI). The placebo group and those that received 2 doses of killed vaccine had pregnancy rates of 90%. The group that received 1 dose of killed vaccine had a pregnancy rate of 86% and the MLV group had a pregnancy rate of 48%. The conclusion from this study was that vaccination of naive heifers with an MLV vaccine had a negative impact on pregnancy success and also resulted in the greatest percentage of abnormal estrous cycles.

How MLV IBR affects reproduction has been described. One study in particular noted mild to marked inflammation of the ovaries as well as necrotic lesions in the corpora lutea of heifers that had been inoculated IV with a commercially available MLV IBR vaccine the day after breeding.[26] The severity was described as being similar to that created by virulent strains. In addition, those that had the most severe ovarian lesions had markedly decreased plasma progesterone concentrations. Although the impact of an MLV BVDV vaccine on reproduction is not conclusive, there is some evidence that the virus can be isolated from ovaries up to several days after vaccination.[24] The concern is that BVDV replication could cause ovarian dysfunction and lead to reduced fertility.[27]

In order to avoid these potential effects the veterinarian has several options. One is to use only inactivated vaccines if vaccinating at or near breeding time. Another option may be to use an MLV only in heifers that have been previously immunized.[28,29] The final option may be to provide sufficient time between vaccination with an MLV and the breeding season, especially if there is a concern about previous vaccination status. It has been recommended to administer MLVs 30 to 60 days before breeding under the assumption that any ovarian effect from the MLV will have subsided before breeding.[30]

Veterinarians should also be aware that there have been reports of abortion associated with using MLV IBR in pregnant animals even though the herds were vaccinated according to label directions.[31,32] It seems that this effect is seen primarily in heifers, especially when vaccinated later in gestation.[31] It is uncertain at this time whether these abortions are related to vaccine or field strains[28] but one report indicated that there was high homology between the vaccine and clinical isolate strains.[32] For these reasons the veterinarian should work closely with the producer to determine whether MLVs should be used during pregnancy.

FURTHER THOUGHTS ON VACCINES

The National Animal Health Monitoring System (NAHMS) 2007 Beef Cow-Calf Study provided information about the use of vaccines in cow-calf operations, especially in replacement heifers and cows. Only 19.4% of operations reported using IBR vaccines in replacement heifers from a period of weaning through breeding, and only 25.1% reported using BVDV during the same time period. Use of IBR and BVDV vaccine in cows was not much higher, with only 24.6% reporting IBR use and 28.1% reporting BVDV use. Although vaccines are widely available and well recognized for their role in herd health programs, there is a need for better adoption, especially in the breeding herd.

PARASITE CONTROL

Intestinal parasites can have a significant impact on growth and reproductive performance of beef cattle.[33–35] Probably the most economically important effect of parasitism is loss of appetite or reduced feed intake.[36] This is thought to occur because of increase gastrin production, secretion of inflammatory chemokines, or possibly abdominal pain associated with infestation.[36] In addition, parasites have been shown to cause immunosuppression, which may decrease an animal's ability to respond to infectious diseases or vaccines.[36]

Because of the naivety of the immune system of younger animals, such as replacement heifers, they tend to be affected more than mature cows by intestinal parasites.[37] Therefore, parasite control in heifers is beneficial and leads to animals that are healthier, grow faster, and reach puberty more rapidly.[37,38]

The appropriate time at which deworming should occur to obtain maximum benefit depends on several considerations, including rainfall, temperature variation, and forage production.[39] Some producers deworm cattle when it is convenient, but that may not be the most effective time.[40] Instead, the epidemiology of local parasites and time the treatment need to be considered so that larval contamination on pastures is reduced.[40] The optimal treatment time may coincide with other events in the cow/calf operation such as spring or fall processing, but that is not always the case.[40] It is the veterinarian's responsibility to advise producers on what the optimal deworming time is for their area.

The other responsibility the veterinarian has is choosing the anthelmintic. This choice may be more complicated now than in the past because of the different classes of anthelmintics that are available as well as the different delivery methods that exist. To complicate the matter, there is also evidence of anthelmintic resistance in the United States and elsewhere.[41] Anthelmintic decisions are therefore more difficult but they are extremely important.

Two concepts veterinarians should familiarize themselves with to optimize parasite control are the Fecal Egg Count Reduction Test (FECRT) and refugia. Describing these in detail is beyond the scope of this article but, briefly, FECRT is the most widely used method for monitoring the effectiveness of anthelmintics and thus providing a way to determine whether resistance is emerging.[42] Refugia is maintaining a population of parasites in the environment that have not experienced anthelmintic pressure so that they can be ingested and contribute anthelmintic-susceptible alleles to future generations of worms.[41] Both of these concepts are intended to limit anthelmintic resistance, which is a matter of increasing concern in the cattle industry.

NUTRITIONAL MANAGEMENT AND BODY CONDITION SCORING

Although nutritional management is discussed by hall elsewhere in this issue, this article reemphasizes its importance. Nutrition is key to optimal reproductive performance as well as the health of the heifer and her offspring. Funston and colleagues[43] provided a summary of several studies showing the benefits of prepartum or postpartum energy or protein on pregnancy rate (**Table 1**) and summarized the positive

Table 1
Effects of prepartum or postpartum dietary energy or protein on pregnancy rates in cows and heifers

	Pregnancy Rate (%)	
Nutrient and Time	Adequate	Inadequate
Energy level before calving	73	60
Energy level after calving	92	66
Protein level before calving	80	55
Protein level after calving	90	69

Data from Refs.[2,4,9,10]

effects that feed levels during gestation had on dystocia, calf survival, and calf scour incidence as well as dam traits (**Table 2**).

The greatest challenge producers face with heifers may be successfully calving them the first time and then getting them rebred. During this time, the heifer is lactating while still trying to meet her own demands for growth, which leads to a high demand for nutrients. A mistake often made by producers is feeding first-calf heifers as if they are mature cows, which may cause the heifers to be underfed. This mistake could have a significant impact on rebreeding success.[44]

Because nutrition is so important to health and longevity, veterinarians should be involved with this aspect of heifer development. Not every veterinarian has the skills necessary to design a feeding program, but they can use body condition scoring (BCS) at key times to ensure that nutrient demands are being met. Although it seems reasonable that producers could use BCS, adoption of this practice is uncommon, with only 14.3% of operations using BCS according 2007 NAHMS data, despite the relationship between BCS and reproduction being well established.[45,46] It is the authors' experience that BCS requires little time commitment but can be of great benefit for the producer.

The BCS system for beef cattle is a scale of 1 to 9, with 1 being emaciated and 9 being obese. **Box 1** provides a description of the BCS system.

The recommended BCS for mature cows at calving is usually around 5 or 6. However, in heifers the recommendation is 6 because of their higher nutrient demands.[47] BCS should be done every 90 to 120 days throughout the year, with more specific times being 30 days before breeding, 90 days after breeding, 100 days before calving, and then at calving.[48] However, if a change in body condition score is needed, a significant change in body weight is required. One study, with Angus and Angus-sired crossbred first-calf beef heifers, determined that a 33-kg weight change resulted in a change of 1 body condition score ($R^2 = 0.72$; $P<.0001$)[49]; however, this depends on the type of animal. The National Research Council's *Nutrient Requirements of*

Table 2
Effects of feed level during gestation on calving and subsequent reproduction[a]

	Gestation Diet of Dam	
Item	Low	High[b]
Calf birth weight (kg)	28.6	31.3
Dystocia (%)	35	28
Calf Survival (%)		
At birth	93	91
Weaning	58	85
Scours (%)		
Incidence	52	33
Mortality	19	0
Dam Traits		
Estrus before breeding season (%)	48	69
Pregnancy (%)	65	75
Precalving pelvic area (cm²)	256	271

[a] Averages from 7 studies.
[b] Diet level fed from up to 150 days before calving; low and high, animals lost or gained weight before calving, respectively.

Box 1
BCS for beef cattle

BCS	Description
1	Emaciated: cow is emaciated with no palpable fat detectable over spinous processes, transverse processes, hip bones, or ribs. Tail-head and ribs project prominently
2	Poor: cow still appears emaciated but tail-head and ribs are less prominent. Individual spinous processes are still sharp to the touch but some tissue cover exists along the spine
3	Thin: ribs are still individually identifiable but not as sharp to the touch. There is obvious palpable fat along spine and over tail-head with some tissue cover over dorsal portion of ribs
4	Borderline: individual ribs are no longer visually obvious. The spinous processes can be indentified individually on palpation but feel rounded rather than sharp. Some fat cover over ribs, transverse processes, and hip bones
5	Moderate: cow has generally good overall appearance. On palpation, fat cover over ribs feels spongy and areas on either side of tail-head now have palpable fat cover
6	High moderate: firm pressure now needs to be applied to feel spinous processes. A high degree of fat is palpable over ribs and around tail-head
7	Good: cow appears fleshy and obviously carries considerable fat. Very spongy fat cover over ribs and around tail-head. Rounds or pones beginning to be obvious. Some fat around vulva and in crotch
8	Fat: cow very fleshy and overconditioned. Spinous processes almost impossible to palpate. Cow has large fat deposits over ribs, around tail-head, and below vulva. Rounds or pones are obvious
9	Extremely fat: cow obviously extremely wasty and patchy and looks blocky. Tail-head and hips buried in fatty tissue and rounds or pones of fat are protruding. Bone structure no longer visible and barely palpable. Animal's motility may even be impaired by large fatty deposits

Adapted from Richards MW, Spitzer JC, Warner MB. Effects of varying levels of postpartum nutrition on body condition at calving on subsequent reproductive performance in beef cattle. J Anim Sci 1986;62:302; with permission.

Table 3
Timeline for health programs designed for replacement beef heifers

60–90 d of Age	Weaning	Before Breeding	Pregnancy Check	100 d Before Calving	Calving
Clostridials	Clostridials	IBR, BVDV[a]	Leptospirosis	BCS	BCS
	IBR[b]	Leptospirosis[a,c]	BCS	—	—
	BVDV[b]	Vibriosis (Campylobacter fetus)[a,c]	—	—	—
	Bovine respiratory syncytial virus[b]	Deworm	—	—	—
	Parainfluenza 3[b]	BCS	—	—	—
	Deworm	Reproductive tract score	—	—	—
		Pelvic measure	—	—	—

[a] Administer vaccine 30–60 days before breeding.
[b] Administer 2 doses 21 days apart. The first dose should ideally occur before weaning.
[c] Administer 2 doses 21 days apart with the final dose occurring a minimum of 30 days before breeding.

Beef Cattle, 7th revised edition, provides additional information for predicting the weight change required to move 1 body condition score. When scheduling a time for BCS, the veterinarian and producer should plan accordingly to ensure plenty of lead time to make changes in condition if necessary.

SUMMARY

Heifer development is an important part of the success of a cow-calf operation and in order for heifers to meet the demands placed on them they must remain healthy. It has been established that health events early in life affect heifer productivity and longevity in the herd and it is up to the veterinarian to design a program that will reduce health risks. **Table 3** shows an example of a health plan for replacement beef heifers based on material presented in this article.

In addition to health, nutrition is an important consideration with regard to the developing heifer and it contributes to cow longevity. First-calf heifers are at greatest risk of being mismanaged nutritionally, which increases the likelihood of them leaving the breeding herd too early. Veterinarians should work with producers to ensure that nutrient demands are being met, especially in this class of animal.

REFERENCES

1. Larson RL. Heifer development: reproduction and nutrition. Vet Clin North Am Food Anim Pract 2007;23(1):53–68.
2. Sanderson MW, Gnad DP. Biosecurity for reproductive disease. Vet Clin North Am Food Anim Pract 2002;18(1):79–98.
3. Leslie K. Health and immune function of dairy calves. WCDS Advances Dairy Technology 2012;24:177–88.
4. Poulsen KP, McGuirk SM. Respiratory disease of the bovine neonate. Vet Clin North Am Food Anim Pract 2009;25:121–37.
5. Manunsell F, Donovan GA. Biosecurity and risk management for dairy replacements. Vet Clin North Am Food Anim Pract 2008;24(1):155–90.
6. Smith DR, Grotelueschen DM. Biosecurity and biocontainment of bovine viral diarrhea virus. Vet Clin North Am Food Anim Pract 2004;20(1):131–49.
7. Ridpath JF. Bovine viral diarrhea virus: global status. Vet Clin North Am Food Anim Pract 2010;26(1):105–21.
8. Evermann JF, Ridpath JF. Clinical and epidemiologic observations of bovine viral diarrhea virus in the Northwestern United States. Vet Microbiol 2002;89:129–39.
9. Kendrick JW. Bovine viral diarrhea virus induced abortion. Theriogenology 1976;5(3):91–3.
10. McClurkin AW, Littledike ET, Cutlip RC. Production of cattle immunotolerant to bovine viral diarrhea virus. Can J Comp Med 1984;48(2):156–61.
11. Arenhart S, Bauermann FV, Oliveira SA, et al. Shedding and transmission of bovine viral diarrhea virus by persistently infected calves. Pesquisa Veterinaria Brasileira 2009;29(9):736–42.
12. Kirkbride CA. Viral agents and associated lesions in a 10-year study of bovine abortions and stillbirths. J Vet Diagn Invest 1992;4:374–9.
13. Anderson ML. Infectious causes of bovine abortion during mid- to late-gestation. Theriogenology 2007;68(3):474–86.
14. Nandi S, Kumar M, Manohar M, et al. Bovine herpes virus infections in cattle. Anim Health Res Rev 2009;10(1):85–98.

15. Grooms DL, Bolin CA. Diagnosis of fetal loss caused by bovine viral diarrhea virus and *Leptospira* spp. Vet Clin North Am Food Anim Pract 2005;21: 463–72.
16. Leonard FC, Quinn PJ, Ellis WA, et al. Duration of urinary excretion of leptospires by cattle naturally or experimentally infected with *Leptospira interrogans* serovar hardjo. Vet Rec 1992;131:435–9.
17. Grooms DL. Reproductive losses caused by bovine viral diarrhea virus and leptospirosis. Theriogenology 2006;66:624–8.
18. Rinehart CL, Zimmerman AD, Buterbaugh RE, et al. Efficacy of vaccination of cattle with the *Leptospira interrogans* serovar Hardjo type hardjoprajitno component of a pentavalent *Leptospira* bacterin against experimental challenge with *Leptospira borgpetersenii* serovar *hardjo* type hardjo-bovis. Am J Vet Res 2012;73(5): 735–40.
19. Bolin CA, Zuerner RL, Trueba G. Effect of vaccination with a pentavalent leptosprial vaccine on *Leptospira interrogans* serovar Hardjo type Hardjo-bovis infection of pregnant cattle. Am J Vet Res 1989;50:161–5.
20. Rodning SP, Marley MS, Zhang Y, et al. Comparison of three commercial vaccines for preventing persistent infection with bovine viral diarrhea virus. Theriogenology 2010;73:1154–63.
21. Saunders JR, Olson SM, Radostits OM. Efficacy of an intramuscular infectious bovine rhinotracheitis vaccine against abortion due to the virus. Can Vet J 1972;13:273–8.
22. Ficken MD, Ellsworth MA, Tucker CM. Evaluation of the efficacy of a modified-live combination vaccine against abortion caused by virulent bovine herpesvirus type 1 in a one-year duration-of-immunity study. Vet Ther 2006;7:275–82.
23. Zimmerman AD, Buterbaugh RE, Herbert JM, et al. Efficacy of bovine herpesvirus-1 inactivated vaccine against abortion and stillbirth in pregnant heifers. J Am Vet Med Assoc 2007;231:1386–9.
24. Chiang BC, Smith PC, Nusbaum KE, et al. The effect of infectious bovine rhinotracheitis vaccine on reproductive efficiency in cattle vaccinated during estrus. Theriogenology 1990;33(5):1113–20.
25. Perry GA, Zimmerman AD, Daly RF, et al. The effects of vaccination on serum hormone concentrations and conception rates in synchronized naïve beef heifers. Theriogenology 2013;79(1):200–5.
26. Van Der Maaten MJ, Miller JM, Whetstone CA. Ovarian lesions induced in heifers by intravenous inoculation with modified live infectious bovine rhinotracheitis virus on the day after breeding. Am J Vet Res 1985;46:1996–9.
27. Grooms DL, Brock KV, Ward LA. Detection of cytopathic bovine viral diarrhea virus in the ovaries of cattle following immunization with a modified live bovine viral diarrhea virus vaccine. J Vet Diagn Invest 1998;10(2):130–4.
28. Miller JM. The effects of IBR virus infection on reproductive function of cattle. Vet Med 1991;86(1):95–8.
29. O'Toole D, Miller MM, Cavender JL, et al. Pathology in practice. J Am Vet Med Assoc 2012;241(2):189–91.
30. Bolton M, Brister D, Burdett D, et al. Reproductive safety of vaccination with Vista 5 L5 SQ near breeding time as determined by the effect on conception rates. Vet Ther 2007;8:177–82.
31. Spire MF, Edwards JF, Leipold HW, et al. Absence of ovarian lesions in IBR seropositive heifers subsequently vaccinated with a modified live IBR virus vaccine. AgriPractice 1996;16:33–8.

32. Texas Veterinary Medical Diagnostic Laboratory: annual report for fiscal year 2010. Available at: http://tvmdl.tamu.edu/wp-content/uploads/2011/12/TVMDL_ 2010AnnualReport1.pdf. Accessed February 21, 2013.
33. Ballweber LR, Smith LL, Stuedemann JA, et al. The effectiveness of single treatment with doramectin or invermectin in the control of gastrointestinal nematodes in grazing yearling stocker cattle. Vet Parasitol 1997;72:53–68.
34. Stromberg BE, Vatthauer RJ, Schlotthauer JC, et al. Production responses following strategic parasite control in a beef cow/calf herd. Vet Parasitol 1997; 68:315–22.
35. Stuedeman JA, Ciordia H, Myers GH, et al. Effect of single strategically timed dose of fenbendazole on cow and calf performance. Vet Parasitol 1989;34:77–86.
36. Stromberg BE, Gasbarre LC. Gastrointestinal nematode control programs with an emphasis on cattle. Vet Clin North Am Food Anim Pract 2006;22:543–65.
37. Bagley CP. Nutritional management of replacement beef heifers: a review. J Anim Sci 1993;71(11):3155–63.
38. Stromberg BE, Moon RD. Parasite control in calves and growing heifers. Vet Clin North Am Food Anim Pract 2008;24(1):105–16.
39. Engelken TJ. Developing replacement beef heifers. Theriogenology 2008;70(3): 569–72.
40. William JC, Loyacano AF. Internal parasites of cattle in Louisiana and other southern states. LSU Research and Extension Research Information Sheet#104, p. 1–20;August 2001.
41. Sutherland IA, Leathwick DM. Anthelmintic resistance in nematode parasites of cattle: a global issue? Trends Parasitol 2011;27(4):176–81.
42. Yazwinski TA, Tucker CA, Hornsby JA, et al. Effectiveness evaluation of several cattle anthelmintics via the fecal egg count reduction test. Parasitol Res 2009; 105:71–6.
43. Funston R, Geary T, Cooke R. Rebreeding the first calf heifer. Cattle Producer's Library CL413. Available at: http://www.ansci.colostate.edu/beef/info/cattlemans library/413.pdf. Accessed February 23, 2013.
44. Dunn TG, Kaltenbach CC. Nutrition and the postpartum interval of the ewe, sow and cow. J Anim Sci 1980;51(Suppl II):29–39.
45. Randel RD. Nutrition and postpartum rebreeding in cattle. J Anim Sci 1990;68: 853–62.
46. Richards MW, Spitzer JC, Warner MB. Effects of varying levels of postpartum nutrition on body condition at calving on subsequent reproductive performance in beef cattle. J Anim Sci 1986;62:300–6.
47. Cochring T, Corah L, Higgins J. Factors predicting the probability of estrus and pregnancy. Rpt of Prog. 514, Manhattan (KS): Kansas State Univ. Available at: http://krex.k-state.edu/dspace/bitstream/handle/2097/6733/cattle87pg55-57. pdf?sequence=1. Accessed February 23, 2013.
48. Encinias AM, Lardy G. Managing your cow herd through body condition scoring. AS-1026. Fargo (ND): North Dakota State University. Available at: http://www.ag. ndsu.edu/pubs/ansci/beef/as1026.pdf. Accessed February 23, 2013.
49. Lalman DL, Keisler DH, Williams JE, et al. Influence of postpartum weight and body condition change on duration of anestrus by undernourished suckled beef heifers. J Anim Sci 1997;75(8):2003–8.

Criteria for Selecting Replacements at Weaning, Before Breeding, and After Breeding

G. Cliff Lamb, MS, PhD

KEYWORDS

- Beef heifer • Selection • Heifer development • Genetics

KEY POINTS

- Selection of heifers to ensure that they calve early during their first breeding season is critical to the lifetime productivity of beef cows and the success of beef operations.
- At weaning, heifers should be considered for replacements based on their dam's previous performance; heifer calving date, age, and weight; and previous exposure to implants.
- Before breeding, heifers should be selected as replacements based on whether they have attained puberty (determined by a prebreeding examination), do not have abnormal pelvic areas, or fail to meet temperament standards.
- After breeding, heifers should be selected as replacements if they conceive early in the breeding season, are capable of achieving 85% of their mature weight by calving, and calve at a body condition of 5.5 to 6.0.
- Selection of replacement heifers will be enhanced with the future commercial development of genetic selection tools for traits such as puberty and antral follicle count.

INTRODUCTION

Infertility (and economic losses) of beef females may be attributed to 3 primary groups: (1) females that fail to become pregnant during the breeding season (usually 60–120 days), (2) females that become pregnant but fail to calve, and (3) females that become pregnant late in the breeding season. Infertility that leads to the failure of a beef female to calve during the subsequent calving season results in the single largest economic loss to beef producers; this is because no economic return will be realized from those cows for at least 1 additional year. Cows that fail to become pregnant during the breeding season do not provide producers with an opportunity to market a calf, becoming an economic liability to beef production systems. Selection of heifers to

Disclosures: The author has nothing to disclose.
North Florida Research and Education Center, University of Florida, 3925 Highway 71, Marianna, FL 32446, USA
E-mail address: gclamb@ufl.edu

Vet Clin Food Anim 29 (2013) 567–578
http://dx.doi.org/10.1016/j.cvfa.2013.07.003
0749-0720/13/$ – see front matter © 2013 Elsevier Inc. All rights reserved.

vetfood.theclinics.com

ensure that they calve early during their first breeding season is critical to the lifetime productivity of beef cows and success of beef operations.[1] Attainment of puberty in heifers before initiation of the breeding season is likely the single most important factor affecting when heifers become pregnant during the breeding season and, subsequently, the lifetime productivity of cows. Age at which heifers attain puberty is directly associated to heifers that become pregnant, fail to become pregnant, or become pregnant late season calving.[2] Thus, cow-calf producers are in need of selection criteria to assess the future productive potential of replacement heifers as early as possible in order to choose the best replacement heifers and to best allocate resources to manage them in preparation for their first breeding season. Therefore, identification and selection of breeding animals that attain puberty at a younger age enhances the overall fertility and subsequent longevity of cows in beef cattle operations.

Fertility of beef cattle is regarded as lowly heritable, but there is considerable evidence that genetic variation exists for fertility traits in heifers that is unaccounted for by differences in weight, nutritional status, growth rate, or management, and can be formulated to be genetically independent of body weight and age.[3-5] The heritability of age at puberty was reviewed by Martin and colleagues,[3] who approximated that, across several studies, the average heritability of age at puberty was 0.40. In specific work by Mialon and colleagues,[6] the heritability of age of puberty was moderate in Charolais cows (0.33). Nonetheless, regardless of the heritability of fertility traits of heifers, there are multiple methods to select heifers during the development phase that ensure that they become productive cows.

SELECTION OF HEIFERS AT WEANING

Replacement heifers represent the next generation of improved genetics for a beef cattle operation and producers must invest significant resources into these females before establishment of pregnancy, but many of these females may fail to become pregnant. Therefore, selection of heifers that have a greater opportunity to become pregnant early in the first breeding season, calve without difficulty within a desired age (usually by 2 years of age), and reinitiate postpartum estrous cycles to become pregnant again during the subsequent breeding season are essential to the economic profitability of beef cattle operations.

Producers should consider genetic variation within and between breeds to ensure that these differences are accounted for during postweaning development. Differences occur among breeds for growth rate and mature size, lean/fat ratio, age at puberty, and milk production.[7] In addition, breeds selected for milk production as well as size reach puberty earlier than do breeds of similar size and growth potential that are not selected for milk production.[7] The negative relationship between milk production and age at puberty may be as great as the positive relationship between mature size and age at puberty. Short and colleagues[8] suggested that breed differences, sire and dam effects within a breed, and heterosis contribute to the genetic control of age at puberty. In addition, age at puberty may be decreased by selecting a breed with a younger age at puberty, selecting within a breed for younger age at puberty, or crossbreeding with another breed that has a similar or younger age at puberty.[8]

There are few management practices that can be applied to potential replacement heifers during the suckling phase and before weaning. With sufficient nutrients, the dam can be expected to nurse her calf to ensure that the calf meets the desired weight at weaning to become a productive female in the herd. However, preweaning recording of dam information is essential for identification of potential replacement heifers. Therefore, it is necessary to maintain a sound record-keeping system that includes individual identification, cow and calf performance, and previous fertility of the dam. Previous fertility may include pregnancy rates, breeding dates, and calving dates. Heifer calves resulting from cows that have good production and reproductive performance are more desirable than calves from cows with a history of less desirable production and reproductive performance characteristics.

In addition to selection based on productivity of the dam, replacement heifers should be selected based on age and weight. Selection of replacements from heifer calves born in the first half of the calving season increases the opportunity for heifers to attain puberty before initiation of the breeding season.[9,10] Age and weight are largely regarded as the primary factors that affect the onset of puberty. In general, regardless of their birth date, calves are typically weaned at the same time; therefore, sorting heifers by weight and frame score is a necessary step in narrowing the pool of replacements at weaning. Heifers that are too large or too small (based on frame score) or too heavy or too light are good candidates to consider culling.

At weaning, producers should also consider the effects of growth-promoting implants and the effects of creep feeding during the suckling phase on future productivity as replacement heifers. Growth-promoting implants are frequently used in suckling calves destined to become replacement heifers.[11,12] Growth-promoting implants contain anabolic agents such as the steroid hormones estrogen or testosterone, or nonsteroidal compounds that have steroid activity, or synthetic steroid compounds. Use of implants in suckled heifer calves has been shown to have detrimental effects on subsequent fertility.[13] Reports have shown that use of growth-promoting implants may inhibit or reduce gonadotropin secretion[14] and delay development of the reproductive tract, puberty, and first ovulation in young heifers.[15] In addition, reviews by Hargrove[11] and Deutscher[12] indicate that growth promotants inhibit development of the mature reproductive endocrine system in suckled heifer calves when receiving growth promotants at or near birth and significantly reduce subsequent pregnancy rates during the breeding season. Suckling heifer calves that are implanted with zeranol, estradiol, or trenbolone acetate have distinct phenotypic characteristics that differ from heifers that do not receive growth-promoting implants.[14] Bartol and colleagues[16] showed that chronic exposure of heifer calves to progesterone or estradiol, beginning on or before postnatal day 45, reduced uterocervical wet weights and altered uterine wall histology. These effects were observed in heifers 15 months after the first steroid exposure. Therefore, it is recommended that heifers destined to become replacement heifers do not receive implants during the suckling phase.

Supplemental feeding of calves during the suckling phase (creep feeding) enhances weaning weights of calves; however, excessive feeding that results in excessive body fat of suckled heifers may influence subsequent development of some desired maternal traits, such as longevity and future number of calves weaned.[17–19] In addition, although creep-fed heifers may be heavier at weaning than heifers not receiving creep feed, the advantage in weight disappears by yearling age.[20]

Therefore, selection criteria to consider when selecting heifers at weaning are:
1. Identify heifers from dams with evidence of good production and reproductive performance using a detailed individual animal recording system
2. Select heifer calves born in the first half of the calving season
3. Select based on age and weight and eliminate heifers in the extremes
4. Previous exposure to growth-promoting implants
5. Previous exposure to creep feeding that may have resulted in heifers that are overconditioned.

SELECTION OF HEIFERS BEFORE BREEDING

Approaching the breeding season, numerous selection criteria may be used to ensure that heifers selected as replacements have the greatest opportunity to become pregnant early in the breeding season and remain productive for many years. In addition, culling heifers that fail to meet specific criteria before the breeding season may decrease the potential losses associated with maintaining undesirable or nonpregnant heifers for an extended period of time. In a 3-year study, we evaluated the economic performance of 1542 pregnant and nonpregnant heifers sold by a commercial heifer development operation using artificial insemination (AI) followed by a 60-day breeding season (**Table 1**). Heifers culled at the time of the prebreeding examinations and finished in a feedlot had a 3-year average net profit of $9, whereas heifers diagnosed as nonpregnant shortly after the breeding season were sold for a net loss of $86. The loss for pregnant heifers that were then diagnosed nonpregnant after wintering on native pasture and sold at a local sale barn was $133 per head. Average profits were $163, $139, and $83, respectively, for heifers sold pregnant after first-service AI, second-service AI, or natural mating. The results emphasize the economic importance of preselection and early culling to reduce losses associated with maintaining open heifers.

The influence of preweaning management and environment on the subsequent reproductive efficiency of 591 weaned Angus × Hereford heifers from 12 sources was evaluated.[21] A prebreeding examination was performed in which heifers were culled for poor average daily weight gain (minimum of 0.64 kg per day), small pelvic area (minimum of 140 cm^2), poor reproductive tract scores, poor disposition, or structural unsoundness. Of the 591 heifers, 14% were culled before the breeding season. The percentage of heifers culled from each source group ranged from 0% to 26%. The difference in culling rates among sources was largely associated with management practices and environmental conditions at each source before the purchase of the heifers. Although heifers may appear to be similar in frame and condition they may not be sufficiently developed to become pregnant early during the breeding season. Therefore, heifers with a decreased likelihood of becoming pregnant early in the breeding season should be identified and culled before initiation of the breeding season.

For a heifer to calve by 2 years of age she must reach puberty by 15 months of age, but in many cases as few as 65% of all beef heifers have attained puberty by 15 months of age.[22–24] In addition, heifers inseminated on their third estrus have a greater first-service conception rate (21%–36%) than those inseminated at puberty.[25,26] Therefore, gains should be targeted to ensure that heifers reach puberty at least 3 weeks before the beginning of breeding. Based on a heifer's genetics and

Table 1
Net profit or loss associated with the sale of heifers at various stages of development

Stage	Year 1 ($/head)	Year 2 ($/head)	Year 3 ($/head)
Prebreeding culls	8	16	4
Postbreeding culls	−33	−144	−84
Precalving culls	−213	−61	−124
First-service AI	160	164	164
Second-service AI	129	88	184
Naturally mated	89	72	86

expected mature size, a target weight should be predetermined to ensure that the development nutrition program is tailored for heifers to achieve the desired breeding weight.[9,10,27] The rate of gain required during the development phase typically ranges from 0.5 to 1.0 kg/d to ensure that the prebreeding weight approaches 60% to 65% of the heifer's expected mature weight. Using the standard set by the Beef Improvement Federation (BIF, 1990) for 9 frame-size classifications for US breeding cattle, producers can estimate body composition and energy requirements per kilogram of gain at various weights during the feeding period.[28] Optimum growth rates for replacement females of various body types are also available. These growth rates represent optimums for heifers that vary in mature size and were developed to maximize female lifetime productivity.[28]

In many cases, heifers may attain puberty and become pregnant at a body weight lower than 60%,[29] but the risk of developing heifers to a reduced percentage of mature body weight may also result in the increased risk of underdeveloped heifers (**Table 2**). Although heifers should be expected to attain puberty at 60% to 65% of their mature weight, this may be affected by genetics, season of birth, and rate of post-weaning gain. Selection of the target weight may be based on the average weight of the heifer group, a percentage of the expected mature weight, or may be extrapolated from the average frame score. Selection criteria of heifers before breeding should include a criterion based on which heifers most effectively meet a specific prebreeding weight before initiation of the breeding season. Heifers that have significantly lower or greater prebreeding weights should be considered for culling before initiation of the breeding season.

A reproductive tract score (RTS) system was developed[30] to assist beef producers with selection of potential replacement heifers before initiation of the breeding season and to estimate pubertal status (**Table 3**). Scores are subjective estimates of sexual maturity, based on ovarian follicular and luteal development and palpable size of the uterus. Heifers with an RTS of 1 are likely the furthest from puberty at the time of examination, whereas those assigned a 2 or 3 are approaching puberty, and those with a score of 4 or 5 have likely attained puberty. Assessing an RTS at 45 to 60 days before initiation of the breeding season allows beef producers the opportunity to select heifers that will have a greater opportunity to become pregnant during the breeding season and cull those heifers that have a decreased opportunity to become pregnant.

Measurement of the pelvic area is also a criterion to consider when selecting heifers before initiation of the breeding season. Pelvic measurements should be used in addition to, but not in place of, selection for size, weight, and fertility.[31] Selection for increased pelvic area does not likely result in increased pelvic dimensions alone, but also results in increased size of the skeleton and the animal.[32] Increased skeletal size of the dam is reflected in higher birth weights and dimensions of the calf; however,

Table 2					
Optimum growth rate for breeding replacement heifers					
	Frame Size				
	1	3	5	7	9
Optimum weight at first estrus (kg)	264	297	331	365	400
Mature weight (kg)	400	467	533	600	667

Data from Fox DG, Sniffen CJ, O'Conner JD. Adjusting nutrient requirements of beef cattle for animal and environmental variations. J Anim Sci 1988;66:1480.

Table 3
RTSs

RTS	Uterine Horns	Ovarian Length (mm)	Ovarian Height (mm)	Ovarian Width (mm)	Ovarian Structures
1	Immature, <20-mm diameter, no tone	15	10	8	No palpable follicles
2	Diameter 20–25 mm, no tone	18	12	10	8-mm follicles
3	Diameter 20–25 mm, slight tone	22	15	10	Follicles 8–10 mm
4	30-mm diameter, good tone	30	16	12	10-mm follicles, CL possible
5	>30-mm diameter	>32	20	15	CL present

Data from Anderson KJ, Lefever DG, Brinks JS, et al. The use of reproductive tract scoring in beef heifers. Agri-Practice 1991;12(4):21.

pelvic measurements may be used to successfully identify abnormally small or abnormally shaped pelvises. Left unidentified, these situations are often associated with extreme dystocia, resulting in cesarean delivery and even death of the calf or dam.[33] In addition, Bullock and Patterson[34] reported that puberty exerts a positive influence on pelvic width and resulting pelvic area in yearling heifers; however, differences seen among heifers as yearlings did not carry through to calving as 2-year-olds. Therefore selection of heifers based on pelvic measurements should include consideration of pubertal status at the time of the examination.

Animal temperament also is critical to selection of future cows to the beef cattle operation. Cattle with excitable temperaments have altered metabolism and partitioning of nutrients in order to sustain the behavioral stress response, which results in decreases in nutrient availability to support body functions.[35,36] Nutritional status largely determines reproductive performance in cattle; therefore, excitable temperament may indirectly impair reproduction in beef heifers by decreasing nutritional balance. Also, the hormones produced during a stress response, particularly cortisol, directly disrupt the physiologic mechanisms that regulate reproduction in beef females, such as ovulation, conception, and establishment of pregnancy. It was recently shown that beef heifers with calm temperaments reached puberty sooner than temperamental cohorts (**Table 4**). Therefore, excitable temperament has detrimental effects on the reproduction of beef females, independently of breed type, and culling more excitable heifers should be considered before the breeding season.

Table 4
Postweaning temperament scores (1, calm; 5, excitable temperament) and blood cortisol concentrations of replacement heifers that attained or did not attain puberty by 12 months of age

Item	Nonpubertal	Pubertal
	Mean ± Standard Error	
Temperament score	2.7 ± 0.14	2.3 ± 0.12
Cortisol (ng/mL)	50.0 ± 3.34	39.7 ± 2.06

Data from Cooke RF, Arthington JD, Austin BR, et al. Effects of acclimation to handling on performance, reproductive, and physiological responses of Brahman-crossbred heifers. J Anim Sci 2009;87:3409–10.

Considerations when selecting heifers before the breeding season are:
1. Heifers that have a decreased opportunity to become pregnant during the breeding season should be culled before the breeding season because they will be a financial liability.
2. Identify heifers that meet specific growth parameters to ensure they have a greater probability of being pubertal.
3. Use RTSs to cull heifers with poor reproductive tract development or retain heifers that are cycling.
4. Use prebreeding pelvic measurements to cull heifers with abnormally small or abnormally shaped pelvic areas.
5. Identify and cull heifers that do not meet specific temperament requirements.

SELECTION OF HEIFERS AFTER BREEDING

As indicated previously, selection of heifers to ensure that they calve early during their first breeding season is critical to the lifetime productivity of beef cows and the success of beef operations.[1] Therefore, identification of heifers that become pregnant early in the breeding season should be the primary focus of the selection criteria after the breeding season. Use of pregnancy diagnosis and embryo or fetal aging is a critical component in accurately determining when heifers become pregnant during the breeding season. There are 3 practical methods that can be used for pregnancy diagnosis in beef herds: (1) rectal palpation, (2) transrectal ultrasonography, or (3) use of a blood sample that is submitted to a laboratory for analyses and results returned to the producer within a few days.

Rectal palpation is an accurate form of pregnancy diagnosis that can be performed after day 35 of pregnancy. Most veterinarians are proficient at pregnancy diagnosis in the form of rectal palpation and it is a simple procedure that requires little time in the cattle handling facility. However, rectal palpation does not provide any information about the viability of the embryo/fetus. Transrectal ultrasonography can be used to detect early pregnancy, as early as 26 days of gestation for heifers and 28 days of gestation for cows, with a high degree of accuracy for determination of embryo or fetal size (**Table 5**).[37] For a skilled technician the procedure is as fast as rectal palpation and may provide additional information in terms of embryo/fetus viability and the incidence

Table 5
Fetal crown-rump length in relation to age in weeks

Fetal Age (wk)	No. of Observations	Crown-Rump Length (mm)		
		Minimum	Maximum	Mean
4	25	6	11	8.9
5	35	8	19	12.8
6	50	16	26	20.2
7	47	23	36	27.7
8	41	36	52	45.5
9	48	39	71	62.4
10	43	61	101	87.4
11	39	95	118	106.5
12	32	107	137	121.8

Data from Hughes EA, Davies DA. Practical uses of ultrasound in early pregnancy in cattle. Vet Rec 1989;124:456–8.

of twins.[38] Use of blood samples is becoming a more popular method of pregnancy diagnosis. Blood samples are taken to evaluate for pregnancy-associated glycoproteins. Heifers may be tested at 30 days or later after breeding and are more than 99% accurate if the cow is diagnosed as pregnant. All three methods of pregnancy diagnosis may be used effectively to establish pregnancy, but the use of blood samples requires multiple samples at various stages during and after the breeding season to establish when heifers may have become pregnant during the breeding season. Transrectal palpation and ultrasound are both procedures that only require a single diagnosis to determine when pregnancies were established.

Transrectal ultrasonography also provides producers with an opportunity to diagnose the sex of the fetus, which can occur between days 55 and 80 of gestation. Many cattle operations are developing strategies to use fetal sexing as either a marketing or purchasing tool. After day 55 of gestation, male and female fetuses can be differentiated by the location of the genital tubercle and development of the genital swellings into the scrotum in male fetuses. We determined the sex of 112 fetuses in Angus heifers with 98.2% accuracy. Depending on the long-term goals of producers, they may prefer to select heifers that will give birth to either male or female calves. Therefore, fetal sex determination may be an excellent tool for selecting replacement heifers after the breeding season.

Following pregnancy examination, weight gains need to focus on having the heifers reach approximately 85% of their expected mature weight by the time they calve. Pregnant heifers should have average daily gains close to 0.5 kg to ensure that heifers reach their first calving with adequate frame, pelvis, and body condition. In addition, it is useful to remember that approximately 70% to 75% of fetal growth occurs during the last trimester of pregnancy and rations should be adjusted accordingly.[27] Once replacement heifers are determined to be pregnant, they also need to be managed to calve in moderate body condition (average body condition score of 5.5–6.0). Heifers calving in moderate condition usually have less dystocia, a shorter postpartum interval, and higher pregnancy rates after their second breeding seasons.

Considerations when selecting heifers after breeding season are:
1. Use pregnancy diagnosis to select heifers that conceive early in the breeding season.
2. Consider using transrectal ultrasonography to select heifers that may give birth to calves of the desired sex.
3. Retain heifers that meet specific average daily gains to ensure that they calve at 85% of their mature weight.
4. Cull heifers that do not maintain a body condition score of 5.5 to 6.0 before calving.

FUTURE SELECTION TOOLS AND SUMMARY

Animal agricultural research is in a transformative period with the advent of genomic tools to improve the accuracy of predicting individual animal genotypes, and incorporation of these tools will enhance knowledge of the mechanisms that cause inter-animal variation in fertility traits, leading to effective selection tools for economically relevant traits such as the onset of puberty and providing an opportunity to select heifers that will have a greater opportunity to become pregnant early in the breeding season.

Several genes in the gonadotropin pathway have been associated with age at puberty and reproductive capacity in cattle[39–42] using fine mapping and candidate gene approaches. The glutamate receptor pathway was identified by Fortes and colleagues,[43] and a polymorphism in the glutamate receptor ionophore AMP1 was associated with ovulation rate, antral follicle count, and conception rate.[40] More recently, researchers at the United States Department of Agriculture Meat Animal Research Center (Clay Center, NE) have been collaborating to identify indicator traits of fertility in beef females, calculate genetic parameters for these traits, and develop methodologies to identify the genes controlling these traits.[4,44–46] With the Bovine SNP50, age at puberty had a genomic heritability of 0.14 and antral follicle count had a genomic heritability of 0.44, and there were favorable genetic correlations between these traits and heifer pregnancy rate (**Table 6**), indicating that age at puberty and antral follicle counts are good indicators of heifer fertility. However, the high costs and impracticality of obtaining onset of puberty data for individual heifers, and conducting high-density genotyping, has limited the number of animals (and thereby experimental power) that can be used in these types of gene-discovery studies. However, as costs of genotyping continue to decrease and genetic testing becomes available, producers will have an opportunity to select heifers as early as birth to determine which heifers to retain as replacements.

Replacement heifers represent a large capital investment for beef producers. Therefore, they need to be selected or culled at critical time points and managed intensively to ensure that they become pregnant early in the breeding season, calve early and without assistance, and rebreed during the subsequent breeding season. The decisions on which heifers to select and the subsequent nutritional management and breeding season management likely affect the productivity of the cow herd for years to come. Therefore, producers should focus on developing a strategy and specific criteria for selecting their heifers to ensure that they meet the needs of each individual program. In addition, producers should also be aware of new commercial genetic selection tools that may become available in the near future to assist in identifying heifers that may have a greater opportunity to become pregnant early in their first breeding season and remain in the herd to become productive cows.

Table 6
Estimated genomic heritabilities and correlations among measures of growth, body condition, puberty, and pregnancy of crossbred heifers[a,b]

Trait	YW	PWG	AFC	AAP	BCS	HPR
YW	**0.54**	0.83	−0.16	0.30	0.73	−0.17
PWG	0.82	**0.46**	−0.26	0.26	0.52	−0.04
AFC	0.08	0.06	**0.44**	0.37	−0.63	−0.55
AAP	−0.01	0.06	0.02	**0.14**	0.15	−0.33
BCS	0.28	0.22	0.03	0.02	**0.09**	−0.07
HPR	0.04	0.05	0.00	0.00	0.12	**0.11**

Abbreviations: AAP, age at puberty; AFC, antral follicle count; BCS, body condition score (1–9) following breeding; HPR, yearling heifer pregnancy rate; PWG, postweaning gain to yearling; YW, yearling body weight.
[a] Parameters estimated from genomic relationship matrix using BovineSNP50 genotypes. Heritability on diagonal, with genomic correlations above and phenotypic correlations below the diagonal.
[b] Two-breed, 3-breed, and 4-breed crosses of Angus, Hereford, Charolais, Gelbvieh, Limousin, Red Angus, and Simmental in Cycle VII, USMARC Germplasm Evaluation Project.
Data from Snelling WM, Cushman A, Fortes MR, et al. How single nucleotide polymorphism chips will advance our knowledge of factors controlling puberty and aid in selecting replacement beef females. J Anim Sci 2012;90:1158.

REFERENCES

1. Short RE, Bellows RA. Relationships among weight gains, age at puberty and reproductive performance in heifers. J Anim Sci 1971;32:127–31.
2. Lesmeister JL, Burfening PJ, Blackwell RL. Date of first calving in beef cows and subsequent calf production. J Anim Sci 1973;36:1–6.
3. Martin LC, Brinks JS, Bourdon RM, et al. Genetic effects on beef heifer puberty and subsequent reproduction. J Anim Sci 1992;70:4006–17.
4. Cushman RA, Allan MF, Kuehn LA. Characterization of biological types of cattle: Indicator traits of fertility in beef cattle. Rev Bras Zool 2008;37:116–21.
5. Cammack KM, Thomas MG, Enns RM. Review: reproductive traits and their heritabilities in beef cattle. Prof Anim Sci 2009;25:517–28.
6. Mialon MM, Renand G, Krauss D, et al. Genetic variability of the length of post-partum anoestrus in Charolais cows and its relationship with age at puberty. Genet Sel Evol 2000;32:403–14.
7. Cundiff LV. The effect of future demand on production programs-biological versus product antagonisms. In: Beef improvement federation proc. Lexington (KY): 1986. p 110–27.
8. Short RE, Staigmiller RB, Bellows RA, et al. Breeding heifers at one year of age: biological and economic considerations. In: Proc. 39th Annu. Beef Cattle Short Course. Gainesville (FL): University of Florida; 1990. p. 93–106.
9. Spire MF. Managing replacement heifers from weaning to breeding. Vet Med 1997;92:182–92.
10. Corah LF, Hixon DL. Replacement heifer development. In: Beef cattle handbook. Ames (IA): MidWest Plan Service; 1999. p. 1–4 [Publication BCH 2100].
11. Hargrove DA. Use of growth promotants in replacement heifers. In: Proc. 39th Annu. Beef Cattle Short Course. Gainesville (FL): University of Florida; 1990. p. 36–48.
12. Deutscher GH. Growth promoting implants on replacement heifers. In: Proc. Tri-State Cow/Calf Symposium. St Francis (KS): 1991.
13. Deutscher GH, Zerfoss LL, Clanton DC. Time of zeranol implantation on growth, reproduction and calving of beef heifers. J Anim Sci 1988;62:875–86.
14. Moran C. The effects of anabolic agents on reproduction and growth of beef heifers [MS thesis]. Dublin (Ireland): National University of Ireland, University College; 1988.
15. Gropp J. Influence of anabolic steroids on performance and side effects in veal calf nutrition. In: Sasiorwski H, editor. Steroids in animal production. Warsaw (Poland): Warsaw Agricultural University Proceedings of International Symposium; 1980. p. 23–31.
16. Bartol FF, Johnson LL, Floyd JG, et al. Neonatal exposure to progesterone and estradiol alters uterine morphology and luminal protein content in adult beef heifers. Theriogenology 1995;43:835–44.
17. Kress DD, Burfening PJ. Weaning weight related to subsequent most probable producing ability in Hereford cows. J Anim Sci 1972;35:327–35.
18. Holloway JW, Totusek R. Relationships between preweaning nutritional management and subsequent performance of Angus and Hereford females through three calf crops. J Anim Sci 1973;37:807–12.
19. Johnsson ID, Obst JM. The effects of level of nutrition before and after eight months of age on the subsequent milk production and calf yield of beef heifers over three lactations. Anim Prod 1984;38:57–68.
20. Martin TG, Lemenager RP, Srinivasan G, et al. Creep feed as a factor influencing performance of cows and calves. J Anim Sci 1981;53:33–9.

21. Lamb GC, Nix DW, Stevenson JS, et al. Prolonging the MGA-prostaglandin alpha interval from 17 to 19 days in an estrus synchronization system for heifers. Theriogenology 2000;53:691–8.
22. Wiltbank JN, Gregory KE, Swiger I A, et al. Effects of heterosis on age and weight at puberty in beef heifers. J Anim Sci 1966;25:744–51.
23. Gregory KE, Laster DB, Cundiff LV, et al. Heterosis and breed maternal and transmitted effects in beef cattle. II. Growth rate and puberty in females. J Anim Sci 1978;47:1042–53.
24. Gregory KE, Laster DB, Cundiff LV, et al. Characterization of biological types of cattle–Cycle III II Growth rate and puberty in females. J Anim Sci 1979;49: 461–71.
25. Byerley DJ, Staigmiller RB, Berardinelli JG, et al. Pregnancy rates of beef heifers bred either on puberal or third estrus. J Anim Sci 1987;65:645–50.
26. Perry RC, Corah LH, Cochran RC, et al. Effects of hay quality, breed, and ovarian development on onset of puberty and reproductive performance of beef heifers. J Prod Agr 1991;4:13–8.
27. Larson RL, Randle RF. Heifer development: nutrition, health and reproduction. In: Youngquist RS, Threlfall WR, editors. Current therapy in large animal theriogenology. St. Louis (MO): Saunders Elsevier; 2007. p. 457–63.
28. Fox DG, Sniffen CJ, O'Conner JD. Adjusting nutrient requirements of beef cattle for animal and environmental variations. J Anim Sci 1988;66:1475–95.
29. Endecott RL, Funston RN, Mulliniks JT, et al. Joint Alpharma-Beef Species Symposium: implications of heifer development systems and lifetime productivity. J Anim Sci 2013;91:1329–35.
30. Anderson KJ, Lefever DG, Brinks JS, et al. The use of reproductive tract scoring in beef heifers. Agri-Practice 1991;12(4):19–26.
31. Bellows RA, Staigmiller RB. Selection for fertility. In: Proc. 39th Annu. Beef Cattle Short Course. Gainesville (FL): University of Florida; 1990. p. 172–89.
32. Morrison DG, Williamson WD, Humes PE. Estimates of heritabilities and correlations of traits associated with pelvic area in beef cattle. J Anim Sci 1986;83: 432–7.
33. Patterson DJ, Perry RC, Kiracofe GH, et al. Management considerations in heifer development and puberty. J Anim Sci 1992;70:4018–35.
34. Bullock KD, Patterson DJ. Pelvic growth in beef heifers and the effects of puberty. In: Proc. Beef Improvement Federation. Sheridan (WY): 1995. p. 171–3.
35. Cooke RF, Arthington JD, Austin BR, et al. Effects of acclimation to handling on performance, reproductive, and physiological responses of Brahman-crossbred heifers. J Anim Sci 2009;87:3403–12.
36. Cooke RF, Arthington JD, Araujo DB, et al. Effects of acclimation to human interaction on performance, temperament, physiological responses, and pregnancy rates of Brahman-crossbred cows. J Anim Sci 2009;87:4125–32.
37. Hughes EA, Davies DA. Practical uses of ultrasound in early pregnancy in cattle. Vet Rec 1989;124:456–8.
38. Lamb GC. Reproductive real-time ultrasound technology: an application for improving calf crop in cattle operations. In: Fields MJ, editor. Factors affecting calf crop: biotechnology of reproduction. FL Boca Raton: CRC Press; 2001. p. 235–53.
39. Marson EP, Ferraz JB, Meirelles FV, et al. Effects of polymorphisms of LHR and FSHR genes on sexual precocity in a *Bos taurus* × *Bos indicus* beef composite population. Genet Mol Res 2008;7:243–51.
40. Sugimoto M, Sasaki S, Watanabe T, et al. Ionotropic glutamate receptor AMPA 1 is associated with ovulation rate. PLoS One 2010;5:e13817.

41. Yang WC, Li SJ, Tang KQ, et al. Polymorphisms in the 5' upstream region of the FSH receptor gene, and their association with superovulation traits in Chinese Holstein cows. Anim Reprod Sci 2010;119:172–7.

42. Líron JP, Prando A, Ripoli MV, et al. Characterization and validation of bovine gonadotropin releasing hormone receptor (GNRHR) polymorphisms. Res Vet Sci 2011;91:391–6.

43. Fortes MR, Reverter A, Zhang Y, et al. Association weight matrix for the genetic dissection of puberty in beef cattle. Proc Natl Acad Sci U S A 2010;107:13642–7.

44. Allan MF, Kuehn LA, Cushman RA, et al. Confirmation of quantitative trait loci using a low-density single nucleotide polymorphism map for twinning and ovulation rate on bovine chromosome 5. J Anim Sci 2009;87:46–56.

45. Allan MF, Thallman RM, Cushman RA, et al. Association of a single nucleotide polymorphism in SPP1 with growth traits and twinning in a cattle population selected for twinning rate. J Anim Sci 2007;85:341–7.

46. Snelling WM, Cushman A, Fortes MR, et al. How single nucleotide polymorphism chips will advance our knowledge of factors controlling puberty and aid in selecting replacement beef females. J Anim Sci 2012;90:1153–65.

Effect of Age at Puberty/ Conception Date on Cow Longevity

George A. Perry, PhD[a],*, Robert Cushman, PhD[b]

KEYWORDS

- Longevity • Heifers • Conception date • Puberty

KEY POINTS

- A cow needs to wean 3 to 5 calves to pay for her development costs. Therefore, longevity of a beef female is important to the sustainability and profitability of any beef operation, and the greatest percentage of cows culled from the herd were for pregnancy status (33%).
- Age at puberty is a critical trait, because pregnancy success during the breeding season has been correlated with the percentage of heifers that reached puberty before or early in the breeding season. Puberty is influenced by both age and weight.
- Survival analysis of heifers indicated that a greater proportion of the heifers that calved in the first 21 days of their first calving season remained in the herd longer when compared to heifers that calved later.
- Heifers that calve early as 2-year olds tend to calve early throughout their life.

Continued

Mention of trade names or commercial products in this publication is solely for the purpose of providing specific information and does not imply recommendation or endorsement by the U.S. Department of Agriculture.

[a] Department of Animal Science, South Dakota State University, North Campus Drive, Brookings, SD 57007, USA; [b] ARS, USDA[1], U.S. Meat Animal Research Center, State Spur 18D, Clay Center, NE 68933, USA

[1] The U.S. Department of Agriculture (USDA) prohibits discrimination in all its programs and activities on the basis of race, color, national origin, age, disability, and where applicable, sex, marital status, familial status, parental status, religion, sexual orientation, genetic information, political beliefs, reprisal, or because all or part of an individual's income is derived from any public assistance program (Not all prohibited bases apply to all programs.). Persons with disabilities who require alternative means for communication of program information (Braille, large print, audiotape, etc.) should contact USDA's TARGET Center at (202) 720-2600 (voice and TDD). To file a complaint of discrimination, write to USDA, Director, Office of Civil Rights, 1400 Independence Avenue, S.W., Washington, D.C. 20250-9410, or call (800) 795-3272 (voice) or (202) 720-6382 (TDD). USDA is an equal opportunity provider and employer.
* Corresponding author.
E-mail address: George.Perry@sdstate.edu

Vet Clin Food Anim 29 (2013) 579–590
http://dx.doi.org/10.1016/j.cvfa.2013.07.011
0749-0720/13/$ – see front matter © 2013 Elsevier Inc. All rights reserved.

vetfood.theclinics.com

Continued

- Long postpartum intervals decrease the proportion of cows that are cycling at the start of the breeding season and thereby decrease the probability of pregnancy during the breeding season. In beef cattle, postpartum interval length is influenced by a variety of factors including suckling, nutrition, age, dystocia, season, genetic variations, stress, and disease.
- There is a moderate genetic correlation between age at puberty and postpartum interval, indicating that there are a common set of genes that are involved with the initiation of reproductive cycles. Furthermore, a negative genetic correlation between age at puberty and heifer pregnancy rate indicate that genetic selection to decrease age at puberty would result in an increase in heifer pregnancy rates.

INTRODUCTION

Calving late as a heifer has long been reported to increase the chance of calving late or not calving the following year,[1] and heifers that calve early tend to remain in those calving groups throughout their life.[1,2] According to a review by Patterson and colleagues,[3] heifers need to calve by 24 months of age to achieve maximum lifetime productivity. Furthermore, heifers that lose a pregnancy or conceive late in the breeding season are likely to not have enough time to rebreed during the subsequent defined breeding season,[3] and any cow that misses a single calving is not likely to recover the lost revenue of that missed calf.[4]

A cow needs to wean 3 to 5 calves to pay for her development costs.[5] Therefore, longevity of a beef female is important to the sustainability and profitability of any beef operation. Considering the importance of longevity, an important question is as follows: Why are females culled from a beef herd? According to the 2007–08 NAHMS survey, the greatest percentage of cows culled from the herd were for pregnancy status (33.0%); other reasons for culling included age or bad teeth (32.1%), economic reasons (14.6%), other reproductive problems (3.9%), producing poor calves (3.6%), temperament (3.6%), injury (2.9%), udder problems (2.7%), bad eyes (1.8%), and other problems (1.8%). Furthermore, 15.6% of cows (animals that have previously calved) culled were less than 5 years of age and 31.8% were 5 to 9 years of age. These females that are culled from a herd before producing 5 calves increase the developmental cost of other heifers and do not contribute to the profitability and sustainability of the operation. Therefore, understanding how puberty and conception date can affect pregnancy success and longevity can have a tremendous impact on the profitability and sustainability of an operation.

FACTORS THAT AFFECT AGE AT PUBERTY

Puberty in the bovine female has been defined as the first ovulation that is accompanied by visual signs of estrus and normal luteal function.[6] Age at puberty is a critical trait when heifers are to be bred during a restricted breeding season and expected to calve at 2 years of age,[7] because pregnancy success during the breeding season has been correlated with the percentage of heifers that reached puberty before or early in the breeding season.[8]

Several studies have reported that heifers reach puberty at a genetically influenced size[9] and that heifers developed to lighter weights will be older when they reach puberty.[8,10] Across several breeds, both age and post-weaning gains have been shown to affect onset of puberty.[7,11] Therefore, timing of puberty depends on both age and weight; however, the age and weight at which puberty occurs vary among breeds as mature size varies across breeds.[8,12,13] Thus, the idea of developing heifers to a specific target weight (usually 65% of mature weight) has become a common management practice. Recent work by Freetly and colleagues[14] reported that, regardless of breed, puberty was obtained between 55% and 60% of mature body weight, indicating that adequate growth and body condition are necessary for the initiation of normal estrous cycles; this is important as several studies have reported that a minimum amount of body condition (total body fat) is necessary for puberty and reproductive success to occur. Leptin is a hormone produced by adipose tissue and regulated by both long-term nutritional history (body condition) and current nutritional status (feed availability).[15] Mean serum concentrations of leptin increased as puberty approached,[16] and changes in diet did not affect concentrations of leptin when percentage of total carcass fat was similar between treatments.[17]

INFLUENCE OF PUBERTY ON CONCEPTION DATE

The percentage of heifers that have reached puberty at the start of the breeding season is variable between herds and years and has been reported to range from 19% to 100%.[18,19] A practical on-farm method to determine pubertal status is reproductive tract scoring.[20] Reproductive tract scoring uses rectal palpation to determine size of the uterine horns and the structures that are present on the ovary (1 = no palpable follicles, 2 = 8 mm follicles, 3 = 8–10 mm follicles, 4 = >10 mm follicles and possibly a corpus luteum [CL], 5 = CL present). The use of reproductive tract scores to determine pubertal status has demonstrated that heifers with infantile tracts (tract score 1) have decreased conception rates following estrous synchronization compared to peripubertal and pubertal heifers.[21] Furthermore, heifers with a tract score of 1 also had later conception dates when inseminated artificially to natural estrus over a 21-day period and placed with bulls for 42 additional days.[22] This later conception date resulted in decreased weaning weight of the calves that were born to these heifers. Additionally, the heifers that had tract scores of 1 but produced a calf as a 2-year-old still had lower conception rates in their second breeding season, again demonstrating that calving late as a heifer can negatively affect subsequent reproductive performance.

Some recent studies have proposed that heifers can be developed to lighter weights before the first breeding season. However, fewer heifers that were developed to 53% of mature weight were cycling before the start of the breeding season compared to heifers developed to 58% of mature weight, but the percentage of heifers pregnant in a 45-d breeding season was not different between treatments.[23] Although this might indicate that heifers can be developed to a lighter weight without negatively affecting reproductive performance, Creighton and colleagues[24] reported that when heifers were developed to 50% of mature weight, 15.7% fewer heifers conceived in the first 30 days of the breeding season compared to heifers developed to 55% of mature weight. Therefore, consideration should be given to the possibility of heifers conceiving later in the breeding season and possibly decreasing longevity of the herd when trying to decrease heifer development costs.

INFLUENCE OF CONCEPTION DATE ON FERTILITY AND LONGEVITY

Heifers that calve early as 2-year-olds tend to calve early throughout their life[1,2]; calving late as a heifer has long been reported to increase the chance of calving late or not calving the following year.[1] Survival analysis of 2 separate groups of heifers indicated that a greater proportion of the heifers that calved in the first 21 days of their first calving season remained in the herd longer when compared to heifers that calved later; this resulted in a greater average herd life for these heifers compared to their contemporary herd mates that calved at a later date (**Fig. 1**).[25] These heifers that calved during the first 21 days were on average born only 2 days earlier than heifers that calved during the second period and only 3 days earlier than heifers that calved during the third period (**Table 1**).[25] There was no difference in the birth weight of the heifers based on the calving period they were in during their first calving season; however, heifers that calved in the first period were the heaviest when they were weaned.[25]

The first postpartum interval from calving to estimated date of conception was significantly longer for heifers that calved in the first period as compared to those that calved in the second or third period; however, this difference disappeared by the second postpartum interval, and there was no difference in postpartum interval from the second to the eighth postpartum interval.[25] It is clear from these data that the cows are not staying completely within their calving periods. If they were, the

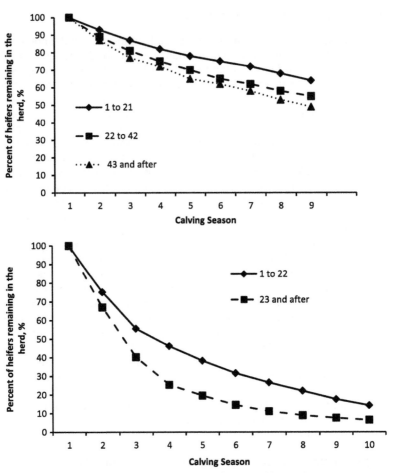

Fig. 1. Influence of calving period on herd survival from 2 different data sets. Data set 1 contains 16,549 heifers. Data set 2 contains 2, 195 heifers. Heifers that calved in the first 21 days of the calving season as 2-year olds remained in the herd longer than heifers that calved later as 2-year olds (*P*<.01). (*Adapted from* Cushman RA, Kill LK, Funston RN, et al. Heifer calving date positively influences calf weaning weights through six parturitions. J Anim Sci 2013 [Epub ahead of print].)

Table 1
Influence of calving period on cow performance traits through the first 9 calves

	Calving Period[a]			P
	1	2	3	
Heifers	11,061	4372	1116	
Birth date, day of year	93.2 ± 1.8[a]	95.2 ± 1.8[b]	96.9 ± 1.8[c]	<.0001
Heifer birth BW, kg	38.6 ± 0.4	38.8 ± 0.4	38.5 ± 0.4	.06
Heifer weaning BW, kg	203.4 ± 3.8[a]	199.3 ± 3.9[b]	195.9 ± 3.9[c]	<.0001
First calf birth date, day of year	70.5 ± 1.6[a]	93.3 ± 1.6[b]	116.1 ± 1.6[c]	<.0001
First calf birth BW, kg	38.0 ± 0.8[a]	38.8 ± 0.8[a]	39.0 ± 0.8[b]	<.0001
First dystocia score[b]	2.90 ± 0.29	2.92 ± 0.29	2.87 ± 0.29	<.69
First post-partum interval,[c] day	113.4 ± 3.2[a]	92.1 ± 3.2[b]	70.5 ± 3.2[c]	<.0001
Second pregnancy rate, %	92.6 ± 0.3[a]	87.6 ± 0.5[b]	83.9 ± 1.2[c]	<.0001
Second calf birth date, day of year	98.0 ± 3.2[a]	99.7 ± 3.2[b]	101.0 ± 3.2[c]	<.0001
Second calf birth BW, kg	38.8 ± 0.9[a]	38.8 ± 0.9[a]	37.7 ± 0.9[b]	<.0001
Second dystocia score	1.27 ± 0.14	1.28 ± 0.14	1.24 ± 0.14	.36
Second post-partum interval, day	82.8 ± 2.6	82.5 ± 2.6	83.9 ± 2.7	.26
Third pregnancy rate, %	92.7 ± 0.3[a]	90.4 ± 0.5[b]	88.4 ± 1.1[c]	<.0001
Third calf birth date, day of year	97.6 ± 2.6[a]	99.3 ± 2.6[b]	101.5 ± 2.7[c]	<.0001
Third calf birth BW, kg	39.6 ± 0.8[a]	39.3 ± 0.8[b]	38.9 ± 0.8[b]	.002
Third dystocia score	1.12 ± 0.08	1.12 ± 0.07	1.11 ± 0.08	.72
Third postpartum interval, day	85.3 ± 3.3	85.3 ± 3.3	85.8 ± 3.4	.84
Fourth pregnancy rate, %	93.7 ± 0.3[a]	91.5 ± 0.5[b]	91.4 ± 1.0[b]	<.0001
Fourth calf birth date, day of year	98.5 ± 3.0[a]	99.8 ± 3.0[b]	102.4 ± 3.0[c]	<.0001
Fourth calf birth BW, kg	41.0 ± 1.0[a]	40.9 ± 1.0[a]	40.3 ± 1.0[b]	.05
Fourth dystocia score	1.12 ± 0.08	1.09 ± 0.08	1.09 ± 0.08	.12
Fourth postpartum interval, day	81.1 ± 2.9	81.4 ± 2.9	81.6 ± 3.0	.84
Fifth pregnancy rate, %	94.4 ± 0.3[a]	91.7 ± 0.6[b]	88.8 ± 1.3[c]	<.0001
Fifth calf birth date, day of year	94.8 ± 2.8[a]	96.5 ± 2.8[b]	99.5 ± 2.8[c]	<.0001
Fifth calf birth BW, kg	43.7 ± 1.0[a]	43.7 ± 1.0[a]	42.9 ± 1.0[b]	.01
Fifth dystocia score	1.04 ± 0.06	1.04 ± 0.06	1.02 ± 0.07	.46
Fifth postpartum interval, d	81.9 ± 3.0	81.7 ± 3.1	81.8 ± 3.2	.93
Sixth pregnancy rate, %	94.3 ± 0.3[a]	92.0 ± 0.6[b]	92.8 ± 1.2[ab]	.002
Sixth calf birth date, day of year	95.2 ± 2.8[a]	96.6 ± 2.8[b]	97.9 ± 2.9[b]	.001
Sixth calf birth BW, kg	41.9 ± 0.9[a]	41.5 ± 0.9[b]	40.8 ± 0.9[c]	.002
Sixth dystocia score	1.08 ± 0.07	1.09 ± 0.07	1.06 ± 0.07	.52
Sixth postpartum interval, day	83.9 ± 3.3[a]	82.8 ± 3.4[a]	79.9 ± 3.5[c]	.009
Seventh pregnancy rate, %	93.7 ± 0.4	93.1 ± 0.7	93.3 ± 1.3	.69
Seventh calf birth date, day of year	96.2 ± 3.0	96.9 ± 3.0	95.1 ± 3.1	.17
Seventh calf birth BW, kg	39.8 ± 1.1[a]	39.2 ± 1.1[b]	38.7 ± 1.1[b]	.002
Seventh dystocia score	1.17 ± 0.09	1.12 ± 0.09	1.19 ± 0.09	.06
Seventh postpartum interval, day	83.1 ± 3.5	83.7 ± 3.6	85.4 ± 3.8	.38
Eighth pregnancy rate, %	92.3 ± 0.5[a]	92.2 ± 0.9[a]	86.8 ± 2.0[b]	.006
Eighth calf birth date, day of year	97.7 ± 3.1	98.6 ± 3.1	98.3 ± 3.3	.40
Eighth calf birth BW, kg	41.1 ± 1.0	40.9 ± 1.0	40.5 ± 1.1	.32

(continued on next page)

Table 1 (continued)				
	Calving Period[a]			
	1	2	3	P
Eighth dystocia score	1.15 ± 0.07	1.13 ± 0.07	1.15 ± 0.07	.72
Eighth postpartum interval, day	87.5 ± 2.9	88.5 ± 3.0	87.7 ± 3.6	.71
Ninth pregnancy rate, %	92.6 ± 0.6	90.4 ± 1.1	91.0 ± 2.1	.17
Ninth calf birth date, day of year	100.7 ± 2.3	102.6 ± 2.7	101.6 ± 3.0	.10
Ninth calf birth BW, kg	41.5 ± 0.8	41.3 ± 0.8	41.3 ± 0.9	.72
Ninth dystocia score	1.07 ± 0.06	1.05 ± 0.06	1.06 ± 0.07	.69

[a] 1 = heifers that gave birth on days 1–21 of their first calving season, 2 = heifers that gave birth on days 23–42 of their first calving season, 3 = heifers that gave birth on or after day 43 of their first calving season.
[b] Scoring system 1 to 7: 1 = no assistance; 2 = little difficulty, assistance given by hand; 3 = little difficulty, mechanical pull; 4 = slight difficulty, mechanical pull; 5 = moderate mechanical pull; 6 = hard mechanical pull; 7 = caesarian section; 8 = abnormal presentation.[56]
[c] Estimated postpartum interval from calving to conception based on consecutive calving dates and assuming a 281 day gestation length.

difference in Julian calving day among the groups would be greater than 2 to 3 days for the second through sixth calf. The estimated postpartum interval from calving to conception was greater in the first postpartum period for those heifers that calved in the first period, but during the second to eighth postpartum interval, their estimated postpartum interval did not differ due to the calving group they calved in as a heifer and averaged about 81 to 83 days.[25]

HOW CONCEPTION DATE CAN AFFECT FERTILITY AND LONGEVITY

To maintain an annual calving interval (≤365 days), conception must occur within 80 days of calving; however, the anestrous period for heifers frequently extends greater than 60 days. In beef cattle, it is generally accepted that long postpartum intervals decrease the proportion of cows that are cycling at the start of the breeding season and thereby decrease the probability of pregnancy during the breeding season. However, the data from Cushman and colleagues[25] indicated that heifers that calved early as a 2-year-old had increased pregnancy rates with their third to sixth calf without a decrease in postpartum interval, indicating that inherent fertility may be improved as well as the ability to initiate reproductive cycles. Furthermore, Snelling and colleagues[26] demonstrated a negative genetic correlation between age at puberty and heifer pregnancy rate, indicating that if genetic selection was used to decrease age at puberty it would result in an increase in heifer pregnancy rates. Therefore, genetic selection could improve longevity in a herd both by improving the ability to initiate reproductive cycles and by improving inherent fertility.

POSTPARTUM INTERVAL

In beef cattle, postpartum interval length is influenced by a variety of factors including suckling, nutrition, age, dystocia, season, genetic variations, stress, and disease.[27–29] Postpartum beef cows that are suckled ad libitum have a longer postpartum anestrous period than cows that are suckled once daily or not suckled at all.[30] This extended anestrous period is a direct function of suckling and presence of a cow's own calf on luteinizing hormone (LH) pulse frequency. Pituitary concentrations of LH returned to normal by day 30 postpartum,[31] and injections of GnRH at day 20 postpartum induced pulses of LH.[32] Cows that were early weaned, suckled by an alien calf, or suckled by their own calf but had their sight and olfactory senses removed had increased LH pulse frequency compared to control cows that were suckled by their own calf.[33] The ability of a cow to recognize her calf influenced the response of anestrous beef cows to once daily suckling. Stagg and colleagues[34] reported that once daily suckling reduced postpartum interval, but cows that were isolated from calves had decreased postpartum interval compared to cows that were penned adjacent to their calves. Therefore, the ability of a cow to recognize her calf prolongs postpartum interval length in addition to the neural stimulation of the suckling stimulus. See the following reviews for a more complete review of the effect of suckling on the postpartum interval in beef cattle.[27–29]

Ruminants have the unique ability to convert low-quality forages into food products (meat and milk), and in times of excess nutrition they deposit energy stores for future maintenance of bodily functions and production. Short and colleagues[27] proposed the following biologic priorities for nutrient utilization (nutrient partitioning) by cattle: (1) basal metabolism, (2) motor activity, (3) growth, (4) basic energy reserves, (5) maintenance of pregnancy, (6) lactation, (7) additional energy reserves, (8) estrous cycles and initiation of pregnancy, and (9) excess reserves. The preceding priorities for nutrient partitioning demonstrate that reproduction (resumption of estrous cycling and pregnancy) is a low priority, particularly for heifers calving at 2 years of age. Since, growth is a higher priority for nutrient partitioning than reproduction and heifers consistently had longer postpartum intervals than multiparous cows[35,36]; the first ovulation postpartum in primiparous cows was often delayed relative to multiparous cows.[37,38] Consequently, as animals reach mature body size, nutrients that were previously partitioned for growth can be used for lower-priority functions including reproduction.

Time to puberty was reduced in heifers experiencing increases in day length.[39–41] Furthermore, cows injected with melatonin had extended intervals from calving to first estrus and ovulation, suggesting that duration of darkness may play a role in postpartum interval length.[37] Supplementation of light to cows in the fall of the year, in some cases, shortened the interval from calving to first estrus and from calving to conception.[42] However, seasonal effects on postpartum interval may be overcome by plane of nutrition. Cows calving late in the summer and fed a high plane of nutrition (approximately twice the low plane) had similar postpartum intervals to cows calving later in the year and fed a high or low plane of nutrition.[43]

Heifers calving at 2 years of age have increased incidence of dystocia compared to older cows. Furthermore, heifers that experienced calving difficulty at 2 years of age weaned fewer calves that were younger and lighter.[44] Dystocia decreased percentage of cows exhibiting standing estrus within 45 days of calving, AI pregnancy rates, and total pregnancy rates among cows[45] and increased the likelihood of being culled from the herd.[46]

However, in the work by Cushman and colleagues,[25] most heifers had the opportunity to ovulate at least one time before conception. Although some influence of postpartum interval on fertility cannot be ignored because some heifers that calve very late might not have the opportunity to initiate estrous cycles before the end of the next breeding season, it does seem likely that other factors are contributing to the decreased lifetime fertility observed among heifers that calved late. In fact, the incidence of anestrus at the start of the breeding season did not differ between low-fertility cows and high-fertility cows,[47,48] whereas low-fertility cows were older at first calving.[47] The increased incidence of early embryonic mortality reported in these low-fertility cows[47,49] combined with the greater age at first calving indicates a direct link between calving date in heifers and intrinsic fertility or possibly even oocyte quality.

GENETIC SELECTION

The genetic parameters of age at puberty were reviewed by Martin and colleagues[50] who reported an average heritability of age at puberty of 0.40. In specific work by Mialon and colleagues,[51] the heritability of age of puberty was moderate in Charolais heifers (0.33). Thus, there are genes that influence the onset of reproductive cycles in beef heifers, and this heritability indicates that advancements could be made in heifer reproductive performance by understanding the gene pathways involved with this trait. These investigators also reported a moderate genetic correlation between age at puberty and postpartum interval, indicating that there were a common set of genes that were involved with the initiation of reproductive cycles.[52] Selection for a decreased age at puberty increased pregnancy rates and decreased calving day in a population of Angus heifers.[53] These data indicate that by decreasing age at puberty, there is a correlated increase in reproductive performance. Thus genes that are influencing the onset of reproductive cycles are also influencing fertility. Although most would argue that this is simply due to an increase in the number of heifers that have initiated reproductive cycles before the first breeding season, there is the possibility of common genes that influence both reproductive cycles and fertility. For instance, in transgenic mice that do not produce the Period 1 protein, there is a decrease not only in the percentage of regularly cycling females but also in the number of pups produced and reproductive longevity.[54]

Both candidate gene and whole genome association studies have been used to try to identify genes associating with age at puberty in beef heifers. Although there has been some success, the whole genome association studies clearly demonstrate that age at puberty is a polygenic trait, controlled by many genes with very small effects of each gene.[26,55] Snelling and colleagues[26] demonstrated a negative genetic correlation between age at puberty and heifer pregnancy rate ($r = -0.33$), indicating that if genetic selection was used to decrease age at puberty it would result in an increase in heifer pregnancy rates. However, care must be used in the application of genetic markers or traditional selection because decreasing age at puberty in beef heifers increases the risk of very young heifers becoming pregnant out of season. Certainly the incorporation of *Bos taurus* germplasm into *Bos indicus* cattle or the use of genetic markers with *Bos indicus* heifers has greater potential due to the greater problems with attainment of puberty in these breeds.

SUMMARY

According to the 2007–08 NAHMS survey, the greatest percentage of cows culled from the herd were for pregnancy status (33.0%). Furthermore, 15.6% of animals culled were less than 5 years of age. These females that are culled from a herd before producing 3 to 5 calves increase the developmental cost of other heifers and do not contribute to the profitability and sustainability of the operation.

The opportunity to pick replacement heifers based on earlier conception can help increase the longevity of animals in a herd. However, management decisions associated with heifers that conceive late becomes an important question. Could they be sold to other producers with a later breeding season? The question remains whether moving those heifers to a different contemporary group would improve their subsequent performance or do many of these cows just have overall decreased fertility? These cows may actually be reproductively insufficient compared to the cows that conceive early. Although the idea of selling heifers that conceived later as yearlings is not novel, to the authors' knowledge there has been no controlled study to examine how these heifers perform relative to their new management groups. As more producers move to breeding extra heifers and selling those that conceive late, the opportunity to investigate subsequent fertility of these later conceiving heifers may provide useful information.

REFERENCES

1. Burrls MJ, Priode BM. Effect of calving date on subsequent calving performance. J Anim Sci 1958;17:527–33.
2. Lesmeister JL, Burfening PJ, Blackwell RL. Date of first calving in beef cows and subsequent calf production. J Anim Sci 1973;36:1–6.
3. Patterson DJ, Perry RC, Kiracofe GH, et al. Management considerations in heifer development and puberty. J Anim Sci 1992;70:4018–35.
4. Mathews KH Jr, Short SD. The beef cow replacement decision. J Agribusiness 2001;19:1191–211.
5. Clark RT, Creighton KW, Patterson HH, et al. Symposium paper: economic and tax implications for managing beef replacement heifers. Prof Anim Sci 2005;17: 164–73.
6. Moran C, Quirke JF, Roche JF. Puberty in heifers: a review. Anim. Reprod. Sci 1989;18:167–82.
7. Ferrell CL. Effects of postweaning rate of gain on onset of puberty and productive performance of heifers of different breeds. J Anim Sci 1982;55:1272–83.
8. Short RE, Bellows RA. Relationship among weight gains, age at puberty and reproductive performance in heifers. J Anim Sci 1971;32:127–31.
9. Taylor CS, Fitzhugh HA Jr. Genetic relationships between mature weight and time taken to mature within a breed. J Anim Sci 1971;33:726–31.
10. Wiltbank JN, Roberts S, Nix J, et al. Reproductive performance and profitability of heifers fed to weigh 272 or 318 kg at the start of the first breeding season. J Anim Sci 1985;60:25–34.
11. Freetly HC, Cundiff LV. Reproductive performance, calf growth, and milk production of first-calf heifers sired by seven breeds and raised on different levels of nutrition. J Anim Sci 1998;76:1513–22.
12. Wiltbank JN, Gregory KE, Swiger LA, et al. Effects of heterosis on age and weight at puberty in beef heifers. J Anim Sci 1966;25:744–51.
13. Varner LW, Bellows RA, Christensen DS. A management system for wintering replacement heifers. J Anim Sci 1977;44:165–71.
14. Freetly HC, Kuehn LA, Cundiff LV. Growth curves of crossbred cows sired by Hereford, Angus, Belgian Blue, Brahman, Boran, and Tuli bulls, and the fraction of mature body weight and height at puberty. J Anim Sci 2011;89:2373–9.
15. Chilliard Y, Delavaud C, Bonnet M. Leptin expression in ruminants: nutritional and physiological regulations in relation with energy metabolism. Domest Anim Endocrinol 2005;29:3–22.
16. Garcia MR, Amstalden M, Williams SW, et al. Serum leptin and its adipose gene expression during pubertal development, the estrous cycle, and different seasons in cattle. J Anim Sci 2002;80:2158–67.
17. Garcia MR, Amstalden M, Morrison CD, et al. Age at puberty, total fat and conjugated linoleic acid content of carcass, and circulating metabolic hormones in beef heifers fed a diet high in linoleic acid beginning at four months of age. J Anim Sci 2003;81:261–8.

18. Lucy MC, Billings HJ, Butler WR, et al. Efficacy of an intravaginal progesterone insert and an injection of $PGf_{2\alpha}$ for synchronizing estrus and shortening the interval to pregnancy in postpartum beef cows, peripubertal beef heifers, and dairy heifers. J Anim Sci 2001;79:982–95.

19. Lamb GC, Larson JE, Geary TW, et al. Synchronization of estrus and artificial insemination in replacement beef heifers using gonadotropin-releasing hormone, prostaglandin f2alpha, and progesterone. J Anim Sci 2006;84:3000–9.

20. Andersen KJ, LeFever DG, Brinks JS, et al. The use of reproductive tract scoring in beef heifers. Agri-Practice 1991;12:106–11.

21. Patterson DJ, Weaber RL, Smith MF, et al. The Missouri show-me-select replacement heifer program. J Anim Sci 2006;84(Suppl 1):187.

22. Holm DE, Thompson PN, Irons PC. The value of reproductive tract scoring as a predictor of fertility and production outcomes in beef heifers. J Anim Sci 2009; 87:1934–40.

23. Funston RN, Deutscher GH. Comparison of target breeding weight and breeding date for replacement beef heifers and effects on subsequent reproduction and calf performance. J Anim Sci 2004;82:3094–9.

24. Creighton KW, Johnson-Musgrave JA, Klopfenstein TJ, et al. Comparison of two development systems for march-born replacement beef heifers. University of Nebraska Beef Report; 2005. p. 3–6.

25. Cushman RA, Kill LK, Funston RN, et al. Heifer calving date positively influences calf weaning weights through six parturitions. J Anim Sci 2013. [Epub ahead of print].

26. Snelling WM, Cushman RA, Fortes MR, et al. Physiology and endocrinology symposium: how single nucleotide polymorphism chips will advance our knowledge of factors controlling puberty and aid in selecting replacement beef females. J Anim Sci 2012;90:1152–65.

27. Short RE, Bellows RA, Staigmiller RB, et al. Physiological mechanisms controlling anestrus and infertility in postpartum beef cattle. J Anim Sci 1990;68: 799–816.

28. Crowe MA, Goulding D, Baguisi A, et al. Induced ovulation of the first postpartum dominant follicle in beef suckler cows using a gnrh analogue. J Reprod Fertil 1993;99:551–5.

29. Yavas Y, Walton JS. Postpartum acyclicity in suckled beef cows: a review. Theriogenology 2000;54:25–55.

30. Williams GL. Suckling as a regulator of postpartum rebreeding in cattle: a review. J Anim Sci 1990;68:831–52.

31. Nett TM, Cermak D, Braden T, et al. Pituitary receptors for gnrh and estradiol, and pituitary content of gonadotropins in beef cows. II. Changes during the postpartum period. Domest Anim Endocrinol 1988;5:81–9.

32. Walters DL, Short RE, Convey EM, et al. Pituitary and ovarian function in postpartum beef cows. III. Induction of estrus, ovulation and luteal function with intermittent small-dose injections of gnrh. Biol Reprod 1982;26:655–62.

33. Griffith MK, Williams GL. Roles of maternal vision and olfaction in suckling-mediated inhibition of luteinizing hormone secretion, expression of maternal selectivity, and lactational performance of beef cows. Biol Reprod 1996;54: 761–8.

34. Stagg K, Spicer LJ, Sreenan JM, et al. Effect of calf isolation on follicular wave dynamics, gonadotropin and metabolic hormone changes, and interval to first ovulation in beef cows fed either of two energy levels postpartum. Biol Reprod 1998;59:777–83.

35. Doornbos DE, Bellows RA, Burfening PJ, et al. Effects of dam age, prepartum nutrition and duration of labor on productivity and postpartum reproduction in beef females. J Anim Sci 1984;59:1–10.

36. Fajersson P, Stanko RL, Williams GL. Distribution and repeatability of anterior pituitary responses to gnrh and relationship of response classification to the postpartum anovulatory interval of beef cows. J Anim Sci 1999;77:3043–9.

37. Sharpe PH, Gifford DR, Flavel PF, et al. Effect of melatonin on postpartum anestrus in beef cows. Theriogenology 1986;26:621–9.

38. Guedon L, Saumande J, Desbals B. Relationships between calf birth weight, prepartum concentrations of plasma energy metabolites and resumption of ovulation postpartum in limousine suckled beef cows. Theriogenology 1999; 52:779–89.

39. Schillo KK, Hansen PJ, Kamwanja LA, et al. Influence of season on sexual development in heifers: age at puberty as related to growth and serum concentrations of gonadotropins, prolactin, thyroxine and progesterone. Biol Reprod 1983;28: 329–41.

40. Hauser ER. Seasonal effects on female reproduction in the bovine (bos taurus) (european breeds). Theriogenology 1984;21:150–69.

41. Schillo KK, Hall JB, Hileman SM. Effects of nutrition and season on the onset of puberty in the beef heifer. J Anim Sci 1992;70:3994–4005.

42. Hansen PJ, Hauser ER. Photoperiodic alteration of postpartum reproductive function in suckled cows. Theriogenology 1984;22:1–14.

43. Montgomery GW, Scott IC, Hudson N. An interaction between season of calving and nutrition on the resumption of ovarian cycles in post-partum beef cattle. J Reprod Fertil 1985;73:45–50.

44. Brinks JS, Olson JE, Carroll EJ. Calving difficulty and its association with subsequent productivity in Herefords. J Anim Sci 1973;36:11–7.

45. Laster DB, Glimp HA, Cundiff LV, et al. Factors affecting dystocia and the effects of dystocia on subsequent reproduction in beef cattle. J Anim Sci 1973;36: 695–705.

46. Rogers PL, Gaskins CT, Johnson KA, et al. Evaluating longevity of composite beef females using survival analysis techniques. J Anim Sci 2004;82:860–6.

47. Warnick AC, Hansen PJ. Comparison of ovulation, fertilization and embryonic survival in low-fertility beef cows compared to fertile females. Theriogenology 2010;73:1306–10.

48. Cushman RA, Miles JR, Rempel LA, et al. Identification of an ionotropic glutamate receptor AMPA1/GRIA1 polymorphism in crossbred beef cows differing in fertility. J Anim Sci 2013;91:2640–6.

49. Maurer RR, Echternkamp SE. Repeat-breeder females in beef cattle: influences and causes. J Anim Sci 1985;61:624–36.

50. Martin LC, Brinks JS, Bourdon RM, et al. Genetic effects on beef heifer puberty and subsequent reproduction. J Anim Sci 1992;70:4006–17.

51. Mialon MM, Renand G, Krauss D, et al. Genetic relationship between cyclic ovarian activity in heifers and cows and beef traits in males. Genet. Sel. Evol 2001;33:273–87.

52. Mialon MM, Renand G, Krauss D, et al. Genetic variability of the length of postpartum anoestrus in Charolais cows and its relationship with age at puberty. Genet. Sel. Evol 2000;32:403–14.

53. Morris CA, Wilson JA, Bennett GL, et al. Genetic parameters for growth, puberty, and beef cow reproductive traits in a puberty selection line. New Zeal J Agr Res 2000;43:83–91.

54. Pilorz V, Steinlechner S. Low reproductive success in Per1 and Per2 mutant mouse females due to accelerated ageing. Reproduction 2008;135:559–68.

55. Fortes MR, Reverter A, Zhang Y, et al. Association weight matrix for the genetic dissection of puberty in beef cattle. Proc Natl Acad Sci U S A 2010;107: 13642–7.

56. Bennett GL. Experimental selection for calving ease and postnatal growth in seven cattle populations. I. Changes in estimated breeding values. J Anim Sci 2008;86:2093–102.

Control of Estrus and Ovulation in Beef Heifers

David J. Patterson, PhD[a],*, Jordan M. Thomas[a],
Neal T. Martin, MS[b], Justin M. Nash, MS[b], Michael F. Smith, PhD[a]

KEYWORDS

- Beef heifer • Estrous synchronization • Reproductive management
- Artificial insemination

KEY POINTS

- Estrous synchronization and artificial insemination contribute to a total heifer development program by concentrating the breeding and resulting calving periods.
- Artificial insemination provides the opportunity to breed heifers to bulls selected for low birth weight or high calving-ease expected progeny difference with high accuracy, a practice that minimizes the incidence and severity of calving difficulty and decreases calf loss that results from dystocia.
- Protocols are now available that facilitate fixed-time artificial insemination without the need to detect estrus.
- Many of the protocols reviewed in this article include the use of progestins. Progestins are used effectively to synchronize estrus in heifers that are pubertal, but may also be used to facilitate the induction of puberty in prepubertal or peripubertal heifers.

INTRODUCTION

Estrous synchronization and artificial insemination (AI) remain the most important and widely applicable reproductive biotechnologies available for cattle.[1] Although hormonal treatment of heifers and cows to synchronize estrous cycles has been a commercial reality now for more than 30 years, beef producers have been slow to adopt this management practice. Perhaps this is because of past failures, which resulted when heifers that were placed on estrous synchronization treatments failed to reach

Disclosure: Portions of this review were previously published by the authors in: *Proceedings, Applied Reproductive Strategies in Beef Cattle*. December 3–4, 2012; Sioux Falls, SD. p. 53–83. Available at: http://www.appliedreprostrategies.com/2012/SiouxFalls/newsroom.html.
[a] Division of Animal Sciences, University of Missouri, Columbia, MO 65211, USA; [b] College of Veterinary Medicine, University of Missouri, Columbia, MO 65211, USA
* Corresponding author.
E-mail address: pattersond@missouri.edu

puberty. In addition, early estrous synchronization programs failed to manage follicular waves, resulting in more days in the synchronized period, which ultimately precluded fixed-time artificial insemination (FTAI) with acceptable pregnancy rates. The development of convenient and economical protocols to synchronize estrus and ovulation to facilitate use of FTAI with resulting high fertility should result in increased adoption of these important management practices.[2] Research has focused on the development of methods that effectively synchronize estrus in replacement beef heifers by decreasing the period of time over which estrous detection is required, thus facilitating the use of FTAI. Although tools are now available for beef producers to successfully use these procedures, transfer of the technology must assume a high priority. Transfer of such technology to beef producers in the United States will require an increase in technical support to facilitate successful use and adoption of these procedures.[3] Veterinarians should position themselves to play a key role in this process.

Improving traits of major economic importance in beef cattle can be accomplished most rapidly through selection of genetically superior sires and widespread use of AI. Procedures that facilitate synchronization of estrus in estrous-cycling heifers and induction of an ovulatory estrus in peripubertal heifers will increase reproductive rates and expedite genetic progress. Estrous synchronization can be an effective means of increasing the proportion of females that become pregnant early in the breeding period, resulting in shorter calving seasons and more uniform calf crops.[4] Females that conceived to a synchronized estrus calved earlier in the calving season, and weaned calves that were on average 13 days older and 21 lb (9.5 kg) heavier than calves from nonsynchronized females.[5]

Effective estrous synchronization programs offer the following advantages: (1) heifers are in estrus at a predicted time that facilitates AI, embryo transfer, or other assisted reproductive techniques; (2) the time required to detect estrus is reduced, thus decreasing labor expense associated with estrous detection; (3) heifers will conceive earlier during the breeding period; (4) AI becomes more practical; and (5) calves will be older and heavier at weaning.

The inability to predict time of estrus for individual heifers in a group often makes it impractical to use AI because of the labor required for detection of estrus. Available procedures to control the estrous cycle of heifers can improve reproductive rates and speed up genetic progress. These procedures include synchronization of estrus in estrous-cycling females, and induction of estrus accompanied by ovulation in heifers that have not yet reached puberty.

The following protocols and terms will be referred to throughout this article.

Protocols for AI performed on the basis of detected estrus:

PG: Prostaglandin $F_{2\alpha}$ (PG; Lutalyse, Estrumate, ProstaMate, InSynch, estroPLAN).

MGA-PG: Melengestrol acetate (MGA; 0.5 mg/h/d) is fed for a period of 14 days with PG administered 17 to 19 days after MGA withdrawal.

GnRH-PG (Select Synch): Gonadotropin-releasing hormone injection (GnRH; Cystorelin, Factrel, Fertagyl, OvaCyst) followed in 7 days with an injection of PG.

MGA-GnRH-PG (MGA Select): MGA is fed for 14 days, GnRH is administered 12 days after MGA withdrawal, and PG is administered 7 days after GnRH.

CIDR Select: A controlled internal drug release (CIDR) device is inserted on day 0 and removed on day 14, GnRH is administered on day 23, and PG is administered on day 30.

14-day CIDR-PG: CIDRs are inserted on day 0 and removed on day 14. PG is administered on day 30.

Protocols for FTAI in beef heifers:

CO-Synch + CIDR: GnRH is administered at CIDR insertion on day 0, followed 7 days later with CIDR removal, and PG. Insemination is performed 54 hours after CIDR removal and PG, with GnRH administered at AI.

CIDR Select: CIDRs are inserted on day 0 and removed on day 14, GnRH is administered on day 23 (9 days after CIDR removal) and PG is administered on day 30. Insemination is performed 72 hours after PG with GnRH administered at AI.

14-day CIDR-PG: CIDRs are inserted on day 0 and removed on day 14 with PG administered on day 30. Insemination is performed 66 hours after PG with GnRH administered at AI.

Terms:

Estrous response: The number of females that exhibit estrus during a synchronized period.

Synchronized period: The period of time during which estrus is expressed after treatment.

Synchronized conception rate: The proportion of females of those exhibiting estrus and inseminated during the synchronized period that become pregnant.

Synchronized pregnancy rate: The proportion of females of the total number treated that become pregnant.

To avoid problems when using estrous synchronization, heifers should be selected for a program when the following conditions are met: (1) replacement heifers are developed to prebreeding target weights that represent at least 65% of their projected mature weight; and (2) reproductive tract scores (RTS) are assigned to heifers no more than 2 weeks before an estrous synchronization treatment begins (scores of 2 or higher on a scale of 1–5), and at least 50% of the heifers are assigned an RTS of 4 or 5.[3]

ESTROUS SYNCHRONIZATION AND AI CONTRIBUTE TO A TOTAL HEIFER DEVELOPMENT PROGRAM

Estrous synchronization and AI contribute to a total heifer development program in several ways. Estrous synchronization improves time management for producers who use AI by concentrating the breeding and resulting calving periods. Managers are able to spend more time observing heifers as they calve because calving occurs over a shorter time period. Calf losses in many cases are reduced because of improved management during the calving period. AI provides the opportunity to breed heifers to bulls selected for low birth weight (BW) or high calving-ease expected progeny difference (EPD) with high accuracy. This practice minimizes the incidence and severity of calving difficulty and decreases calf loss that results from dystocia. In addition, heifers that conceive during a synchronized period typically wean calves that are older and heavier at weaning time.[5] Finally, heifer calves that result from AI can be an excellent source of future replacements, facilitating more rapid improvement in the genetic makeup of an entire herd.

Progestins were used to induce estrus in peripubertal heifers[6] and were originally combined with estrogen to mimic changes that occur in concentrations of blood hormones around the time of puberty. Increased progesterone is thought to be a prerequisite for the development of normal estrous cycles. Progesterone increases during the initiation of puberty in the heifer,[7] and before resumption of normal ovarian cyclicity in postpartum suckled beef cows.[8,9] Progestins stimulate an increase in follicular growth that results subsequently in increased production of estrogen by ovarian follicles.[10–13] MGA and CIDR initiate estrous cyclicity in peripubertal beef heifers[14,15] and are associated with increased luteinizing hormone (LH) pulse frequency during the treatment period.[16,17] Recent studies suggest that the stimulatory effects of progestins on LH secretion are greatest after removal of the steroid.[17,18] Furthermore, improvements in pubertal induction response following treatment with a progestin occur with an increase in age.[18] The increase in pulsatile release of LH that occurs in response to progestin treatment in peripubertal heifers results in a decrease in estrogen receptors within neuronal systems that mediate negative feedback actions of estradiol on GnRH secretion.[19]

Because puberty is a heritable trait, induced puberty in replacement heifers over several generations might result in situations whereby attainment of puberty would be difficult without hormone treatment.[20] This consideration cannot be overlooked. However, there is a need for treatments to induce puberty in cattle that are later-maturing but of sufficient age and weight at the time of treatment to permit successful application.[14] The decision to use this practice within a herd perhaps differs with various types of beef operations. For instance, the common goal of most managers of commercial cow-calf herds is to maximize weaning rate. In other words, the investment in time and resources in a heifer from weaning to breeding requires that management efforts be made to facilitate puberty onset and maximize the likelihood of early pregnancy. In this scenario, a method to induce puberty in heifers could serve as a valuable tool to improve reproductive performance of heifers retained for breeding purposes. On the other hand, seed stock managers should weigh the economic importance of puberty onset in their herds, as well as their customers', and the associated potential and resulting implication of masking its true genetic expression.

MGA-BASED PROGRAMS

This section reviews methods to control estrous cycles of cattle using MGA. Three methods are outlined for using the MGA program to facilitate estrous synchronization in beef heifers. The choice of which system to use depends largely on a producer's goals. MGA is the common denominator in each of the 3 systems presented here. MGA is an orally active progestin. When consumed on a daily basis, MGA will suppress estrus and prevent ovulation.[21,22] MGA may be fed with a grain or a protein carrier, and either top-dressed onto other feed or batch-mixed with larger quantities of feed. MGA is fed at a rate of 0.5 mg/animal/d in a single daily feeding. The duration of feeding may vary among protocols, but the level of feeding is consistent and critical to success. Animals that fail to consume the required amount of MGA on a daily basis may return to estrus prematurely during the feeding period; this may be expected to reduce the estrous response during the synchronized period. Therefore, adequate bunk space (60 linear centimeters per head) must be available so that all animals consume feed simultaneously.[2]

Animals should be observed for behavioral signs of estrus on each day of the feeding period, and may be done as animals approach the feeding area and before feed distribution. This practice ensures that all females receive adequate intake. Heifers will exhibit estrus beginning 48 hours after MGA withdrawal, and this will continue for 6 to 7 days. It is generally recommended that females exhibiting estrus during this period not be inseminated or exposed for natural service, because of the reduced fertility experienced by females at the first heat after MGA withdrawal.

Method 1: MGA with Natural Service

The simplest method involves using bulls to breed synchronized groups of females. This practice is useful in helping producers make a transition from natural service to AI. In this process, heifers receive the normal 14-day feeding period of MGA and are then exposed to fertile bulls about 10 days after MGA withdrawal (**Fig. 1**).

This system works effectively, although careful consideration of bull to female ratios is advised. It is recommended that 15 to 20 synchronized females be exposed per bull. Age and breeding condition of the bull and results of breeding-soundness examinations should be considered.

Method 2: MGA + Prostaglandin

This method of estrous synchronization involves the combination of MGA with PG. PG is a luteolytic compound normally secreted by the uterus of the cow. PG can induce luteal regression but cannot inhibit ovulation. When PG is administered in the presence of a functional corpus luteum (CL) during days 6 to 16 of the estrous cycle, premature regression of the CL begins and the cow returns to estrus.

In this program, PG should be administered 19 days after the last day of MGA feeding. This treatment places all animals in the late luteal stage of the estrous cycle at the time of PG injection, which shortens the synchronized period and maximizes conception rate (**Fig. 2**). Although a 19-day interval is optimal, 17- to 19-day intervals produce acceptable results and provide flexibility for extenuating circumstances.[23–25] Five available PG products for synchronization of estrus in cattle can be used after the MGA treatment: Estrumate, estroPLAN, InSynch, Lutalyse, or ProstaMate. Label-approved dosages differ with each of these products; directions for proper administration must be carefully read and followed before their use.

Management Considerations Related to Long-Term Feeding of MGA to Heifers

Long-term feeding of MGA to beef heifers and associated effects on fertility may be a concern in specific production systems. It is not uncommon for heifers to be placed on MGA for extended periods of time, and subsequently exposed for breeding after placement in backgrounding programs that necessitate long-term MGA administration. There have been no reports[26] of any negative effects of either long-term or repeated intervals of feeding MGA to beef heifers, other than the expected reduced conception rate when cattle were bred at the synchronized estrus 3 to 7 days after the last day of MGA feeding. A study was designed (**Fig. 3**)[27] to compare estrous response and fertility during synchronized estrous periods among beef heifers that were fed MGA for 87 days (long-term, LT) or 14 days (short-term, ST) before PG. Heifers were stratified by age and weight to LT-MGA or ST-MGA treatments

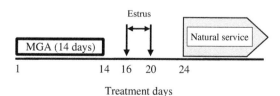

Fig. 1. Melengestrol acetate (MGA) and natural service. (*Adapted from* Patterson DJ, Wood SL, Kojima FN, et al. Current and emerging methods to synchronize estrus with melengestrol acetate. In: 49th Annual Beef Cattle Short Course Proceedings "Biotechnologies of Reproductive Biology". Gainesville (FL): University of Florida; 2000. p. 66; with permission.)

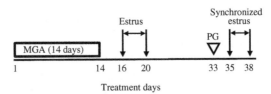

Fig. 2. The MGA–prostaglandin $F_2\alpha$ (PG) protocol. (*Data from* Refs.[23–25].)

(**Table 1**), and received 0.5 mg MGA per head per day for 87 or 14 days, respectively. Heifers in each group were administered PG 17 days after MGA withdrawal. Heifers in both groups that failed to exhibit estrus within 6 days after the first injection of PG were administered a second injection of PG 11 days later (see **Fig. 3**).

Transrectal ultrasonography was used to examine ovaries of all heifers at the end of treatment with MGA and at the time PG was administered. Heifers that failed to exhibit estrus after the first injection of PG were reexamined before the second PG injection. All heifers were exposed for natural service for an additional 45 days after the AI period. More ST-treated heifers exhibited estrus after the first injection of PG than LT-treated heifers (**Table 2**; $P<.05$). Total response after the 2 injections of PG, however, did not differ between treatments. Furthermore, there were no significant differences between treatments in synchronized conception or pregnancy rates, or pregnancy rates at the end of the breeding period (see **Table 2**). A higher incidence of luteinized follicular cysts (**Table 3**) was observed among heifers in the LT-treatment group compared with heifers in under ST treatment (LT, 11/30 [37%]; ST, 0/31 [0%]). This observation may explain differences in estrous response between treatments following the first injection of PG. These data indicate that long-term feeding of MGA may result in a higher than normal incidence of luteinized follicular cysts and an associated reduction in estrous response after PG. The data indicate, however, that reinjection with PG resulted in satisfactory breeding performance among heifers that were fed MGA for extended periods of time.

Method 3: MGA Select

Studies with heifers showed that both synchrony of estrus and total estrous response were improved when PG is administered 19 days after MGA withdrawal in comparison with those of heifers injected on day 17 after MGA withdrawal.[24,25] A modified

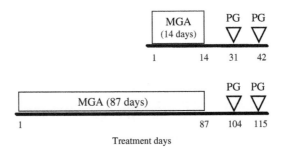

Treatment days

Fig. 3. Comparison of short-term and long-term MGA treatments. (*From* Patterson DJ, Kearnan JM, Bradley NW, et al. Estrus response and fertility in yearling beef heifers after chronic treatment with an oral progestogen followed by prostaglandin F2α. University of Kentucky Beef Cattle Research Report. Progress Report 353. 1993. p. 32; with permission.)

Table 1
Ages and weights of heifers at the time PG was administered

Treatment	No. of Heifers	Age (d)	Weight (kg)
Short-term, 14 d	31	427	392
Long-term, 87 d	30	423	386

Data from Patterson DJ, Kojima FN, Smith MF. A review of methods to synchronize estrus in replacement heifers and postpartum beef cows. J Anim Sci 2003;81(E Suppl 2):E166–77.

MGA-PG protocol for inducing and synchronizing a fertile estrus in beef heifers was evaluated (**Fig. 4**).[28] The first modification changed the day of PG injection from day 31 to day 33 of treatment. The second modification was the addition of GnRH on day 26 of treatment. The addition of GnRH on day 26 of the MGA-PG protocol induced luteal tissue formation and initiated a new follicular wave on approximately day 28 in estrous-cycling beef heifers (**Fig. 5B**). The proportion of heifers with synchronized follicular waves on day 33 was increased significantly in comparison with heifers that did not receive GnRH (see **Fig. 5**).[28]

Differences in estrous response and synchrony of estrus during the synchronized period among heifers assigned to the treatments illustrated in **Fig. 6** were reported.[29] This difference in estrous response and degree of synchrony was based on the percentage of heifers that were pubertal at the time treatment with MGA began. **Fig. 6** illustrates these differences.[29] **Fig. 6A** shows the distribution of estrus whereby only 30% of the heifers were pubertal at the time treatment with MGA began, whereas **Fig. 6B** illustrates the distribution of estrus for heifers whereby 56% of the heifers were pubertal at the same time. The increased degree of estrous cyclicity of heifers shown in **Fig. 6B** was associated with a reduced variance in the interval to estrus among MGA-GnRH-PG–treated heifers, which means that more heifers exhibited estrus over a shorter period of time. Pregnancy rates resulting from AI remained high for both MGA-GnRH-PG and MGA-PG treated heifers and were not different

Table 2
Estrous response and fertility of heifers treated long-term or short-term with MGA

Response Variable	Short-Term MGA, 14 d			Long-Term MGA, 87 d		
	First PG[a]	Second PG[a]	Total	First PG[a]	Second PG[a]	Total
Estrous response	24/31 (77%)[b]	4/7 (57%)	28/31 (90%)	16/30 (53%)[c]	10/14 (71%)	26/30 (87%)
Synchronized conception	15/24 (63%)	3/4 (75%)	18/28 (64%)	12/16 (75%)	6/10 (60%)	18/26 (69%)
Synchronized pregnancy	—		18/31 (58%)	—		18/30 (60%)
Final pregnancy	—		28/31 (90%)	—		27/30 (90%)

[a] First PG refers to animals that responded to PG administered 17 days after MGA withdrawal. Second PG refers to animals that failed to respond to the first injection of PG that were reinjected 11 days later.
[b,c] Percentages within row and between treatments with unlike superscripts differ (P<.05).
Data from Patterson DJ, Kojima FN, Smith MF. A review of methods to synchronize estrus in replacement heifers and postpartum beef cows. J Anim Sci 2003;81(E Suppl 2):E166–77.

Table 3
Ovarian morphology of heifers treated long-term or short-term with MGA

Treatment	Normal	Abnormal[a]
Short-term	31/31 (100%)	0/31 (0%)
Long-term	19/30 (63%)	11/30 (37%)

[a] Abnormal = presence of luteinized follicular cysts, 20–45 mm diameter.
Data from Patterson DJ, Kojima FN, Smith MF. A review of methods to synchronize estrus in replacement heifers and postpartum beef cows. J Anim Sci 2003;81(E Suppl 2):E166–77.

from one another (67% and 60%, respectively [see **Fig. 6**A] and 75% and 72%, respectively [see **Fig. 6**B]).

Additional Considerations

An additional consideration for Methods 2 and 3 (MGA-PG and MGA Select) pertains to heifers that fail to exhibit estrus after the last PG injection. In this case, nonresponders may be reinjected with PG 11 to 14 days after the last injection of PG was administered. These females would then be observed for signs of behavioral estrus for an additional 6 to 7 days. This procedure would maximize efforts to inseminate as many females as possible within the first 2 weeks of the breeding period. Females that were inseminated during the first synchronized period should not be reinjected with PG. The decision to use Method 3 in heifers should be based on careful consideration of the heifer's age, weight, and pubertal status.[29–33] In addition, FTAI may be used with Method 2. In this case, all heifers would be inseminated beginning 72 hours after the administration of PG, and GnRH would be administered to all heifers at the time AI was performed.

DEVELOPMENT OF THE 7-DAY CIDR-PG PROTOCOL FOR HEIFERS

The initial studies[15] conducted in the United States involving CIDR (1.38 g progesterone)-based protocols for use in synchronizing estrus in beef heifers are summarized in **Table 4**. These data were submitted to the Food and Drug Administration in support of the original approval for the CIDR in beef heifers and cows. Three

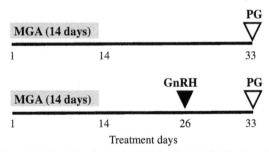

Fig. 4. A modified long-term MGA protocol. Heifers were fed MGA for 14 days; 19 days after MGA withdrawal, PG was administered to all heifers. Gonadotropin-releasing hormone (GnRH) was administered to one-half of the heifers 7 days before PG. (*Adapted from* Wood SL, Lucy MC, Smith MF, et al. Improved synchrony of estrus and ovulation with addition of GnRH to a melengestrol acetate-prostaglandin F2α estrus synchronization treatment in beef heifers. J Anim Sci 2001;79:2211; with permission.)

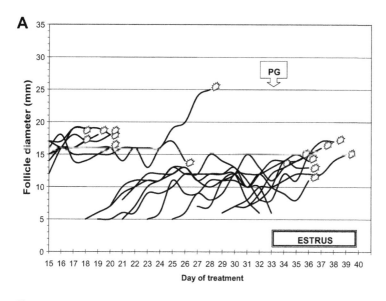

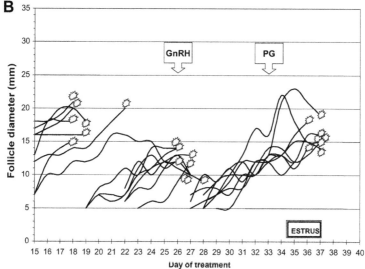

Fig. 5. (A, B) Patterns of dominant follicle development in control (MGA-PG; A) and GnRH-treated (MGA-GnRH-PG; B) heifers. Administration of GnRH (B) caused the synchronized development of a dominant follicle before PG injection. Follicular development in MGA-PG–treated heifers was poorly synchronized. (Adapted from Wood SL, Lucy MC, Smith MF, et al. Improved synchrony of estrus and ovulation with addition of GnRH to a melengestrol acetate-prostaglandin F2α estrus synchronization treatment in beef heifers. J Anim Sci 2001;79:2213; with permission.)

treatments were involved in the study: (1) an untreated control; (2) PG only; and (3) 7-day CIDR-PG. The 7-day CIDR-PG–treated heifers had CIDRs inserted for 7 days with PG administered on day 6 of CIDR treatment. The 7-day CIDR-PG protocol yielded greater pregnancy rates compared with control or PG-treated heifers.

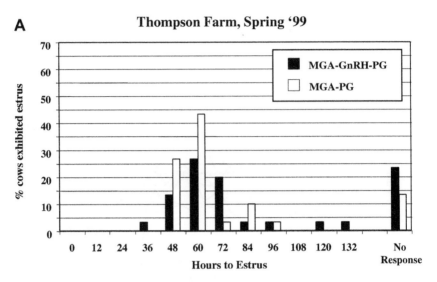

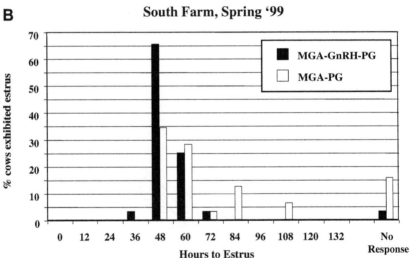

Fig. 6. (*A, B*) Percentage of heifers observed in estrus for MGA-PG and MGA-GnRH-PG–treated heifers. Estrous cyclicity rates were 30% and 56% for heifers at locations 1 (*A*) and 2 (*B*), respectively, at the time treatment with MGA began. (*Adapted from* Wood-Follis SL, Kojima FN, Lucy MC, et al. Estrus synchronization in beef heifers with progestin-based protocols. I. Differences in response based on pubertal status at the initiation of treatment. Theriogenology 2004;62:1523; with permission.)

Treatment with CIDR increased synchronization rates within the first 3 days following PG, resulting in enhanced pregnancy rates. The improved pregnancy rate in prepubertal beef heifers treated with the CIDR was noteworthy because prepubertal heifers in the control or PG treatments never attained pregnancy rates that were similar to those of the 7-day CIDR-PG–treated heifers. The drawback of the protocol was that PG was administered on day 6 after CIDR insertion, which required an additional day of handling the heifers.

Table 4
Synchronization, conception, and pregnancy rate for beef heifers

Item	Synchronization Rate No.	%	Conception Rate No.	%	Pregnancy Rate No.	%
Prepubertal						
Control	8/107	7	6/8	75	6/7	6
PG	11/101	11	6/11	50	6/101	6
CIDR PG	50/105	48	29/50	58	29/105	28
Cyclic						
Control	25/44	17	13/25	52	13/144	9
PG	56/151	37	29/56	52	29/151	19
CIDR-PG	93/116	80	57/93	61	57/116	49
Total						
Control	33/151	22	19/33	58	19/151	13
PG	67/252	27	35/67	52	35/252	14
CIDR-PG	143/221	65	86/143	60	86/221	39

Data from Lucy MC, Billings HJ, Butler WR, et al. Efficacy of an intravaginal progesterone insert and an injection of PG F2$_\alpha$ for synchronizing estrus and shortening the interval to pregnancy in postpartum beef cows, peripubertal beef heifers, and dairy heifers. J Anim Sci 2001;79:982–95.

Dejarnette (Mel DeJarnette, personal communication) compared timing of estrus, estrous response, and pregnancy rate resulting from AI during the synchronized period among heifers that were assigned to a 7-day CIDR treatment and received PG on day 6 or 7 of the treatment schedule. Although heifers that received PG on day 6 (1 day before CIDR removal) exhibited estrus earlier than heifers that received PG on day 7 (at CIDR removal), there were no differences between groups for the response variables considered. Therefore, to simplify treatment administration, PG is in most cases now administered coincident with the time of CIDR removal.

THE MULTISTATE CIDR TRIAL

A multistate trial[34] involving heifers at 12 locations in 6 states was conducted to determine whether: (1) administration of an estrous synchronization protocol followed by FTAI could yield pregnancy rates similar to those of a protocol requiring detection of estrus; and (2) whether an injection of GnRH at CIDR insertion enhanced pregnancy rates in beef heifers. Four treatments were involved in the study (**Fig. 7**). Heifers in treatment 1 were observed for signs of behavioral estrus and inseminated based on observed estrus through 72 hours after PG. Eighty-four hours following the administration of PG, all heifers that failed to exhibit estrus to that point were inseminated by appointment, with GnRH administered at AI. Heifers in treatment 2 were handled the same way as heifers in treatment 1; however, all heifers in treatment 2 received an injection of GnRH at CIDR insertion. Heifers in treatments 3 and 4 received the same treatment schedules as heifers in treatments 1 and 2, respectively; however, heifers in treatments 3 and 4 both were inseminated by appointment 60 hours after PG with GnRH administered at AI. Although no differences in pregnancy rates were detected among treatments, heifers that were inseminated in the estrous-detection treatments had numerically higher pregnancy rates than heifers in the FTAI treatment group (**Table 5**).

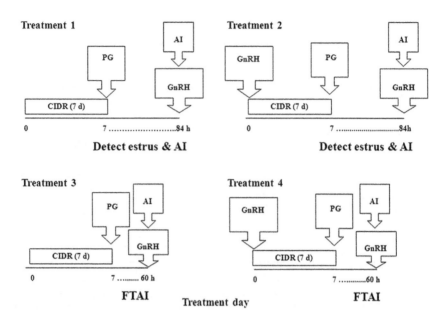

Fig. 7. Treatment schedules for heifers in the multistate controlled internal drug release (CIDR) trial. (*Data from* Lamb GC, Larson JE, Geary TW, et al. Synchronization of estrus and artificial insemination in replacement beef heifers using gonadotropin-releasing hormone, prostaglandin F, and progesterone. J Anim Sci 2006;84:3002.)

HOW DO MGA-BASED AND CIDR-BASED PROTOCOLS COMPARE?
Substituting EAZI-BREED CIDR Inserts for MGA in the MGA Select Protocol in Beef Heifers

In recent years, there have been reports that pregnancy rates resulting from MGA-based estrous synchronization protocols have declined in yearling-age beef heifers.[35] These instances of reduced fertility are generally associated with heifers, in which estrous cyclicity rates are high, and heifers generally weigh more and are in higher body condition before treatment with MGA than are lighter-weight, lower-conditioned heifers.

A study was designed[36] to compare long-term progestin-based estrous synchronization protocols in beef heifers. Presynchronization with MGA (MGA Select) or CIDR (CIDR Select: 14-day treatment with MGA or CIDR, followed 12 or 9 days later, respectively, with an injection of GnRH, and PG 7 days after GnRH) was compared on the

Table 5								
Pregnancy rates following AI among beef heifers in the multistate CIDR trial								
	Treatments[a]							
	1		2		3		4	
Item	No.	%	No.	%	No.	%	No.	%
Prepubertal	19/36	53	32/54	59	22/36	61	28/44	64
Cycling	195/341	57	201/317	63	189/353	54	185/346	54

[a] Refer to **Fig. 7** for a description of the 4 treatment protocols.

Data from Lamb GC, Larson JE, Geary TW, et al. Synchronization of estrus and artificial insemination in replacement beef heifers using gonadotropin-releasing hormone, prostaglandin F, and progesterone. J Anim Sci 2006;84:3000–9.

basis of estrous response, timing of AI, and pregnancy rate in beef heifers. No differences in estrous response were detected between MGA Select and CIDR Select heifers; however, CIDR Select–treated heifers showed an improvement in synchrony of estrus, conception, and pregnancy rates during the synchronized period. These improvements associated with the CIDR Select treatment were attributed to a reduced interval to estrus[37] and improved synchronization of follicular waves after CIDR removal rather than at the end of MGA feeding.

A widely held hypothesis is that GnRH is less effective at synchronizing follicular waves in heifers than are cows; a hypothesis supported in part by the multistate CIDR trial,[34] wherein no difference in synchrony of estrus or pregnancy rate between heifers treated by CIDR + PG and Select Synch + CIDR was observed, suggesting that response to GnRH in heifers at CIDR insertion may be of limited value. More recently, studies were designed (**Table 6**)[38] to evaluate the follicular response to GnRH among pubertal beef heifers on specific days of the estrous cycle. Response was based on ovulation or luteinization of a dominant follicle and subsequent initiation of a new follicular wave in response to GnRH. These data (see **Table 6**) support the concept that presynchronization before initiation of the GnRH + PG protocol may be of greater importance in heifers, and therefore significant in relation to success initially reported with the CIDR Select protocol.[36]

The CIDR Select protocol was used successfully in conjunction with either heat detection and AI[39] or FTAI when AI was performed 72 hours after PG and GnRH was administered at the time of AI (**Fig. 8**).[39,40] On-farm field trials are summarized in **Table 7**, reporting results after use of the CIDR Select protocol in conjunction with breeding programs requiring heat detection or FTAI. It is interesting that pregnancy rates following administration of the CIDR Select protocol were comparable, whether heifers were inseminated on the basis of observed estrus (see **Table 7**) or at predetermined fixed times (see **Table 7**).

A subsequent study[41] compared CIDR-PG and MGA-PG protocols in beef heifers. The study compared: (1) estrous synchronization response following progestin removal, and PG administered 17 or 19 days after progestin withdrawal; and (2) AI pregnancy rates during the synchronized period. More CIDR-treated heifers than MGA-treated heifers exhibited estrus within 120 hours after progestin removal. Intervals to estrus after progestin removal were shorter for CIDR-treated heifers than for MGA-treated heifers, and more CIDR-treated heifers exhibited estrus and were inseminated within 60 hours after PG in comparison with MGA-treated heifers. Pregnancy rates did not differ between MGA-treated (66%) and CIDR-treated heifers (62%).

Table 6
Response to GnRH in estrous-cycling beef heifers based on the day of the estrous cycle GnRH was administered

Day of Treatment	First GnRH (n, % Responding)	Second GnRH (n, % Responding)
Day 2	0/7 = 0%	3/7 = 43%
Day 5	8/8 = 100%	8/8 = 100%
Day 10	0/6 = 0%	5/6 = 83%
Day 15	5/8 = 63%	1/8 = 13%
Day 18	5/8 = 63%	2/8 = 25%

Data from Atkins JA, Busch DC, Bader JF, et al. Gonadotropin-releasing hormone-induced ovulation and luteinizing hormone release in beef heifers: effect of day of the cycle. J Anim Sci 2008;86:83–93.

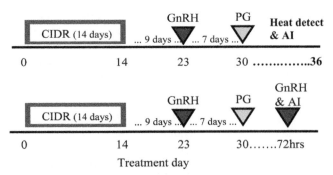

Fig. 8. Estrous synchronization schedules involving use of the CIDR Select protocol in breeding programs for beef heifers that require heat detection or fixed-time AI (FTAI).

Use of CIDR as a progestin source was equally effective as MGA in synchronizing estrus in beef heifers.[41]

More recently, 2 experiments were conducted[42] to evaluate long-term MGA-based and CIDR-based estrous synchronization protocols, based on their potential for use in facilitating FTAI in estrous-cycling and prepubertal beef heifers. Heifers in the first experiment (**Fig. 9**) were fitted with HeatWatch estrous-detection transmitters at the time of progestin removal for continuous estrous detection, and in both experiments the synchronized period was designated as 0 to 144 hours following PG. HeatWatch transmitters were maintained on all heifers until AI was performed. **Fig. 10** illustrates the pattern of estrous distribution following withdrawal of MGA from feed or removal of CIDR for the respective treatments. The variance associated with interval to estrus after progestin withdrawal/removal was significantly reduced among 14-day CIDR-PG–treated in comparison with MGA-PG–treated heifers.

Estrous response after PG was greater for 14-day CIDR-PG (92%) than for MGA-PG (85%) treated heifers (**Table 8**). The distribution of estrus after PG is depicted in **Fig. 11**. The mean interval to estrus after PG did not differ between heifers treated by MGA-PG (57.4 ± 2.5 hours) and 14-day CIDR-PG (56.2 ± 2.5 hours) (**Table 9**). There was, however, a significant difference in the mean interval to estrus after PG between estrous-cycling (62.4 ± 2.4 hours) and prepubertal heifers (52.4 ± 4.4 hours) assigned to the MGA-PG protocol, but no difference between estrous-cycling and prepubertal heifers assigned to 14-day CIDR-PG (55.4 ± 2.4 and 57.0 ± 4.4 hours, respectively).

The variance associated with interval to estrus after PG was reduced among 14-day CIDR-PG–treated than for MGA-PG–treated heifers. Variance for interval to estrus after PG differed between treatments for estrous-cycling and prepubertal heifers; however, the variance for interval to estrus after PG did not differ within treatment for estrous-cycling and prepubertal heifers (see **Table 9**).

Table 7
Pregnancy rates after administration of the CIDR Select protocol in field trials involving AI performed after observed estrus or FTAI performed 72 hours after PG

Breeding Program	No. Pregnant	No. Inseminated	Pregnancy Rate (%)
Estrous detection and AI	499	830	60
Fixed-time AI	518	853	61

Data from Patterson DJ, Schafer DJ, Busch DC, et al. Review of estrus synchronization systems: MGA. In: Proceedings Applied Reproductive Strategies in Beef Cattle. St. Joseph: 2006. p. 63–103.

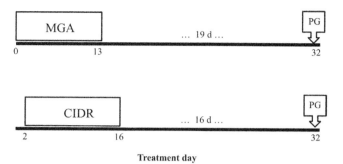

Fig. 9. Treatment schedule for heifers assigned to the MGA-PG and 14-day CIDR-PG treatment protocols. Heifers assigned to MGA-PG received MGA in a 1.0-kg feed supplement for 14 days and were administered PG on day 32. Heifers assigned to 14-day CIDR-PG received a CIDR insert from day 2 of treatment to day 16, and PG on day 32. (*From* Mallory DA, Wilson DJ, Busch DC, et al. Comparison of long-term progestin-based estrus synchronization protocols in beef heifers. J Anim Sci 2010;88:3569; with permission.)

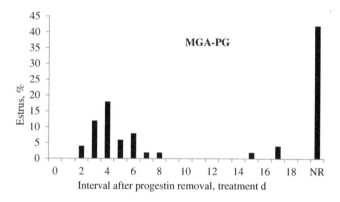

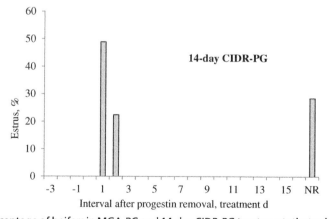

Fig. 10. Percentage of heifers in MGA-PG and 14-day CIDR-PG treatments that exhibited estrus after withdrawal/removal of progestin: MGA-PG (*black bars*) and 14-day CIDR-PG (*gray bars*). NR, no estrous response. Heifers assigned to MGA-PG received MGA in a 1.0-kg feed supplement for 14 days and were administered PG on day 32. Heifers assigned to 14-day CIDR-PG received a CIDR insert from day 2 of treatment to day 16, and PG on day 32. (*Adapted from* Mallory DA, Wilson DJ, Busch DC, et al. Comparison of long-term progestin-based estrus synchronization protocols in beef heifers. J Anim Sci 2010;88:3571; with permission.)

Table 8
Estrous response for estrous-cycling and prepubertal heifers assigned to MGA-PG or 14-day CIDR-PG treatment protocols

Item	MGA-PG	14-d CIDR-PG
Estrous response after PGF$_{2\alpha}$		
Proportion	170/200	180/196
Percent	85[a]	92[b]
Estrous-cycling		
Proportion	135/154	138/151
Percent	88[x]	91
Prepubertal		
Proportion	35/46	42/45
Percent	76[c,y]	93[d]

See **Fig. 11** for a description of the treatment protocols.
  Estrous-cycling = heifers assigned an RTS of 4 or 5; Prepubertal = heifers assigned an RTS of 2 or 3.
  [a,b] Means within rows with different superscripts are different ($P = .01$).
  [c,d] Means within rows with different superscripts are different ($P = .03$).
  [x,y] Means within columns with different superscripts tend to differ ($P = .06$).
  Data from Mallory DA, Wilson DJ, Busch DC, et al. Comparison of long-term progestin-based estrus synchronization protocols in beef heifers. J Anim Sci 2010;88:3568–78.

HOW DO SHORT-TERM AND LONG-TERM CIDR-BASED PROTOCOLS COMPARE IN SYNCHRONIZING OVULATION BEFORE FTAI IN BEEF HEIFERS?

Collectively, these studies were then followed by a report citing improvements in synchrony of estrus and ovulation among CIDR Select–treated heifers in comparison with Select Synch + CIDR–treated contemporaries (**Fig. 12**).[43] There was more variance associated with the interval from PG to estrus and ovulation between prepubertal

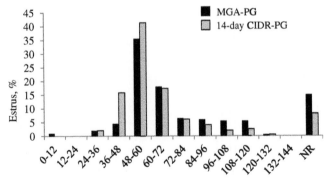

Interval after PG administration, **h**

Fig. 11. Percentage of heifers in MGA-PG and 14-day CIDR-PG treatments that exhibited estrus after PG: MGA-PG (*black bars*) and 14-day CIDR-PG (*gray bars*). NR, no estrous response. Heifers assigned to MGA-PG received MGA in a 1.0-kg feed supplement for 14 days and were administered PG 19 days later. Heifers assigned to 14-day CIDR-PG received a CIDR insert for 14 days and were administered PG 16 days later. (*Adapted from* Mallory DA, Wilson DJ, Busch DC, et al. Comparison of long-term progestin-based estrus synchronization protocols in beef heifers. J Anim Sci 2010;88:3573; with permission.)

Table 9
Mean and variance for interval from PG to estrus for estrous-cycling and prepubertal heifers assigned to MGA-PG or 14-day CIDR-PG treatment protocols

Item	MGA-PG	14-d CIDR-PG
Interval from $PGF_{2\alpha}$ to estrus, hours (least-squares mean ± SE)	57.4 ± 2.5	56.2 ± 2.5
Estrous-cycling	62.4 ± 2.4[a,x]	55.4 ± 2.4[b]
Prepubertal	52.4 ± 4.4[y]	57.0 ± 4.4
Variance for interval to estrus after $PGF_{2\alpha}$	466[c]	282[d]
Estrous-cycling	432[c]	272[d]
Prepubertal	615[e]	316[f]

See **Fig. 9** for a description of the treatment protocols.
[a,b] Means within rows with different superscripts are different ($P = .04$).
[c,d] Variances within rows with different superscripts are different ($P<.01$).
[e,f] Variances within rows with different superscripts are different ($P<.05$).
[x,y] Means within columns with different superscripts are different ($P = .04$).
Data from Mallory DA, Wilson DJ, Busch DC, et al. Comparison of long-term progestin-based estrus synchronization protocols in beef heifers. J Anim Sci 2010;88:3568–78.

and estrous-cycling heifers synchronized with the Select Synch + CIDR protocol compared with CIDR Select.[43] These data[43] suggested that the CIDR Select protocol may facilitate FTAI more effectively than Select Synch + CIDR in mixed groups of prepubertal and estrous-cycling beef heifers.

Pregnancy rates resulting from FTAI were then compared following administration of either one of two CIDR-based protocols (**Fig. 13**).[39] Heifers were assigned to one of two treatments within RTS (1–5, 1 = immature and 5 = cycling) by age and weight. Heifers assigned to CIDR Select received a CIDR insert from days 0 to 14 followed by GnRH 9 days after CIDR removal and PG 7 days after GnRH treatment. Heifers assigned to CO-Synch + CIDR were administered GnRH and received a CIDR insert, and PG and CIDR removal 7 days later (see **Fig. 13**).

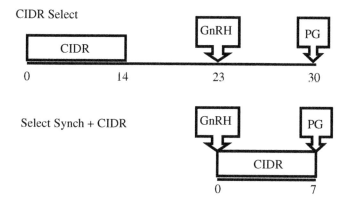

Treatment days

Fig. 12. Comparison of CIDR Select and select Synch + CIDR protocols. (*Adapted from* Leitman NR, Busch DC, Bader JF, et al. Comparison of protocols to synchronize estrus and ovulation in estrous cycling and prepubertal beef heifers. J Anim Sci 2008;86:1810; with permission.)

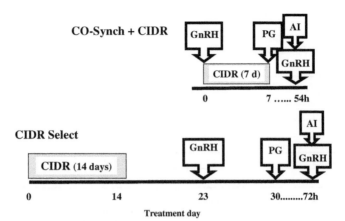

Fig. 13. Treatment schedule for heifers assigned to the CIDR Select and CO-Synch + CIDR protocols. (*Adapted from* Busch DC, Wilson DJ, Schafer DJ, et al. Comparison of CIDR-based estrus synchronization protocols before FTAI on pregnancy rate in beef heifers. J Anim Sci 2007;85:1935; with permission.)

AI was performed at predetermined fixed times for heifers in both treatments at 72 or 54 hours after PG for the CIDR Select and CO-Synch + CIDR groups, respectively. All heifers were administered GnRH at the time of insemination. Pregnancy rates resulting from FTAI (**Table 10**) were significantly greater following the CIDR Select protocol (62%) compared with the CO-Synch + CIDR protocol (47%). In summary, the CIDR Select protocol resulted in a greater and more synchronous estrous response and significantly greater FTAI pregnancy rates compared with the CO-Synch + CIDR protocol.[39]

HOW DO THE CIDR SELECT (CIDR-GNRH-PG) AND 14-DAY CIDR-PG PROTOCOLS COMPARE ON THE BASIS OF ESTROUS RESPONSE, SYNCHRONY OF ESTRUS, AND PREGNANCY RATES RESULTING FROM AI DURING THE SYNCHRONIZED PERIOD?

Recent studies raised questions regarding the utility of GnRH in estrous synchronization protocols for beef heifers.[29,34,44,45] These questions arose from studies wherein the administration of GnRH at the beginning of an estrous synchronization protocol in beef heifers failed to demonstrate an increase in pregnancy rates resulting from FTAI; however, the standard deviation of pregnancy rates was increased when GnRH was not included. These data suggest that incorporation of GnRH into an FTAI protocol may increase the uniformity of pregnancy rates in beef heifers across locations when compared with protocols based on estrous detection alone.[34]

Table 10
Pregnancy rates of heifers in response to FTAI and at the end of the breeding season (means ± SE)

Item	Pregnancy Rate to Fixed-Time AI		Pregnancy Rate at End of Breeding Season	
	Proportion	%	Proportion	%
CIDR Select	67/108	62[a]	97/108	90
CO-Synch + CIDR	51/109	47[b]	99/109	91

[a,b] Means within a column with different superscripts are different, $P<.05$.
Data from Busch DC, Wilson DJ, Schafer DJ, et al. Comparison of CIDR-based estrus synchronization protocols prior to fixed-time AI on pregnancy rate in beef heifers. J Anim Sci 2007;85:1933–9.

A study was designed to compare the CIDR Select and 14-day CIDR-PG protocols to determine the need for adding a GnRH injection to synchronize estrus in beef heifers that were prepubertal or estrous-cycling at the initiation of treatment (**Fig. 14**).[45] Treatments were compared based on estrous response and distribution of estrus after PG, and of synchronized AI conception and pregnancy rates.

Fig. 15 illustrates differences in estrous response after PG between treatments. Heifers assigned to the CIDR-PG protocol had a more highly synchronized estrus compared with heifers assigned to the CIDR Select protocol; moreover, regardless of treatment, the prepubertal heifers had a more highly synchronized estrus compared with the estrous-cycling heifers. Improved synchrony of estrus observed among prepubertal heifers may be a result of a more highly synchronized estrous response following CIDR removal when compared with estrous-cycling heifers. Stage of cycle differences among estrous-cycling heifers at CIDR insertion would perhaps explain the potential for reduced synchrony of estrus following CIDR removal in comparison with the prepubertal heifers. Both the estrous-cycling and prepubertal heifers assigned to the CIDR-PG protocol had a more highly synchronized estrus than their counterparts assigned to the CIDR Select protocol.

It is known from previous studies that there is no difference in estrous response following CIDR removal when comparing estrous-cycling or prepubertal heifers treated with a 14-day CIDR protocol.[43] Presynchronization with a progestin[43] before GnRH and PG was hypothesized to be more effective in synchronizing estrus in comparison with 7-day CIDR-based or GnRH-PG estrous synchronization protocols. This hypothesis was tested and accepted.

The significant improvement in synchrony of estrus for heifers treated by 14-day CIDR-PG in comparison with CIDR Select is difficult to explain. Although response to GnRH in heifers is reported to be inconsistent when compared with cows,[46–48] these data indicate that the addition of GnRH to a 14-day CIDR-PG protocol reduced the synchrony of estrus after PG, despite similarities between treatments in estrous response.

In addition, conception rate to AI (**Table 11**) tended to be greater for heifers assigned to the 14-day CIDR-PG protocol than for CIDR Select heifers, but was not influenced by estrous cyclicity status. Heifers assigned to 14-day CIDR-PG, however, had a higher pregnancy rate to AI compared with heifers assigned to CIDR Select.

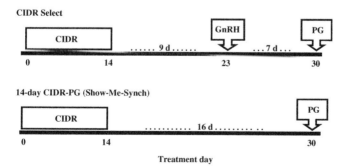

Fig. 14. Treatment schedule for heifers assigned to the CIDR Select and 14-day CIDR-PG protocols. Heifers assigned to CIDR Select received a CIDR insert from days 0 to 14, GnRH on day 23, and PG on day 30. Heifers assigned to 14-day CIDR-PG received a CIDR insert from days 0 to 14, and PG on day 30. (*Adapted from* Leitman NR, Busch DC, Wilson DJ, et al. Comparison of controlled internal drug release insert-based protocols to synchronize estrus in prepubertal and estrous-cycling beef heifers. J Anim Sci 2009;87:3977; with permission.)

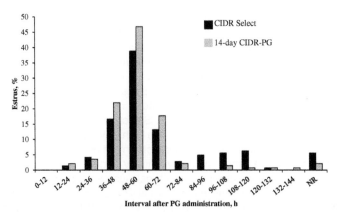

Fig. 15. Percentage of heifers in the CIDR Select and 14-day CIDR-PG treatments that exhibited estrus after PG: CIDR Select (*black bars*) and 14-day CIDR-PG (*gray bars*). NR, no estrous response. See **Fig. 14** for a description of the treatment protocols. (*Adapted from* Leitman NR, Busch DC, Wilson DJ, et al. Comparison of controlled internal drug release insert-based protocols to synchronize estrus in prepubertal and estrous-cycling beef heifers. J Anim Sci 2009;87:3979; with permission.)

Pregnancy rate to AI (see **Table 11**) was not influenced by estrous cyclicity status. These data point to the effectiveness of both protocols in inducing cyclicity in prepubertal or peripubertal heifers, and successfully preparing heifers for breeding and subsequent pregnancy.

Table 11
Estrous response and interval to estrus after PG, and AI conception rates and pregnancy rates for heifers assigned to CIDR Select or 14-day CIDR-PG

Item	CIDR Select	14-d CIDR-PG
Estrous response after PG		
Proportion	136/144	138/141
%	94	98
Interval from PG to estrus, h (least-squares mean ± SE)	61.5 ± 1.7[a]	54.4 ± 1.7[b]
Variance for interval to estrus after PG	508[a]	262[b]
Conception rate to AI		
Proportion	78/135[c]	92/137[d]
%	58	67
Pregnancy rate to AI		
Proportion	78/143[e]	92/140[f]
%	55	66
Pregnancy rate at the end of the breeding season		
Proportion	116/143	113/140
%	81	81

See **Fig. 16** for a description of the treatment protocols.
[a,b] Means and/or variances within rows with different superscripts are different ($P \leq .01$).
[c,d] Means within rows with different superscripts tend to differ ($P = .09$).
[e,f] Means within rows with different superscripts are different ($P = .05$).
Data from Leitman NR, Busch DC, Wilson DJ, et al. Comparison of controlled internal drug release insert-based protocols to synchronize estrus in prepubertal and estrous-cycling beef heifers. J Anim Sci 2009;87:3976–82.

HOW DO THE CIDR SELECT (CIDR-GNRH-PG) AND 14-DAY CIDR-PG PROTOCOLS COMPARE BASED ON PREGNANCY RATES RESULTING FROM FTAI IN HEIFERS?

Pregnancy rates resulting from FTAI were compared in heifers after treatment with the CIDR Select and 14-day CIDR-PG treatment protocols (**Fig. 16**).[49] Pregnancy rates resulting from FTAI tended to differ between treatments, with the advantage to heifers assigned to the 14-day CIDR-PG protocol (**Table 12**). Pretreatment estrous cyclicity status did not affect FTAI pregnancy rate; however, there was a trend toward higher FTAI pregnancy rates among estrous-cycling heifers assigned to the 14-day CIDR-PG protocol compared with those assigned to CIDR Select.

Timing of insemination for heifers assigned to the 14-day CIDR-PG protocol in this study was based on previous reports.[42,44,45] Peak estrous response in those studies occurred 48 to 60 hours after PG, and the peak AI date was 3 days after PG. Mean intervals to estrus after PG for the 3 experiments were 59.3 ± 2.8, 54.4 ± 1.7, and 56.2 ± 2.5 hours, respectively.[42,44,45] Based on the consistency of these results,[49] timing of insemination at 66 hours following the administration of PG was chosen. Timing of insemination after the CIDR Select protocol (72 hours) was based on previous studies.[39,43]

These data clearly indicate that the 14-day CIDR-PG protocol effectively synchronizes estrus before FTAI in beef heifers and provides an alternative to the CIDR Select protocol in facilitating expanded use of AI.[49–51] This study further supported previously published reports[45] indicating that GnRH is not required to synchronize estrus before FTAI among heifers that are presynchronized with a 14-day CIDR treatment. Modification of the CIDR Select protocol to the 14-day CIDR-PG protocol (Show-Me-Synch) allows producers to minimize trips through the chute, and reduces costs associated with estrous synchronization and FTAI.

COMPARING REPRODUCTIVE TRACT SCORES WITH FTAI PREGNANCY RATES

The Show-Me-Select Replacement Heifer Program has resulted in improved reproductive efficiency of beef herds in Missouri, and offers a unique opportunity to track

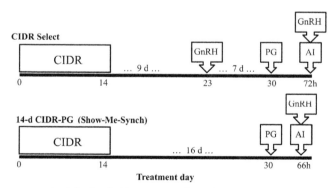

Fig. 16. Treatment schedule for heifers assigned to the CIDR Select and 14-day CIDR-PG (Show-Me-Synch) treatment protocols. Heifers assigned to the CIDR Select protocol received an EAZI-Breed CIDR insert from day 0 to day 14, GnRH on day 23, PG on day 30 followed by FTAI at 72 hours after PG administration. Heifers assigned to 14-day CIDR-PG (Show-Me-Synch) received a CIDR insert from day 0 to 14 and PG on day 30 followed by FTAI 66 hours after PG administration. (*Adapted from* Mallory DA, Nash JM, Ellersieck MR, et al. Comparison of long-term progestin-based protocols to synchronize estrus before fixed-time artificial insemination in beef heifers. J Anim Sci 2011;89:1359; with permission.)

Table 12
Al pregnancy and final pregnancy rates for heifers assigned to CIDR Select or 14-day CIDR-PG (Show-Me-Synch) treatment protocols

Item	CIDR Select	14-d CIDR-PG (Show-Me-Synch)
Pregnancy rate to AI		
Proportion	98/192	124/200
%	51[a]	62[b]
Estrous-cycling	83/158	102/162
%	53[c]	63[d]
Prepubertal	15/34	22/38
%	44	58
Pregnancy rate at the end of the breeding season		
Proportion	164/192	166/200
%	85	83
Estrous-cycling	135/158	134/162
%	85	83
Prepubertal	29/34	32/38
%	85	84

[a,b] Means within rows with different superscripts tended to differ ($P = .07$).
[c,d] Means within rows with different superscripts tended to differ ($P = .06$).
Data from Mallory DA, Nash JM, Ellersieck MR, et al. Comparison of long-term progestin-based protocols to synchronize estrus before fixed-time artificial insemination in beef heifers. J Anim Sci 2011;89:1358–65.

reproductive data on large numbers of heifers throughout the state. The objectives of the program are detailed in the article by Patterson and colleagues elsewhere in this issue. As part of the program, prebreeding examinations (RTS) are performed by licensed veterinarians before the breeding season. In addition, pregnancy diagnoses must be performed within 90 days of the start of breeding and reconfirmed after the end of the breeding season. In recent years, program participants have increased the use of FTAI programs in their herds. Data collected from 2010 to 2012 were used to evaluate relationships between RTS and pregnancy outcome after FTAI. The reproductive tract scoring system ranges from 1 to 5: 1 = infantile; 2 and 3 = non-cycling/prepubertal; 4 and 5 = cycling/pubertal. A summary of RTS and FTAI pregnancy rate for 8308 heifers evaluated from 2010 to 2012 is provided in **Table 13**.

Table 13
Pregnancy rates resulting from FTAI based on reproductive tract score (FTAI; fall 2010 to spring 2012): Missouri Show-Me-Select Replacement Heifer Program[a]

	RTS and Fixed-Time AI Pregnancy Rate				
	1	2	3	4	5
No. of heifers	22	298	2448	2496	3044
FTAI pregnancy rate (%)	5	34	48	52	57

[a] Pregnancy rates resulting from FTAI based on RTS. These data include pregnancy rates for 8308 heifers that were inseminated beginning during the fall of 2010 through spring of 2012.
Data from Thomas JM, Nash JM, Martin NT, et al. The Missouri Show-Me-Select Replacement Heifer Program: tracking reproductive performance of heifers and AI sires. J Anim Sci, in press.

These data support the practice of establishing prebreeding criteria for identification of heifers that are good candidates for an FTAI program.

In addition, these same data were used to compare pregnancy rates of heifers after FTAI that were compared on the basis of RTS and estrous synchronization protocol. These data are summarized in **Table 14**. Although the protocols appear to perform similarly for heifers that are estrous cycling at the time RTS is performed, it appears there is an advantage for heifers assigned to the 14-day CIDR-PG protocol that were prepubertal or peripubertal before treatment administration.

SUMMARY

Expanded use of AI and/or adoption of emerging reproductive technologies for beef heifers and cows require precise methods of estrous-cycle control. Effective control of the estrous cycle requires the synchronization of both luteal and follicular functions. Efforts to develop more effective estrous synchronization protocols have focused on synchronizing follicular waves by injecting GnRH followed 7 days later by injection of PG (Ovsynch, CO-Synch, Select Synch). A factor contributing to reduced synchronized pregnancy rates among heifers treated with the preceding protocols is the extreme variability in response to GnRH based on the day of the cycle GnRH is administered or the heifer's pubertal status, whereas 5% to 15% of cows treated with the preceding protocols exhibit estrus on or before PG injection. New protocols for inducing and synchronizing a fertile estrus in replacement beef heifers and postpartum beef cows in which progestins are used provide new opportunities for beef producers to synchronize estrus and ovulation and to facilitate FTAI. **Table 15** provides a summary of the various estrous synchronization protocols for use in replacement beef heifers, including estrous response for the respective treatments and the synchronized pregnancy rate that resulted. These data suggest that new methods of inducing and synchronizing estrus for replacement beef heifers now create the opportunity to significantly expand the use of AI in the United States cowherd.

RESOURCES FOR VETERINARIANS

The Beef Reproduction Task Force and Beef Reproduction Leadership Team provide an annual updated list of recommended protocols to synchronize estrus in replacement beef heifers and postpartum beef cows. A list of recommended protocols may be accessed at: http://beefrepro.unl.edu/resources.html.

Table 14
Pregnancy rates resulting from FTAI based on RTS and estrous synchronization protocol (FTAI; fall 2010 to spring 2012): Missouri Show-Me-Select Replacement Heifer Program[a]

Protocol	RTS and Fixed-Time AI Pregnancy Rate (%)				
	1	2	3	4	5
7-d CO-Synch + CIDR	0	33	42	50	53
MGA-PG	0	22	36	41	57
14-d CIDR-PG	6	34	50	53	57

7-day CO-Synch + CIDR: n = 398; MGA-PG: n = 717; 14-day CIDR-PG: n = 7193.
[a] Pregnancy rates resulting from FTAI based on RTS. These data include pregnancy rates for 8308 heifers that were inseminated beginning during the fall of 2010 through spring of 2012.
Data from Thomas JM, Nash JM, Martin NT, et al. The Missouri Show-Me-Select Replacement Heifer Program: tracking reproductive performance of heifers and AI sires. J Anim Sci, in press.

Table 15
Comparison of estrous response and fertility in beef heifers after treatment with various estrous synchronization protocols

Treatment	Estrous Response		Synchronized Pregnancy Rate	
AI based on detected estrus				
MGA-PG 14–19 d	1129/1302	87%	768/1302	59%
MGA Select	433/499	87%	280/499	56%
CIDR-PG (d6)	200/285	70%	112/830	39%
CIDR Select	896/974	92%	577/974	59%
14-d CIDR-PG	394/422	93%	241/422	57%
Heat detection and FTAI				
CIDR-PG (d7): 84 h			282/517	55%
Select Synch + CIDR: 84 h			289/504	57%
14 d CIDR + PG: 72 h			48/77	62%
14 d MGA + PG: 72 h			52/79	66%
AI performed at predetermined fixed times with no estrous detection				
7-d CIDR-PG	FTAI @ 60 h		258/525	49%
CO-Synch + CIDR	FTAI @ 60 h		282/531	53%
CO Synch + CIDR	FTAI @ 54 h		51/109	47%
CIDR Select	FTAI @ 72 h		616/1051	58%
14-d CIDR-PG (Show-Me-Synch)	FTAI @ 66 h		1729/2656	65%

In addition, a complete curriculum pertaining to estrous synchronization and AI is available through the University of Missouri Division of Animal Sciences Web site at: http://animalsciences.missouri.edu/extension/beef/estrous_synch/.

The curriculum includes 3 separate courses with the following topics:

Course 1:
- Physiologic principles that underlie estrous synchronization
- An overview of commercially available estrous synchronization products

Course 2:
- Specific estrous synchronization protocols currently recommended for beef heifers and cows

Course 3:
- Management considerations for implementing an estrous synchronization program
- A description of the impact of estrous synchronization on reproductive management

Finally, veterinarians and beef producers may obtain support in scheduling protocols to synchronize estrus in heifers through the Iowa State University Beef Center at: http://www.iowabeefcenter.org/estrus_synch.html.

ACKNOWLEDGMENTS

Research summarized in this manuscript was supported by National Research Initiative Competitive Grant no. 00-35203-9175 and 2005-55203-15750 from the

USDA National Institute of Food and Agriculture. The authors gratefully acknowledge Pfizer Animal Health (New York, NY) for providing Lutalyse and EAZI BREED CIDR Cattle inserts; Merial (Athens, GA) for providing Cystorelin; TEVA Animal Health for providing OvaCyst; ABS Global, Accelerated Genetics, Genex Cooperative, Inc., and Select Sires, Inc., for providing semen; and Circle A Ranch at Lineville, IA, SL Lock at Genex Cooperative, Inc., and DS McAtee and JJD Schreffler at the University of Missouri Thompson Farm for their dedicated support of this research.

REFERENCES

1. Seidel GE Jr. Reproductive biotechnologies for profitable beef production. Sheridan (WY): Proc Beef Improvement Federation; 1995. p. 28–39.
2. Patterson DJ, Kojima FN, Smith MF. A review of methods to synchronize estrus in replacement heifers and postpartum beef cows. J Anim Sci 2003;81(E Suppl 2): E166–77 Online. Available at: http://www.asas.org/symposia/03esupp2/jas2402.pdf. Accessed June 19, 2003.
3. Patterson DJ, Wood SL, Randle RF. Procedures that support reproductive management of replacement beef heifers. Proc Am Soc Anim Sci 2000. 1999. Available at: http://www.asas.org/jas/symposia/proceedings/0902.pdf. Accessed August 3, 2000.
4. Dziuk PJ, Bellows RA. Management of reproduction in beef cattle, sheep and pigs. J Anim Sci 1983;57(Suppl 2):355.
5. Schafer DW, Brinks JS, LeFever DG. Increased calf weaning weight and weight via estrus synchronization. Beef Program Report. Fort Collins (CO): Colorado State University; 1990. p. 115–24.
6. Gonzalez-Padilla E, Ruiz R, LeFever D, et al. Puberty in beef heifers. III. Induction of fertile estrus. J Anim Sci 1975;40:1110–8.
7. Berardinelli JG, Dailey RA, Butcher RL, et al. Source of progesterone prior to puberty in beef heifers. J Anim Sci 1979;49:1276–81.
8. Prybil MK, Butler WR. The relationship between progesterone secretion and the initiation of ovulation in postpartum beef cows. J Anim Sci 1978;47(Suppl 1): 383.
9. Rawlings NC, Weir L, Todd B, et al. Some endocrine changes associated with the postpartum period of the suckling beef cow. J Reprod Fertil 1980;60: 301–8.
10. Henricks DM, Hill JR, Dickey JF. Plasma ovarian hormone levels and fertility in beef heifers treated with melengestrol acetate (MGA). J Anim Sci 1973;37: 1169–75.
11. Wetteman RP, Hafs HD. Pituitary and gonadal hormones associated with fertile and nonfertile inseminations at synchronized and control estrus. J Anim Sci 1973;36:716–21.
12. Sheffel CE, Pratt BR, Ferrell WL, et al. Induced corpora lutea in the postpartum beef cow. II. Effects of treatment with progestogen and gonadotropins. J Anim Sci 1982;54:830–6.
13. Garcia-Winder M, Lewis PE, Deaver DR, et al. Endocrine profiles associated with the life span of induced corpora lutea in postpartum beef cows. J Anim Sci 1986;62:1353–62.
14. Patterson DJ, Corah LR, Brethour JR. Response of prepubertal *Bos taurus* and *Bos indicus* × *Bos taurus* heifers to melengestrol acetate with or without gonadotropin-releasing hormone. Theriogenology 1990;33:661–9.

15. Lucy MC, Billings HJ, Butler WR, et al. Efficacy of an intravaginal progesterone insert and an injection of PG F2α for synchronizing estrus and shortening the interval to pregnancy in postpartum beef cows, peripubertal beef heifers, and dairy heifers. J Anim Sci 2001;79:982–95.

16. Smith RK, Day ML. Mechanism of induction of puberty in beef heifers with melengestrol acetate. In: Ohio Beef Cattle Res Ind Rep. Columbus (OH): 1990. p. 137–42.

17. Imwalle DB, Patterson DJ, Schillo KK. Effects of melengestrol acetate on onset of puberty, follicular growth, and patterns of luteinizing hormone secretion in beef heifers. Biol Reprod 1998;58:1432–6.

18. Hall JB, Staigmiller RB, Short RE, et al. Effect of age and pattern of gain on induction of puberty with a progestin in beef heifers. J Anim Sci 1997;75:1606–11.

19. Anderson LH, McDowell CM, Day ML. Progestin-induced puberty and secretion of luteinizing hormone in heifers. Biol Reprod 1996;54:1025–31.

20. Burfening PJ. Induction of puberty and subsequent reproductive performance. Theriogenology 1979;12:215–21.

21. Imwalle DB, Fernandez DL, Schillo KK. Melengestrol acetate blocks the preovulatory surge of luteinizing hormone, the expression of behavioral estrus and ovulation in beef heifers. J Anim Sci 2002;80:1280–4.

22. Patterson DJ, Wood SL, Kojima FN, et al. Current and emerging methods to synchronize estrus with melengestrol acetate. In: 49th Annual Beef Cattle Short Course Proceedings "Biotechnologies of Reproductive Biology". Gainesville (FL): Univesity of Florida; 2000. p. 45–66.

23. Brown LN, Odde KG, LeFever DG, et al. Comparison of MGA-PGF2α to Syncro-Mate B for estrous synchronization in beef heifers. Theriogenology 1988;30:1.

24. Deutscher GH. Extending interval from seventeen to nineteen days in the melengestrol acetate-prostaglandin estrous synchronization program for heifers. Prof Anim Sci 2000;16:164–8.

25. Lamb GC, Nix DW, Stevenson JS, et al. Prolonging the MGA-prostaglandin F2α interval from 17 to 19 days in an estrus synchronization system for heifers. Theriogenology 2000;53:691–8.

26. Zimbelman RG, Lauderdale JW, Sokolowski JH, et al. Safety and pharmacologic evaluations of melengestrol acetate in cattle and other animals. A review. J Am Vet Med Assoc 1970;157:1528–36.

27. Patterson DJ, Kearnan JM, Bradley NW, et al. Estrus response and fertility in yearling beef heifers after chronic treatment with an oral progestogen followed by prostaglandin F2α. University of Kentucky Beef Cattle Research Report. Progress Report 353. 1993. p. 31–3.

28. Wood SL, Lucy MC, Smith MF, et al. Improved synchrony of estrus and ovulation with addition of GnRH to a melengestrol acetate-prostaglandin F2α estrus synchronization treatment in beef heifers. J Anim Sci 2001;79:2210–6.

29. Wood-Follis SL, Kojima FN, Lucy MC, et al. Estrus synchronization in beef heifers with progestin-based protocols. I. Differences in response based on pubertal status at the initiation of treatment. Theriogenology 2004;62:1518–28.

30. Zimbelman RG. Maintenance of pregnancy in heifers with oral progestogens. J Anim Sci 1963;22:868.

31. Zimbelman RG, Smith LW. Control of ovulation in cattle with melengestrol acetate. I. Effect of dosage and route of administration. J Reprod Fertil 1966;11(2):185–91.

32. Patterson DJ, Kiracofe GH, Stevenson JS, et al. Control of the bovine estrous cycle with melengestrol acetate (MGA): a review. J Anim Sci 1989;67:1895–906.

33. Federal Register. New animal drugs for use in animal feeds. Melengestrol Acetate 1997;62(58):14304–5.

34. Lamb GC, Larson JE, Geary TW, et al. Synchronization of estrus and artificial insemination in replacement beef heifers using gonadotropin-releasing hormone, prostaglandin F, and progesterone. J Anim Sci 2006;84:3000–9.

35. Utter SD, Corah LR. Influence of dietary energy levels on reproductive function and fertility in yearling beef heifers. Kansas State University Cattlemen's Day Proceedings. Manhattan (KS): Kansas State University; 1994. p. 104–6.

36. Kojima FN, Bader JF, Stegner JE, et al. Substituting EAZI-BREED CIDR inserts (CIDR) for melengestrol acetate (MGA) in the MGA Select protocol in beef heifers. J Anim Sci 2004;82(Suppl 1):255.

37. Macmillan KL, Peterson AJ. A new intravaginal progesterone releasing device for cattle (CIDR-B) for oestrous synchronization, increasing pregnancy rates and the treatment of post-partum anoestrus. Anim Reprod Sci 1993;33:1–25.

38. Atkins JA, Busch DC, Bader JF, et al. Gonadotropin-releasing hormone-induced ovulation and luteinizing hormone release in beef heifers: effect of day of the cycle. J Anim Sci 2008;86:83–93.

39. Busch DC, Wilson DJ, Schafer DJ, et al. Comparison of CIDR-based estrus synchronization protocols prior to fixed-time AI on pregnancy rate in beef heifers. J Anim Sci 2007;85:1933–9.

40. Patterson DJ, Schafer DJ, Busch DC, et al. Review of estrus synchronization systems: MGA. In: Proceedings Applied Reproductive Strategies in Beef Cattle. Missouri: St. Joseph; 2006. p. 63–103.

41. Tauck SA, Wilkinson JR, Olsen JR, et al. Comparison of controlled internal drug release device and melengestrol acetate as progestin sources in an estrous synchronization protocol for beef heifers. Theriogenology 2007;68:162–7.

42. Mallory DA, Wilson DJ, Busch DC, et al. Comparison of long-term progestin-based estrus synchronization protocols in beef heifers. J Anim Sci 2010;88: 3568–78.

43. Leitman NR, Busch DC, Bader JF, et al. Comparison of protocols to synchronize estrus and ovulation in estrous cycling and prepubertal beef heifers. J Anim Sci 2008;86:1808–18.

44. Leitman NR, Busch DC, Mallory DA, et al. Comparison of long-term CIDR-based protocols to synchronize estrus in beef heifers. Anim Reprod Sci 2009;114: 345–55.

45. Leitman NR, Busch DC, Wilson DJ, et al. Comparison of controlled internal drug release insert-based protocols to synchronize estrus in prepubertal and estrous-cycling beef heifers. J Anim Sci 2009;87:3976–82.

46. Macmillian KL, Thatcher WW. Effects of an agonist on gonadotropin-releasing hormone on ovarian follicles in cattle. Biol Reprod 1991;45:883–9.

47. Pursley JR, Mee MO, Wiltbank MC. Synchronization of ovulation in dairy cows using PGF2α and GnRH. Theriogenology 1995;44:915–24.

48. Moreira F, de la Sota RL, Diaz T, et al. Effect of day of the estrous cycle at the initiation of a timed artificial insemination protocol on reproductive responses in dairy heifers. J Anim Sci 2000;78:1568–76.

49. Mallory DA, Nash JM, Ellersieck MR, et al. Comparison of long-term progestin-based protocols to synchronize estrus before fixed-time artificial insemination in beef heifers. J Anim Sci 2011;89:1358–65.

50. Mallory DA, Lock SL, Woods DC, et al. Efficacy of using gender selected semen in fixed-time AI protocols in dairy heifers. J Anim Sci, in press.

51. Thomas JM, Nash JM, Martin NT, et al. The Missouri Show-Me-Select Replacement Heifer Program: tracking reproductive performance of heifers and AI sires. J Anim Sci, in press.

Application of Sex-selected Semen in Heifer Development and Breeding Programs

George E. Seidel Jr, PhD

KEYWORDS

- Sexed semen • Heifers • Economics • Fertility

KEY POINTS

- Measuring DNA content of individual sperm with a flow cytometer/cell sorter is the only feasible method for sexing mammalian sperm.
- With excellent management, skilled inseminators, and appropriate handling of semen, fertility of sexed semen is 70% to 90% of fertility of unsexed control semen in the same herds.
- The accuracy of sexing sperm routinely is set at about 90% of the desired sex, sorting at higher accuracy is more costly.
- It is unlikely that a different method for practical application for sexing sperm will be found in the next 3 to 5 years, but incremental improvements of sexing procedures are constantly being developed.

BRIEF HISTORY OF SEXED SEMEN

Being able to choose the sex of offspring of people has been a goal for millennia; for example, Democritus in Greece mentioned this issue and made recommendations nearly 2500 years ago. This also has been a goal of cattle producers for centuries. However, only recently have scientific principles been applied to the problem; dozens of methods of sexing sperm have been attempted over the past 60 years. These include centrifugation, electrophoresis, manipulating pH, separation by the swimming speed of sperm, using antibodies, etc. Unfortunately, all of these methods have failed to date, either because they are not effective, severely damage sperm, or otherwise are problematic, despite hundreds of studies and hundreds of mostly useless patents.

Disclosures: The author has nothing to disclose.
Animal Reproduction and Biotechnology Laboratory, Colorado State University, 3107 Rampart Road, Fort Collins, CO 80523-1683, USA
E-mail address: gseidel@colostate.edu

However, there is one efficacious method, which despite limitations and imperfections, is about 90% accurate and is available commercially for cattle.[1] This method, measuring DNA content of individual sperm by a process termed flow cytometry and then sorting the sperm based on DNA content, was pioneered by about a dozen scientists and first convincingly demonstrated to alter the sex ratio of offspring by a team headed by Lawrence Johnson at a US Department of Agriculture laboratory in Beltsville, Maryland. Currently, this is the only method available that is efficacious in any practical sense, and it is unlikely to be replaced commercially by any other method in the next several years, and maybe not for decades.

HOW ARE SPERM SEXED?

Bovine X-chromosome–bearing sperm (which result in females) contain about 4% more genetic material (DNA) than Y-chromosome–bearing sperm (which result in males). Sperm are incubated for about half an hour with a DNA-binding dye that emits fluorescent light when stimulated by a particular wavelength of ultraviolet light, which usually is provided by a laser. The sperm then flow past the laser and fluorescence detectors in a device called flow cytometer/cell sorter. The fluorescence of each individual sperm is evaluated by computer into 3 categories: probably X-sperm, probably Y-sperm, or unable to distinguish if X or Y.[2] As illustrated in **Fig. 1**, droplets are formed at the tip of the nozzle of the cell sorter, and those droplets containing putative X-sperm are given a positive charge, those droplets containing putative Y-sperm are given a negative charge, and those droplets containing no sperm or sperm with indistinguishable sex chromosomes are not charged at all. The droplets exit the nozzle at about 80 km per hour and pass by strong positive and negative electric fields (see **Fig. 1**). Because opposite electrical charges attract, the positively charged X-sperm droplets veer toward the negative electric field, the negatively charged droplets veer toward the positive electric field, and the uncharged droplets fall straight. In this way, droplets can be sorted into 3 test tubes. In the process, the sperm become highly diluted, so they must be concentrated by centrifugation and removal of the excess fluid, after which they are packaged in straws and frozen.[2] This complicated process damages the sperm slightly, so they are slightly less fertile than unsexed sperm.

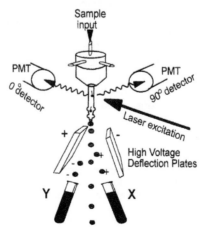

Fig. 1. Sorting by charge. (*From* Johnson LA, Welch GR, Rens W. Beltsville sperm sexing technology: High speed sperm sorting gives improved sperm output for in vitro fertilization and AI. J Anim Sci 1999:77(Suppl 2):213–20.)

For practical reasons, the equipment for sexing and sorting sperm usually is located near where bulls are housed, although it is possible to ship freshly collected semen to a sperm-sexing facility and obtain satisfactory fertility if the shipping time is less than about 15 hours. Frozen semen also can be sexed; however, it must then be used within a few hours, which usually is done via in vitro fertilization. Refreezing semen that previously was frozen is very detrimental to fertility in most situations.

The sperm sorters are remarkable in speed and efficiency.[2] The droplet formation rates can exceed 80,000 droplets per second. For statistical reasons, only about one-third of the droplets contain a sperm because attempting to get a sperm in each droplet results in many droplets with 2 or even 3 sperm, which makes those droplets unsortable. The fluorescence detectors make 180,000 consecutive measurements each second to evaluate the sperm as they pass by at 80 km per hour. These measurements are used to evaluate the sex chromosome composition of each sperm. For a variety of technical reasons, the sex cannot be determined accurately for over half the sperm.

There is one major fringe benefit of sexing sperm, which is that dead or dying sperm (around 10% in normal ejaculates) are discarded along with the unsexable sperm. In the end, only around 15% of sperm usually are collected; about half are ineligible because they would result in the "wrong" sex, although both X-sperm and Y-sperm can be collected at the same time; over half of the rest are discarded because they cannot be sexed accurately with current technology; and the dead or dying sperm also are discarded. The end result is that usually 5000 to 10,000 X-sperm or Y-sperm are collected per second, which would be 18 to 36 million sperm per hour. A few percentage are lost during centrifugation after sexing, so we would end up with about 3 to 6 straws of sexed semen per hour if packaged at 10 million sperm per straw, which is in the low range of normal numbers for beef bulls.

The sperm sorters cost hundreds of thousands of dollars each, and for the process to work economically, sexed sperm usually are packaged at 2 million sperm per straw, or less than one-fifth the normal number; this obviously contributes to lower fertility than with the larger number of sperm typically used with unsexed semen.

RECOMMENDATIONS FOR THAWING AND INSEMINATION OF SEXED SEMEN

Because the sexing process damages sperm slightly, plus only having 2 million sexed sperm per insemination dose, it is critical to optimize sexed semen handling, thawing, and insemination procedures. The situation is even more critical because sexed semen is packaged in 0.25-ml straws rather than the usual 0.5-ml straws. There are advantages to the smaller straws if handled properly; however, the smaller straws are more vulnerable to mishandling, that is they result in higher fertility if handled well, but lower fertility than the larger straws if mishandled. Thus, the 3-second rule is exceedingly important, no more than 3 seconds from transfer from one liquid nitrogen tank to another. Straws need to be thawed according to recommendations of the supplier of semen, generally in 95°F to 98°F water for 30 seconds, and then used within 10 min.

Sexed semen can be used successfully with appointment breeding protocols,[3] but that is risky as results can be very poor with some bulls and some synchronization procedures. If such protocols are used, it is best to breed about 6 hours later than what is recommended with unsexed semen. However, results are much more reliable if sexed semen is used only for situations in which insemination is timed relative to standing estrus. Results will be best if insemination is done around 18 hours after standing estrus is first detected, rather than the normally recommended 12 hours. A scheme that has worked very well with heifers in the author's experience is to breed once daily including only those seen in estrus between 12 and 24 hours earlier.[4]

PREGNANCY RATES AND SEXING ACCURACY

Pregnancy rates are compromised with sexed semen for 2 reasons: sperm are damaged slightly due to the complex sexing procedures and fewer sperm are used per insemination dose. If management is excellent, inseminators are well trained, and heifers are bred only if seen in estrus 12 to 24 hours before insemination, pregnancy rates are almost always 70% to 90% of those using control, unsexed semen in the same herd with the same bulls and inseminators; this is clearly illustrated by the data in **Table 1**. Results are typically 45% to 50% pregnant with sexed semen when controls are 60% to 65%. Often the difference is 10% points, for example, 60% control and 50% sexed. However, 10 percentage points is really 20% more pregnant; in this example, 10% of 50%.

Semen usually is sexed at 90% accuracy, and the sexes of calves at birth almost always are in that statistical range if averaged over sufficient numbers.[5] However, if only 4 or 5 calves result from sexed semen in a particular herd, it is not unusual to have 1 or 2 of the "wrong" sex. It is possible to sex bull semen at 95% accuracy, but this is prohibitively expensive compared with 90% because fewer sexed sperm are obtained per unit time. There is also a 75% accurate product produced by one bull stud, which lowers the cost considerably because more sperm can be collected per unit time with 75 rather than 90% accuracy.

COSTS AND NORMALITY OF CALVES RESULTING FROM USING SEXED SPERM

Currently, the extra costs charged for sexed semen usually are in the range of $15 to $20 per straw. As procedures become more efficient, the cost per dose might eventually be as low as $10. However, the added cost of purchasing sexed semen is minor relative to the cost of the lower fertility.

Most economic analyses indicate that calves of the desired sex must be worth $200 to $300 more at birth than calves of the other sex.[6] This takes into account the added cost of the sexed semen, the lower fertility, the 10% inaccuracy, etc. Sometimes it is difficult to quantify costs and benefits of sexed semen, for example, when expanding herd size without buying outside animals for biosecurity purposes.

There have been a few small scale studies and one large scale study on the normality of calves resulting from using sexed semen. All indications from these studies are that resulting calves are completely normal,[5] although there is a suggestion that the bull calves born as the "wrong" sex when selecting for heifers have higher neonatal death rates than expected.[7] The extra deaths in these bull calves represent a very small percentage of total calves (around 1%) and probably represent a statistical quirk of concentrating the aneuploid sperm that occur normally in the population.

Table 1
Pregnancy Rates (2 months) with sexed semen: Angus heifers- 2 bulls and 4 inseminators- 1 herd

No. Sperm	No. Heifers	% Pregnant
20×10^6 unsexed	126	67[a]
4.5×10^6 sexed	126	51[b]
1.5×10^6 sexed	123	54[b]

[a,b] $P < .05$.

SUGGESTED APPLICATIONS OF SEXED SEMEN

There are literally dozens of reasons for wanting more calves of one sex than the other, but nearly all have the common theme that one sex is worth more economically, either to sell or to increase herd profitability in other ways. As suggested earlier, if the difference in economic value of the sexes is less than $200, use of sexed semen is likely to be unprofitable. If that difference exceeds $300, sexed semen is likely to be profitable, with the caveat that management needs to be excellent, inseminators skilled, semen purchased from a reliable company, etc.

Currently most sexed semen is used by dairy farmers to have heifers have heifer calves. In many cases, this is done in the context of herd expansion, which also might be appropriate in some situations for beef cattle. There are 2 main advantages to expanding herds without purchasing outside cattle: (1) biosecurity issues are minimized, such as preventing introduction of insidious diseases such as Johne's disease and (2) one can build on already successful breeding programs. A third advantage is that it may be less costly to raise than purchase replacement females.

There are 2 special advantages to having heifers produce female replacements. First, the best genetics of any progressive herd are in the youngest animals; otherwise the breeding program is regressing. The second advantage is that female calves, on average, weigh about 2 kg less at birth than male calves, thus decreasing dystocia.

Of course, obtaining female calves for replacements from proved, older cows can be exceedingly valuable as well, especially for seedstock producers. On the other hand, for some matings, the males will be more valuable than the females, and if that is the case, sexed semen to produce males is the obvious choice. All of these arguments are amplified when cows or heifers are superovulated and inseminated with sexed semen to produce embryos for transfer. This obvious application results in greatly reduced fertility; typically with 50% to 60% of normal embryo production compared with using unsexed semen.[8] However, this still usually is worth doing if one sex of embryos is of little value because one does not waste resources on recipients gestating pregnancies of little value.

Steer calves are worth more for meat production than heifer calves, both because they weigh more at weaning and because they sell for more per pound due to more efficient growth. However, this difference in value usually is only on the order of $100 at weaning, a difference too small to justify use of sexed semen with current costs and fertility. However, if sexed semen is used to produce replacements from heifers and selected older cows, the remaining cows not needed for this purpose can be bred with unsexed semen from terminal cross sires, which produce more appropriate calves of both sexes for fattening than using genetics for maternal traits. This is starting to be recognized as an advantage in dairy herds, particularly of the Jersey breed; sexed semen from dairy sires is used to produce replacements, and unsexed beef semen is used to inseminate the remainder of cows to produce terminal-cross calves for beef production.

A final potential application of sexed semen for beef production is to produce beef without a cow herd by having each female replace herself by having a female calf. Calves would be weaned at 3 to 4 months of age and their mothers then fattened for 2 to 3 months and slaughtered before 30 months of age. After reaching puberty, their calves would then be bred to sexed semen to continue the cycle. With such a system, all animals are growing at all times, and the huge cost of maintaining a cow herd is eliminated; for much of the year most nutrients go for cow maintenance rather than for growth with conventional beef cattle herds.

Of course, such a beef production system will not be sustainable without adding some replacements because some bull calves will be produced, there will be some neonatal death, not all heifers will become pregnant, etc. However, if such a system only works for 70% of animals, the other 30% can come from a greatly reduced, more traditional herd.

A great intrinsic advantage of a system as just described compared with more conventional systems is that much more beef will be produced per unit of feed, land, energy, water, etc. Furthermore, there will be less manure, greenhouse gasses, and other environmental intrusions than with conventional beef production. This system does require somewhat intensive management, and it has not been tried to date, although each component such as early weaning and use of sexed semen has been demonstrated to be effective in certain situations.

FUTURE DIRECTIONS

Eventually it is likely that someone will invent a method of sexing semen that is faster than the current procedure of evaluating each sperm individually, in series. Currently, most sperm sorting systems consist of 2 nozzles, so 2 streams are evaluated simultaneously. Some research has been done on 4-nozzle systems, but these have been difficult to control by one technician; systems of 4 banks of 4 nozzles, somewhat like a 16-cylinder engine have been envisaged, but all of these systems still are evaluating sperm individually. They require constant monitoring of each nozzle and considerable computer power.

Unfortunately, no one has developed a suitable alternative to currently used methodology. The problem originates because nature has gone to great lengths to make X-chromosome–bearing and Y-chromosome–bearing sperm identical so that a 50:50 sex ratio results. For example, during spermatogenesis, the cells that will form X-chromosome–bearing and Y-chromosome–bearing sperm are connected with each other via intercellular bridges, so that they are exposed to identical environments. The connections are broken only after the finished sperm are released from the testes.

Despite the theoretical and empirical constraints, a better method of sexing sperm likely will be found eventually. Meanwhile, there will be incremental improvements to current methodology to make systems faster and gentler.

An approach not involving artificial insemination is being used considerably with dairy cattle, in vitro fertilization plus embryo transfer. Because the sperm are placed next to eggs in very small volumes, fewer sexed sperm are needed.[9] With fertilization by injecting 1 sperm into the egg, very few sexed sperm are needed, an approach already used with people and horses.

The ultimate in sex ratio control would be to modify males so they only produce X-chromosome–bearing or Y-chromosome–bearing sperm. Experiments along these lines already have been done with mice; one strain was produced that results in a 2:1 sex ratio of males to females with natural mating,[10] and 100% of one sex or the other is theoretically possible. However, it will be very expensive to develop bulls with such characteristics.

REFERENCES

1. Garner DL, Seidel GE Jr. History of commercializing sexed semen for cattle. Theriogenology 2008;69:886–95.
2. Seidel GE Jr, Garner DL. Current status of sexing mammalian sperm. Reproduction 2002;124:733–43.

3. Schenk JL, Cran DG, Everett RW, et al. Pregnancy rates in heifers and cows with cryopreserved sexed sperm: effects of sperm numbers per inseminate, sorting pressure and sperm storage before sorting. Theriogenology 2009;71:717–28.

4. Seidel GE Jr, Schenk JL. Pregnancy rates in cattle with cryopreserved sexed sperm: effects of sperm numbers per inseminate and site of sperm deposition. Anim Reprod Sci 2008;105:129–38.

5. Tubman LM, Brink Z, Suh TK, et al. Characteristics of calves produced with sperm sexed by flow cytometry/cell sorting. J Anim Sci 2004;82:1029–36.

6. Seidel GE Jr. Economics of selecting for sex: the most important genetic trait. Theriogenology 2003;59:585–98.

7. DeJarnette JM, Nebel RC, Marshall CE. Evaluating the success of sex-sorted semen in US dairy herds from on-farm records. Theriogenology 2009;71:49–58.

8. Schenk JL, Suh TK, Seidel GE Jr. Embryo production from superovulated cattle following insemination of sexed sperm. Theriogenology 2006;65:299–307.

9. Barcelo-Fimbres M, Campos-Chillon LF, Seidel GE Jr. In vitro fertilization using nonsexed and sexed bovine sperm: sperm concentration, sorter pressure, and bull effects. Reprod Domest Anim 2011;46:495–502.

10. Herrmann BG, Koschorz B, Wertz K, et al. A protein kinase encoded by the t complex responder gene causes non-Mendelian inheritance. Nature 1999;402: 141–6.

Postbreeding Heifer Management

Sandy K. Johnson, PhD[a],*, Richard N. Funston, PhD[b]

KEYWORDS

- Primiparous • Body condition • Nutrition • Pregnancy • Ionophore

KEY POINTS

- When a short breeding season is used on replacement heifers, the last heifer to calve has more time to resume estrous cycles and conceive as a 2-year-old.
- Body energy reserves at calving and nutrient status from calving through breeding are two major factors influencing pregnancy rate in beef cattle.
- A body condition score of 5 or 6 should be achieved by calving and maintained through rebreeding.
- Reducing energy or protein in late gestation does not reduce calving difficulty but may affect calf health and survival and a heifer's ability to rebreed.
- Diet changes, new environment, transportation, and other stressors may affect embryo survival.
- Early pregnancy detection provides information for increased management opportunities.
- Ionophores can conserve forage, control coccidiosis, and be beneficial to reproduction.

INTRODUCTION

Postbreeding management of primiparous heifers often receives less emphasis than prebreeding management; however, it is equally important. During this time, nutrient demands of the growing heifer increase to include advancing fetal growth, overcoming stress from calving, and first lactation. Failure to become pregnant after the birth of the first calf is one of the primary reasons for culling in a beef cattle operation. The economic consequences of nonpregnant 2-year-old cows have long been recognized and are discussed in more detail elsewhere in this series by Hughes. Nutrition is the primary management factor that influences the postpartum interval (PPI) and subsequent pregnancy rates. Feed also represents the single largest expense in a cow-calf operation. Finding the optimum reproductive rate for a given production environment can be a fine balance, particularly with the first-calf heifer. This article addresses management strategies to optimize second-calf pregnancy rates in primiparous heifers.

The authors have nothing to disclose.
[a] Department of Animal Sciences and Industry, Northwest Research and Extension Center, Kansas State University, PO Box 786, 105 Experiment Farm Road, Colby, KS 67701, USA;
[b] Department of Animal Science, West Central Research and Extension Center, University of Nebraska, 402 West State Farm Road, North Platte, NE 69101-7751, USA
* Corresponding author.
E-mail address: sandyj@ksu.edu

CONCEPTS
PPI

The period from calving until the cow conceives is critical in a cow's production cycle; minimizing this time period maximizes reproductive and economic efficiency of a beef cattle operation. Factors affecting the PPI have been reviewed[1–4] and include impacts of nutrition, suckling, parity, season, breed, dystocia, disease, and presence of a bull. PPI is longer in primiparous than multiparous cows[5] and, even if calving occurs before the mature cow herd, fewer primiparous cows have resumed estrous cycles by the beginning of the breeding season than mature cows.[6]

Cows that are in estrus early in the breeding season have more opportunities to become pregnant during a limited time. A short breeding season for replacement heifers is of particular advantage to the last heifers to calve, providing more days to achieve a positive energy balance before the first day of the breeding season. With an extended breeding season for replacements, a heifer may not have calved before the breeding season begins. An additional advantage of a short breeding season is the shortened calving season, creating a more uniform calf crop that is more valuable at weaning. To have a successful, short breeding season, cattle must conceive early in the breeding season.

The ability to minimize the PPI is limited by uterine involution, which is the time needed for repair of the reproductive tract so another pregnancy can be established. However, uterine involution does not affect the length of postpartum anestrus[7] because it is generally completed by the time the inhibitory effects of suckling and negative energy balance allow the first postpartum ovulation. Size differences between the previously gravid and nongravid horn can still be distinguished up to 4 weeks postpartum,[8] but size may not reflect when cellular changes occur. Before day 20 postpartum, fertilization rates and pregnancy rates are low, but not zero, and sperm transport may be a barrier to fertilization.[3] Malnutrition, disease, and calving difficulty can delay uterine involution in beef cows.

Body Condition Score

Body condition can greatly affect net income on a cow-calf operation because it is correlated with several reproductive events such as PPI, services per conception, calving interval, milk production, weaning weight, calving difficulty, and calf survival (**Table 1**).[9] Body condition score (BCS; 1 = emaciated to 9 = obese) is generally a reflection of nutritional management; however, disease and parasitism can contribute to decreased BCS even if apparent nutrient requirements are met.

Table 1
Relationship of body condition score (BCS) to beef cow performance and income

BCS	Pregnancy Rate (%)	Calving Interval (d)	Calf ADG (kg)	Calf WW (kg)	Calf Price ($/45.5 kg)	$/Cow Exposed[a]
3	43	414	0.73	170	96	154
4	61	381	0.80	209	86	241
5	86	364	0.84	234	81	358
6	93	364	0.84	234	81	387

Abbreviations: ADG, average daily gain; WW, weaning weight.
[a] Income per calf × pregnancy rate.
Data from Kunkle W, Sands R, Rae D. Effect of body condition on productivity in beef cattle. In: Fields M, Sands R, editors. Factors affecting calf crop. Boca Raton (FL): CRC Press; 1994. p. 174.

Nutritional Management

The relationship of nutrition to successful beef cattle reproduction has been reviewed.[10–12] Hess and colleagues[12] summarized key findings as follows:

1. Prepartum nutrition is more important than postpartum nutrition in determining the length of postpartum anestrus.
2. Inadequate dietary energy during late pregnancy lowers reproduction even when dietary energy is sufficient during lactation.
3. A BCS greater than or equal to 5 ensures that body reserves are adequate for postpartum reproduction.
4. Further declines in reproduction occur when lactating cows are in negative energy balance.

Nutrient demands during late gestation include continuing heifer growth as well as fetal growth. Fetal birth weight increases by 60% during the last 70 days of gestation.[13] Timely provision of adequate dietary energy and protein to meet this demand is a key step to having adequate body condition at calving. The importance of prepartum protein and energy level on reproductive performance has been consistently shown (**Table 2**).[11] Reproduction has low priority among partitioning of nutrients and consequently cows with thin BCSs often do not rebreed.

In addition to affecting subsequent cow reproduction, nutrient intake during gestation affects dystocia, calf health, and calf survival (**Table 3**).[14] Inadequate protein and energy to the dams results in calves that are more susceptible to cold stress, weak, and slow to suckle, increasing the risk for passive transfer failure.[15]

If heifers are thin at calving, achieving a positive energy balance postpartum is essential for timely return to estrus and pregnancy. Lalman and colleagues[16] provided increasing amounts of energy to thin (BCS 4), primiparous heifers postpartum and decreased PPI as dietary energy increased (**Table 4**). Body condition at calving also influences response to postpartum nutrient intake. Primiparous cows fed to achieve a BCS 4, 5, or 6 at calving were targeted to gain either 0.9 or 0.45 kg/d postpartum.[17] The magnitude of response to energy level was greater for BCS 4 heifers than those with greater BCS on the proportion of heifers initiating estrous cycles early in the breeding season. However, even with increased postpartum energy, the pregnancy rates of thin, primiparous cows may not be acceptable.

Fat

Inadequate dietary energy intake and poor BCS can negatively affect reproductive function. Supplemental lipids have been used to increase diet energy density and

Table 2
Effect of prepartum or postpartum dietary energy or protein on pregnancy rates in cows and heifers

	Adequate	Inadequate
Nutrient and Time	Percent Pregnant	
Energy level before calving[a]	73	60
Energy level after calving[b]	92	66
Protein level before calving[c]	80	55
Protein level after calving[d]	90	69

[a,b,c,d] Combined *data from* Refs.[2,4,8,9] respectively; and Randel R. Nutrition and postpartum rebreeding in cattle. J Anim Sci 1990;68:854–55.

Table 3
Effects of feed level during gestation on calving and subsequent reproduction[a]

Item	Gestation Diet of Dam	
	Low	High[b]
Calf birth weight (kg)	28.6	31.4
Dystocia (%)	35	28
Calf Survival (%)		
At Birth	93	91
Weaning	58	85
Scours (%)		
Incidence	52	33
Mortality	19	0
Dam Traits		
Estrus (before breeding season; %)	48	69
Pregnancy (%)	65	75

[a] Average of 7 studies; cows and heifers combined.
[b] Diet level fed from up to 150 days before calving; low and high, animals lost or gained weight before calving, respectively.
    Data from Bellows RA. Managing the first-calf heifer. In: Proceedings of the International Beef Symposium. Great Falls (MT): Montana State University; 1995. p. 81.

avoid the negative associative effects[18] that are sometimes experienced with cereal grains[19] in high-roughage diets.

Supplemental lipids may also have direct positive effects on beef cattle reproduction independently of energy contribution. Lipid supplementation has been shown to positively affect reproductive function in several important tissues including the hypothalamus, anterior pituitary, ovary, and uterus. The target tissue and reproductive response seem to depend on the types of fatty acids contained in the fat source. Lactating dairy cows commonly receive fat supplements, primarily to increase diet energy density. Associated positive and negative effects on reproduction have been reported.[20,21] The effects of fat supplementation on beef reproduction have been reviewed[22] and are summarized later.

Table 4
Influence of postpartum diet on weight change, BCS change, and PPI

Item	Diet			
	Low	Maintenance	Maintenance/High	High
Calving weight (kg)	379	374	376	373
Calving BCS	4.27	4.26	4.18	4.10
PPI[a] (d)	134	120	115	114
PPI weight change[a] (kg)	5.6	18.2	31.6	35.2
PPI BCS change[a]	−0.32	0.37	1.24	1.50

[a] Linear effect, $P<.01$.
    Data from Lalman D, Keislesr D, Williams J, et al. Influence of postpartum weight and body condition change on duration of anestrus by undernourished suckled beef heifers. J Anim Sci 1997;75:2004.

Fat supplementation prepartum
Results from feeding supplemental fat prepartum are inconclusive. However, supplementation response seems to depend on postpartum diet. Beef animals apparently have the ability to store certain fatty acids, supported by studies in which fat supplementation discontinued at calving resulted in a positive effect on reproduction. Postpartum diets containing adequate levels of fatty acids may mask any beneficial effect of fat supplementation. There seems to be no benefit, and in some cases feeding supplemental fat postpartum can have a negative effect, particularly when supplemental fat was also fed prepartum. Fat supplementation has been reported to both suppress and increase prostaglandin F2α (PGF$_{2\alpha}$) synthesis. When dietary fat is fed at high levels for extended periods of time, PGF$_{2\alpha}$ synthesis may be increased and compromise early embryo survival. Hess and colleagues[12] summarized research on supplementing fat during late gestation and concluded that feeding fat to beef cows for approximately 60 days before calving may result in a 6.4% improvement in pregnancy rate in the next breeding season.

Fat supplementation postpartum
Supplementing fat postpartum seems to be of limited benefit from studies reviewed by Funston.[22] Many of the studies reported approximately 5% total fat in the experimental diet, so it is not known whether more or less fat would have elicited a different response (either positive or negative). If supplementing fat can either increase or decrease PGF$_{2\alpha}$ production, the amount of fat supplemented might affect which response is elicited. First-service conception rates decreased from 50% in controls to 29% in young beef cows fed high-linoleate safflower seeds (5% DMI as fat) postpartum.[13] The same laboratory has also reported[23] an increase in PGF$_{2\alpha}$ metabolite when high-linoleate safflower seeds are fed postpartum and a decrease in several hormones important for normal reproductive function.[24,25]

Summary of fat supplementation
At present, research is inconclusive on how to supplement fat to improve reproductive performance beyond energy contribution. Most studies have attempted to achieve isocaloric and isonitrogenous diets. Several studies had only sufficient animal numbers to detect large differences in reproductive parameters such as conception and pregnancy rate. Research on feeding supplemental fat has resulted in varied (positive, negative, no effect) and inconsistent reproductive results. Postpartum fat supplementation seems to be of limited benefit and adding a fat source high in linoleic acid postpartum may have a negative effect on reproduction.

As is the case for any technology or management strategy that improves specific aspects of ovarian physiology and cyclic activity, improvements in pregnancy rates, weaned calf crop, or total weight of calf produced depend on an array of interactive management practices and environmental conditions. Until these relationships are better understood, producers are advised to strive for low cost and balanced rations. If a supplemental fat source can be added with little or no change in the ration cost, producers are advised to do so.

Minerals and Vitamins

Minerals and vitamins are important for all physiologic processes in the beef animal, including reproduction. Both deficiencies and excesses can contribute to suboptimal reproduction. Management guidelines for mineral supplementation in cow-calf operations have been provided.[26] The increased use of grain by-products in cattle rations requires that traditional mineral programs be reevaluated, making allowances for high phosphorus and sulfur contents and altered calcium/phosphorus ratios found in grain by-products. Overfeeding phosphorus is costly, of potential environmental concern, and does not positively influence reproduction in beef[27] or dairy cattle.[28] Inadequate consumption of certain trace elements combined with antagonistic interactions of other elements can reduce reproductive efficiency.[29]

Most vitamins (C, D, E, and B complex) are either synthesized by rumen microorganisms, synthesized by the body (vitamin C), or are available in common feeds and not of concern under normal growing conditions. However, vitamin A deficiency occurs naturally in cattle grazing winter range or consuming low-quality crop residues and forages.[30] Drought can extend periods when low-quality forages are fed and increase the need for vitamin A supplementation. The role of vitamin A in reproduction and embryo development was reviewed by Clagett-Dame and Deluca.[31] Vitamin A supplementation before and after calving has been shown to improve pregnancy rates.[32,33]

Nutrition and Calving Difficulty

Feeding a balanced diet during the last trimester of pregnancy decreases calving difficulty. Heifers fed diets deficient in energy or protein in the last trimester experience more calving difficulty; conceive later in the breeding season; and have increased sickness, death, and lower weaning weights in their calves (see **Table 3**).

Beef producers may be concerned that excessive dietary nutrients during the last trimester of pregnancy may negatively influence calf birth weight and dystocia. Providing either adequate or inadequate amounts of dietary energy and protein and their effects on calving difficulty, reproductive performance, and calf growth have been reviewed[34] and are summarized in **Tables 5** and **6**. Reducing energy prepartum

Table 5
Supplemental prepartum energy effects on calving difficulty, subsequent reproductive performance, and calf growth

Researcher	Prepartum Supplementation	Effect	Birth Weight	Dystocia	Other
Christenson et al, 1967	HE vs LE for 140 d	HE	+	+	+ Milk, + estrus activity
Dunn et al, 1969	ME vs LE for 120 d	ME	+	+	—
Bellows et al, 1972	HE vs LE for 82 d	HE	+	NC	NC weaning weight
Laster & Gregory, 1973	HE vs ME vs LE for 90 d	HE	+	NC	—
Laster, 1974	HE vs ME vs LE for 90 d	HE	+	NC	—
Corah et al, 1975	ME vs LE for 100 d	ME	+	NC	+ Estrus activity, + calf vigor and + weaning weight
Bellows & Short, 1978	HE vs LE for 90 d	HE	+	NC	+ Estrus activity, + pregnancy rate Decreased PPI
Anderson et al, 1981	HE vs LE for 90 d	HE	NC		NC milk, NC weaning weight
Houghton et al, 1986	ME vs LE for 100 d	ME	+	NC	+ Weaning weight

Abbreviations: +, increased response; HE, high energy (>100% NRC); LE, low energy (<100% NRC); ME, moderate energy (approximately 100% NRC); NRC, National Research Council; NC, no change.

Data from Houghton P, Corah L. A review of calving difficulty in beef cattle. Kansas State University Report of Progress 1987;525:28.

Table 6
Summary of studies on feeding supplemental protein during gestation on calving difficulty, subsequent reproductive performance, and calf growth

Study	Supplementation	Effect	Birth Weight	Dystocia	Other
Wallace & Raleight, 1967	HP vs LP for 104–137 d prepartum	HP	+	DEC	+ cow weight, + conception rates
Bond & Wiltbank, 1970	HP vs MP throughout gestation	HP	NC		NC calf survivability
Bellows et al, 1978	HP vs LP for 82 d prepartum	HP	+	+	+ cow weight, + cow gain, + weaning weight, DEC conception rate
Anthony et al, 1982	HP vs LP for 67 d prepartum	HP	NC	NC	NC PPI
Bolze, 1985	HP vs MP vs LP for 112 d prepartum	HP	NC	NC	NC weaning weight, NC milk, NC conception rate, DEC PPI

Abbreviations: DEC, decrease; HP, high protein (more than 100% NRC); LP, low protein (less than 100% NRC); MP, moderate protein (approximately 100% NRC).
Data from Houghton P, Corah L. A review of calving difficulty in beef cattle. Kansas State University Report of Progress 1987;525:31.

does not affect dystocia rates, even though birth weights were altered in some experiments. Of the 9 trials summarized, 6 showed that increased energy intake during the last trimester did not increase calving difficulty.

In addition, beef producers may be concerned that crude protein levels may influence calf birth weight and subsequent calving difficulty. Houghton and Corah[34] summarized studies investigating the effects of prepartum protein intake on calving difficulty (see **Table 6**). Reducing prepartum dietary crude protein does not decrease calving difficulty, but it may compromise calf health and cow reproductive performance.

Excess Protein and Energy

Caution should be used with feeding excess nutrients before or after calving. Not only is it costly but cows and heifers with BCSs greater than 7 have lower pregnancy rates and more calving difficulty than beef females with BCSs of 5 to 6. Excess protein and energy can negatively affect pregnancy rates. Overfeeding protein during the breeding season and early gestation, particularly if energy is limiting, may be associated with decreased pregnancy rates.[35] This decrease in fertility may result from decreased uterine pH during the luteal phase of the estrous cycle in cattle receiving high levels of degradable protein. The combination of high levels of degradable protein and low dietary energy in early-season grasses may contribute to low conception rates. Negative effects of excess rumen degradable protein on reproduction are well documented in dairy literature.[36]

Supplementing feedstuffs high in undegradable intake protein (UIP) during late gestation and/or early postpartum has shown positive reproductive responses in cows grazing low-quality forages[37,38]; however, considering the broader set of data, results are inconclusive and may depend on the UIP level[39] and energy density of the diet.[40] Further research is needed to understand how UIP stimulates or inhibits reproductive processes and under what conditions.

A recent study[41] challenges dogma regarding the BCS required at calving for successful conception rates. Two-year-old and 3-year-old cows were retrospectively grouped by BCS 30 days before calving into 3 groups whose average BCSs were 4.3 (n = 186), 5.0 (n = 108), and 5.8 (n = 57). Days to body weight nadir, days to first postpartum ovulation, and pregnancy rates were similar among BCS groups. Cows studied by Mulliniks and colleagues[41] were managed as 1 group before and after calving so body condition manipulation before calving did not affect the results. In contrast, other studies[17,42] used prepartum ration changes to achieve the desired BCS differences at calving.

Interpretation of this study[41] must be tempered with the knowledge that dams of these heifers were successfully managed in the same production system for 10 years. Cows had access to sufficient grazing resources, as shown by similar body weight changes even in years when precipitation was limiting. The implications of this observation across a wide variety of management systems are unknown; however, considered with recent demonstrations of successful moderate heifer development systems,[43,44] it questions the common solution of providing more feed (and cost) to correct all young cow reproductive deficiencies.

MANAGEMENT CONSIDERATIONS
Breeding to Pregnancy Diagnosis

Many heifer development systems for spring calving herds rely on a period of drylot development before shifting to pasture grazing. The transition from a drylot diet to grazing may come at the end of an artificial insemination (AI) program, at the same time as early embryonic development. Stress during this transition may affect embryonic mortality.

If heifers must be moved after AI, consideration should be given to when the move occurs because transportation stress can affect pregnancy rates. Mean conception date was earlier when heifers were transported 300 miles 1 to 4 days after AI compared with 8 to 12 or 29 to 33 days after AI.[45] Additional studies in heifers[46] and cows[47] investigated transportation 1 hour before or after AI and 14 days after AI. Concentrations of cortisol increased with AI and with transportation 14 days after AI, but pregnancy rates were not affected.

Nutritional stress can also reduce embryo quality and survival. Changing from a gaining or maintenance diet before insemination to 80% of maintenance for 6 days to 2 weeks after insemination produced developmentally delayed embryos[48] and lower embryo survival, and pregnancy rates[49] occurred. Embryonic loss is greatest during early gestation, with most losses occurring from day 8 to 16, corresponding with the time period between when the embryo reaches the uterus and maternal recognition of pregnancy.[50] Pregnancy rate to AI through the second service was higher in heifers gaining weight for 21 days after AI compared with heifers either maintaining or losing weight.[51] Heifers maintaining or losing weight after AI had similar pregnancy rates.

Grazing is a learned behavior and it has been suggested that grazing experience during development may improve yearling heifer performance.[52] Increased energy required for grazing and the novelty of new surroundings and feedstuffs could combine to create a short-term energy deficit for heifers transitioning from drylot to pasture. Weight loss was 1.6 ± 0.08 kg/d the first week on spring pasture for drylot-developed heifers.[53] Pregnancy rate was similar compared with range-developed heifers; however, the breeding season did not begin until after an adaption period. A heifer development system that included a postweaning grazing period reduced the number of steps taken on the first day of turnout compared with heifers developed in a drylot.[54] Drylot-developed heifers receiving supplementation in the first month of grazing following AI had higher pregnancy rates than nonsupplemented heifers.[54] Supplementation on pasture did not increase pregnancy rates to AI when heifers were developed on range compared with heifers receiving no supplement or that were drylot developed.[54] Improving heifer average daily gain on summer pasture has traditionally received minimal consideration in discussions of heifer development systems. Heifers with less gain (little to no supplement) during winter development had greater gains on summer pasture compared with heifers with higher gain (or supplemented) during winter development.[13,55,56]

Pregnancy Detection

Early pregnancy detection should not be overlooked as a management tool for producers. In addition to traditional palpation, increasing availability of ultrasound and commercial serum pregnancy tests provide more options for producers and veterinarians.[57] Pregnancy can be accurately detected with ultrasound as early as 25 days after breeding, but speed and accuracy are improved by waiting until day 30 or later.[58] Heifers conceiving early in the breeding period have greater lifetime productivity[59] (discussed by Perry elsewhere in this series) in the herd and should be favored in selection if drought or market conditions require herd reduction.

Pregnancy Diagnosis to Calving

Continued gain is needed through calving for heifer and fetal growth, particularly for more moderate development systems. Body weights and BCS at pregnancy diagnosis and 90 days before calving should be used to monitor development. Forage intake in pregnant heifers decreases as gestation advances,[60] which could affect gain and energy intake during the third trimester. Recommendations have been made for heifers to achieve 85% of mature weight and a condition score of 5 to 6 by calving.[61] However, heifers developed to 53% of mature body weight at breeding that reached 77% of mature body weight at calving had pregnancy rates through 4 calving seasons ranging from 92% to 96%.[62] Although dietary restriction during early heifer development may reduce cost and capitalize on compensatory gain, continued restriction during subsequent winter (gestation) periods increases the proportion of nonpregnant heifers and reduces herd retention rate.[44,63] Two-year-old heifers failing to rebreed weighed less at calving and breeding than those that successfully became pregnant the second time.[63]

CALVING TO REBREEDING
Calving Difficulty

First-calf heifers experience more calving difficulty compared with the mature cow. Bellows[14] indicated that cows experiencing calving difficulty take longer to resume estrus than cows not experiencing calving difficulty. Sire selection and genetic components of dystocia are reviewed elsewhere in this series by Van Eenennaam and his colleagues.

Time of intervention, when obstetric assistance is needed, also affects resumption of estrous cycles. Dams provided with early assistance had a higher percentage in estrus by the beginning of the breeding season, increased fall pregnancy rate, and improved calf gains compared with late assistance dams (**Table 7**).[64,65] Therefore, early assistance, when needed, is important to ensure that heifers return to estrus as soon as possible.

Table 7
Effect of time of calving assistance or duration of labor on dam breeding and calf performance

Item	Time of Assistance/Duration of Labor	
	Early/Short	Late/Prolonged
PPI (d)	49	51
In heat at beginning of breeding season (%)	91[a]	82[b]
Services/conception	1.15	1.24
Fall pregnancy (%)	92[c]	78[d]
Calf average daily gain (kg)	0.76[a]	0.79[b]
Calf weaning weight (kg)[a]	183	179

[a,b] Means differ $P<.10$.
[c,d] Means differ $P<.05$.

Data from Bellows RA, Short RE, Staigmiller RB, et al. Effects of induced parturition and early obstetrical assistance in beef cattle. J Anim Sci 1988;66:1077–9; and Doornbos D, Bellows R, Burfening P, et al. Effects of dam age, prepartum nutrition and duration of labor on productivity and postpartum reproduction in beef females. J Anim Sci 1984;59:7–8.

Stimulating Estrus

Ionophores

Ionophores can influence reproductive performance during the postpartum period.[66] Cows and heifers fed an ionophore have a shorter PPI provided adequate energy is provided in the diet (**Table 8**).[11] This effect is more evident in less intensively managed herds with a moderate (60–85 days) to longer PPI. If measured, pregnancy rates generally were not different in the studies summarized by Randel[11]; however, in most cases the number of observations was low. In a more recent study replicated over 2 years and 12 pastures, monensin was provided to crossbred cows early postpartum, reducing days to conception and increasing calving percentage compared with cows not receiving monensin.[67] Adding an ionophore may also reduce feed costs through reduced intake and improved feed efficiency on lower quality forages and improved rate of gain with higher quality feedstuffs offered ad libitum.[66]

Calf removal

Suckling stimulus has a negative effect on estrous activity during the postpartum period; however, animals in a positive energy balance and adequate BCS generally overcome this negative stimulus before the breeding season. Calf removal, either

Table 8
Effect of ionophore feeding on PPI in beef cows and heifers

Study	Ionophore PPI (d)	Control PPI (d)	Difference (d)
1	30	42	12
2	59	69	10
3	67	72	5
4	65	86	21
5	92	138	46

Data from Randel R. Nutrition and postpartum rebreeding in cattle. J Anim Sci 1990;68:857.

Table 9
Studies that evaluated reproductive performance (resumption of cyclic activity and pregnancy rates) in postpartum cows exposed to males (EXP) or isolated from males (ISO)

Exposure Type and Length (d)	Cyclic Activity (%)		Pregnancy (%)		Reference
	EXP	ISO	EXP	ISO	
ASE/DPC (20 d)	—	—	58.5	50.0	Ungerfeld, 2010
BE/DPC (60 d)	81[a]	41[b]	67	63	Berardinelli et al, 2001
BE/DPC-EPB (63 d)	87[a]	19[b]	87[a]	56[b]	Anderson et al, 2002
BE/DPC-EPB (60 d)	85.1[a]	31.3[b]	66.3[a]	51.5[b]	Berardinelli et al, 2007
BE/DPC (35 d)	100[a]	70.4[b]	85[a]	60[b]	Tauck & Berardinelli, 2007
BE/DPC (50 d)	82[a]	38.5[b]	54.5[a]	15.4[b]	Gokuldas et al, 2010
BE/FCB (42 d)	86[a]	76[b]	58	77	Tauck & Berardinelli, 2007
TBU (64 d)	15	33	89.5[a]	55[b]	Tauck & Berardinelli, 2007

Abbreviations: ASE, androgenized steers exposure; BE, bull exposure; DPC, direct physical contact; EPB, excretory products of bulls; FCB, fence-line contact with bulls; TBU, treatment with bull urine.
  [a,b] Different letters in the same row and for each experiment differ, $P<.05$.
  Data from Fiol C, Ungerfeld R. Biostimulation in cattle: stimulation pathways and mechanisms of response. Trop Subtrop Agroecosystems 2012;15(Suppl 1):S38. Available at: http://www.veterinaria.uady.mx/ojs/index.php/TSA/article/view/1342/656. Accessed March 15, 2013.

temporary or permanent, can increase the number of cows returning to estrus during the breeding season.[11,68] Some synchronization programs remove calves for 48 hours,[69] which can induce estrus in postpartum cows and first-calf heifers. It is important to provide the calves with a clean, dry pen with grass hay and water and to make sure that calves have found their mothers before going to pasture.

Induction of estrus with hormones
An intravaginal insert containing progesterone, can shorten the PPI provided nutrition and BCS are adequate.[70,71] Several protocols for synchronization of estrus and ovulation incorporate a progestin and have resulted in pregnancies in previously noncycling females.[72] Ovulation induction with gonadotropin-releasing hormone was limited in primiparous cows until BCSs were greater than or equal to 5.[6]

Bull exposure
Bull exposure requires exposing cows to surgically altered bulls not capable of a fertile mating. Reproductive performance of postpartum cows in response to bull exposure has been reviewed[73] and is summarized in **Table 9**. Exposure length, proximity, timing of exposure, and nutritional status have affected response. Primiparous cows exposed to bulls at 15, 35, or 55 days postpartum had shorter PPIs than nonexposed cows, but PPIs were similar regardless of the date exposure began.[74] The PPI was reduced in cows exposed to as many as 1 bull per 29 females.[75] Exposure to androgenized steers[76] or cows[75] produces similar results.

SUMMARY

The interaction of nutrition and reproduction in young beef cows has been studied extensively. Diets that meet the high nutrient demands of late gestation and early lactation require attention and monitoring. Adequate nutrition limits calving difficulty, increases health and vigor of the calf, and allows a timely second pregnancy. Heifers that conceive in a short breeding season have more time to achieve positive energy balance before the second breeding season. A BCS of 5 or 6 should be achieved by calving and maintained through the breeding season to minimize PPI. Several interventions can assist in shortening the PPI but none take the place of timely nutritional management. Advances in understanding of nutrition and reproduction interactions may provide opportunities for strategic supplementation to optimize reproduction for a given production system.

REFERENCES

1. Casida LE. The postpartum interval and its relation to fertility in the cow, sow and ewe. J Anim Sci 1971;32(Suppl 1):66–72.
2. Inskeep EK, Lishman AW. Factors affecting postpartum anestrus in beef cattle. In: Hawk H, editor. Beltsville symposium on animal reproduction, no. 3. Montclair (NJ): Allanheld, Osmun; 1979. p. 277–89.
3. Short RE, Bellows RA, Staigmiller RB, et al. Physiological mechanisms controlling anestrus and infertility in postpartum beef cattle. J Anim Sci 1990;68: 799–816.
4. Yavas Y, Wallon J. Induction of ovulation in postpartum suckled beef cows: a review. Theriogenology 2000;54:1–23.
5. Dunn TG, Kaltenbach CC. Nutrition and the postpartum interval of the ewe, sow and cow. J Anim Sci 1980;51(Suppl 2):21–39.
6. Stevenson J, Johnson S, Milliken G. Incidence of postpartum anestrus in suckled beef cattle: treatments to induce estrus, ovulation and conception. Prof Anim Sci 2003;19:124–34.
7. Kiracofe G. Uterine involution: its role in regulating postpartum interval. J Anim Sci 1980;51(Suppl 2):16–27.
8. Sheldon M. The postpartum uterus. Vet Clin Food Anim Pract 2004;20:569–91.
9. Kunkle W, Sands R, Rae D. Effect of body condition on productivity in beef cattle. In: Fields M, Sands R, editors. Factors affecting calf crop. Boca Raton (FL): CRC Press; 1994. p. 167–78.
10. Wettemann R, Lents C, Ciccioli N, et al. Nutritional- and suckling-mediated anovulation in beef cows. J Anim Sci 2003;81:E48–59.
11. Randel R. Nutrition and postpartum rebreeding in cattle. J Anim Sci 1990;68: 853–62.
12. Hess BW, Lake SL, Scholljegerdes EJ, et al. Nutritional controls of beef cow reproduction. J Anim Sci 2005;83(Suppl E):E90–106.
13. Bauman DE, Currie B. Partitioning of nutrients during pregnancy and lactation: a review of mechanisms involving homeostasis and homeorhesis. J Dairy Sci 1980;63:1514–29.
14. Bellows RA. Managing the first-calf heifer. In: Proceedings of the International Beef Symposium. Great Falls (MT): Montana State University; 1995. p. 74–85.
15. Sanderson MW, Chenoweth PJ. Controlling neonatal calf morbidity and mortality: prepartum management. Compend Contin Educ Pract Vet 2001;23(9): S95–9.
16. Lalman D, Keisler D, Williams J, et al. Influence of postpartum weight and body condition change on duration of anestrus by undernourished suckled beef heifers. J Anim Sci 1997;75:2003–8.
17. Spitzer J, Morrison D, Wettemann R, et al. Reproductive responses and calf birth and weaning weights as affected by body condition at parturition and postpartum weight gain in primiparous beef cows. J Anim Sci 1995;73:1251–7.

18. Coppock C, Wilks D. Supplemental fat in high-energy rations for lactating cows: effects on intake, digestion, milk yield, and composition. J Anim Sci 1991;69: 3826–37.
19. Bowman J, Sanson D. Starch- or fiber-based energy supplements for grazing ruminants. Proc 3rd Grazing Livest Nutr Conf Proc West Sec Amer Soc Anim Sci 1996;42:1–18.
20. Grummer R, Carroll D. Effects of dietary fat on metabolic disorders and reproductive performance of dairy cattle. J Anim Sci 1991;69:3838–52.
21. Staples C, Burke J, Thatcher W. Influence of supplemental fats on reproductive tissues and performance of lactating cows. J Dairy Sci 1998;81:856–71.
22. Funston R. Fat supplementation and reproduction in beef females. J Anim Sci 2004;82(Suppl E):E154–61.
23. Grant M, Hess B, Bottger J, et al. Influence of supplementation with safflower seeds on prostaglandin F metabolite in serum of postpartum beef cows. Proc West Sec Amer Soc Anim Sci 2002;53:436–9.
24. Scholljegerdes E, Hess E, Van Kirk E, et al. Effects of supplemental high-linoleate safflower seeds on ovarian follicular development and hypophyseal gonadotropins and GnRH receptors. J Anim Sci 2003;81(Suppl 1):236.
25. Scholljegerdes E, Hess B, Van Kirk E, et al. Effects of dietary high-linoleate safflower seeds on IGF-I in the hypothalamus, anterior pituitary gland, serum, liver, and follicular fluid of primiparous beef cattle. J Anim Sci 2004;82(Suppl 2):48.
26. Olson KC. Management of mineral supplementation programs for cow-calf operations. Vet Clin Food Anim Pract 2007;23:69–90.
27. Dunn T, Moss G. Effects of nutrient deficiencies and excesses on reproductive efficiency of livestock. J Anim Sci 1992;70:1580–93.
28. Lopez H, Kanitz F, Moreira V, et al. Reproductive performance of dairy cows fed two concentrations of phosphorus. J Dairy Sci 2004;87:146–57.
29. Greene L, Johnson A, Paterson J, et al. Role of trace minerals in cow-calf cycle examined. Feedstuffs 1998;70:34.
30. Lemenager R, Funston R, Moss G. Manipulating nutrition to enhance (optimize) reproduction. McCollum F, Judkins F, editors. Proc 2nd Grazing Livest Nutr Conf Oklahoma Agric Exp Sta MP-133. 1991. p. 13–31.
31. Clagett-Dame M, DeLuca H. The role of vitamin A in mammalian reproduction and embryonic development. Annu Rev Nutr 2002;22:347–81.
32. Bradfield D, Behrens WC. Effects of injectable vitamins on productive performance on beef cattle. Proc West Sect Am Soc Anim Sci 1968;19:1–5.
33. Meacham TN, Bovard KP, Priode BM, et al. Effect of supplemental vitamin A on the performance of beef cows and their calves. J Anim Sci 1970;31:428–33.
34. Houghton P, Corah L. A review of calving difficulty in beef cattle. Kansas State University Report of Progress 1987;525:22–35.
35. Elrod C, Butler W. Reduction of fertility and alteration of uterine pH in heifers fed excess ruminally degradable protein. J Anim Sci 1993;71:694–701.
36. Ferguson J. Nutrition and reproduction in dairy herds. Intermountain Nutrition Conference Proceedings, Utah State University Publication No 169. 2001. p. 65–82.
37. Hawkins D, Petersen M, Thomas M, et al. Can beef heifers and young postpartum cows be physiologically and nutritionally manipulated to optimize reproductive efficiency? J Anim Sci 2000;77:1–10.
38. Mulliniks J, Cox S, Kemp M, et al. Protein and glucogenic precursor supplementation: a nutritional strategy to increase reproductive and economic output. J Anim Sci 2011;89:3334–43.

39. Kane K, Hawkins D, Pulsipher G, et al. Effect of increasing levels of undegradable intake protein on metabolic and endocrine factors in estrous cycling beef heifers. J Anim Sci 2004;82:283–91.

40. Martin JL, Cupp AS, Rasby RJ, et al. Utilization of dried distillers grains for developing beef heifers. J Anim Sci 2007;85:2298–303.

41. Mulliniks J, Cox S, Kemp M, et al. Relationship between body condition score at calving and reproductive performance in young postpartum cows grazing native range. J Anim Sci 2012;90:2811–7.

42. Ciccioli N, Wettemann R, Spicer L, et al. Influence of body condition at calving and postpartum nutrition on endocrine function and reproductive performance of primiparous beef cows. J Anim Sci 2003;81:3107–20.

43. Funston R, Larson D. Heifer development systems: dry-lot feeding compared with grazing dormant winter forage. J Anim Sci 2011;89:1595–602.

44. Roberts AJ, Geary TW, Grings EE, et al. Reproductive performance of heifers offered ad libitum or restricted access to feed for a one hundred forty-day period after weaning. J Anim Sci 2009;87:3043–52.

45. Harrington T, King M, Mihura H, et al. Effect of transportation time on pregnancy rates of synchronized yearling beef heifers. Colorado State University Beef Program Report. Fort Collins (CO): Colorado State University; 1995. p. 81–6.

46. Yavas Y, De Avila D, Reeves J. Trucking stress at breeding does not lower conception rate of beef heifers. Theriogenology 1996;45:623–32.

47. Merrill M, Ansotegui R, Burns P, et al. Effects of flunixin meglumine and transportation on establishment of pregnancy in beef cows. J Anim Sci 2007;85:1547–54.

48. Bridges G, Kruse S, Funnell B, et al. Changes in body condition on oocyte quality and embryo survival. Proceedings Applied Reproductive Strategies in Beef Cattle. Sioux Falls (SD): South Dakota State University; 2012. p. 269–83.

49. Dunne L, Diskin M, Boland M, et al. The effect of pre- and post-insemination plane of nutrition on embryo survival in beef heifers. Anim Sci 1999;69:411–7.

50. Diskin MG, Parr MH, Morris DG. Embryonic death in cattle: an update. Reprod Fertil Dev 2012;24:244–51.

51. Arias R, Gunn P, Lemenager R, et al. Effects of post-AI nutrition on growth performance and fertility of yearling beef heifers. Proc West Sec Am Soc Anim Sci 2012;63:117–21.

52. Olson K, Jaeger J, Brethour J. Growth and reproductive performance of heifers overwintered in range or drylot environments. J Prod Agr 1992;5:72–6.

53. Salverson RR, Patterson HH, Perry GA, et al. Evaluation of performance and costs of two heifer development systems. Proc West Sect Am Soc Ani Sci 2005;56:409–12.

54. Perry G, Larimore E, Bridges G, et al. Management strategies for improving lifetime reproductive success in beef heifers. Proceedings Applied Reproductive Strategies in Beef Cattle. Sioux Falls (SD): South Dakota State University; 2012. p. 249–66.

55. Lemenager R, Smith W, Martin T, et al. Effects of winter and summer energy levels on heifer growth and reproductive performance. J Anim Sci 1980;51:837–42.

56. Short RE, Bellows RA. Relationships among weight gains, age at puberty and reproductive performance in heifers. J Anim Sci 1971;32:127–31.

57. Lucy M. Pregnancy determination by palpation and beyond. Proceedings Applied Reproductive Strategies in Beef Cattle. Sioux Falls (SD): South Dakota State University; 2012. p. 309–16.

58. Fricke PM, Lamb GC. Potential applications and pitfalls of reproductive ultrasonography in bovine practice. Vet Clin Food Anim Pract 2005;21:419–36.

59. Lesmeister J, Burfening P, Blackwell R. Date of first calving in beef cows and subsequent calf production. J Anim Sci 1973;36:1–6.

60. Patterson H, Klopfenstein T, Adams D, et al. Supplementation to meet metabolizable protein requirements of primiparous beef heifers: I. Performance, forage intake, and nutrient balance. J Anim Sci 2003;81:800–11.

61. Bolze R, Corah LR. Selection and development of replacement heifers. C841. Manhattan (KS): Kansas State University; 1993.

62. Funston R, Deutscher G. Comparison of target breeding weight and breeding date for replacement beef heifers and effects on subsequent reproduction and calf performance. J Anim Sci 2004;82:3094–9.

63. Endecott R, Funston R, Mulliniks J, et al. Implications of beef heifer development systems and lifetime productivity. J Anim Sci 2012;91:1329–35.

64. Bellows R, Short R, Staigmiller R, et al. Effects of induced parturition and early obstetrical assistance in beef cattle. J Anim Sci 1988;66:1073–80.

65. Doornbos D, Bellows R, Burfening P, et al. Effects of damage, prepartum nutrition and duration of labor on productivity and postpartum reproduction in beef females. J Anim Sci 1984;59:1–10.

66. Sprott L, Goehring T, Beverly J, et al. Effects of ionophores on cow herd production: a review. J Anim Sci 1988;66:1340–6.

67. Bailey C, Goetsch A, Hubbell D, et al. Effects of monensin on beef cow reproduction. Can J Anim Sci 2008;88:113–5.

68. Williams GL. Suckling as a regulator of postpartum rebreeding in cattle: a review. J Anim Sci 1990;68:831–52.

69. Smith M, Burrell W, Shipp L, et al. Hormone treatments and use of calf removal in postpartum beef cows. J Anim Sci 1979;48:1285–94.

70. Day M. Hormonal induction of estrus cycles in anestrous *Bos taurus* beef cows. Anim Reprod Sci 2004;82–83:487–94.

71. Perry G, Smith M, Geary T, et al. Ability of intravaginal progesterone inserts and melengestrol acetate to induce estrous cycles in postpartum beef cows. J Anim Sci 2004;82:695–704.

72. Stevenson J, Lamb G, Johnson S, et al. Supplemental norgestomet, progesterone, or melengestrol acetate increases pregnancy rates in suckled beef cows after timed insemination. J Anim Sci 2003;81:571–86.

73. Fiol C, Ungerfeld R. Biostimulation in cattle: stimulation pathways and mechanisms of response. Trop Subtrop Agroecosystems 2012;15(Suppl 1):S29–45. Available at: http://www.veterinaria.uady.mx/ojs/index.php/TSA/article/view/1342/656. Accessed March 15, 2013.

74. Berardinelli JG, Joshi PS. Introduction of bulls at different days postpartum on resumption of ovarian cycling activity in primiparous beef cows. J Anim Sci 2005;83:2106–10.

75. Burns PD, Spizter JC. Influence of biostimulation on reproduction in postpartum beef cows. J Anim Sci 1992;70:358–62.

76. Ungerfeld R. Short-term exposure of high body weight heifers to testosterone-treated steers increases pregnancy rate during early winter bull breeding. Anim Reprod 2009;6:446–9.

Raised Replacement Heifers
Some Economic Considerations

Harlan Hughes, PhD

KEYWORDS

- Raised replacement heifers • Economic considerations • Replacement rate
- Economic costs • Future profitability • Cost analysis • Cost summary

KEY POINTS

- The management decision to raise replacement heifers needs to be based on the economic costs of raising and developing the replacement heifers.
- A 6-step process that calculates the economic cost of developing a raised pregnant replacement heifer is recommended.

INTRODUCTION

There are 3 general reasons why a beef producer wants to raise replacement heifers. The first reason is to maintain a perpetual beef cow herd. As older and/or less productive cows are culled, young females generally need to be added back into the herd. North Dakota's herd performance (CHAPS) data suggest that producers typically replace around 15.1% of the cow herd annually.[1] The 15.1% replacement rate is the average for herds between 2007 and 2011 herds. These herds tend to be more intensely managed herds and may not be typical. My integrated resource management (IRM) data for the mountain states suggest that those producers typically replace from 12% to 14% of their cow herds annually. This replacement rate may be more typical.

The second reason that beef producers want to raise replacement heifers is to increase the size of their cow herds. The typical driving force stimulating added replacement heifers is increasing calf prices. As cattle prices increase, producers' interest in holding back added replacement heifers also increases.

The third reason for raising replacement heifers is to repopulate the herd after depopulating in a drought. Whatever the reason for considering raised replacement heifers, it is important that producers use the proper cost measures to determine their cost of raising replacement heifers.

Disclosures. The author has nothing to disclose.
North Dakota State University, Fargo, North Dakota, USA
E-mail address: harlan.hughes@gte.net

Vet Clin Food Anim 29 (2013) 643–652
http://dx.doi.org/10.1016/j.cvfa.2013.07.013
0749-0720/13/$ – see front matter © 2013 Elsevier Inc. All rights reserved.

The 3 common cost measures applicable to a raised replacement heifer enterprise are:

1. Accounting costs, including depreciation
2. Cash costs (out-of-pocket costs), including interest and principle payments but excluding depreciation
3. Economic costs, where all resources consumed are valued at an opportunity cost (ie, resources are valued at their value in the next best use)

Opportunity cost has farm-raised feeds priced in at the local market price rather than at cost of raising the feed. Opportunity cost also includes an interest charge on the capital invested in the heifer calves regardless of who finances the heifer calves. No principle payments are included in economic costs, just an interest charge for the average investment. Principle payment just determines who owns the asset and is a cash cost only.

Each cost measure is designed for a specific management purpose:

- If a producer wants to know past profitability of his or her replacement heifer enterprise, the producer would use accounting costs to make that evaluation. Farm-raised feeds fed would typically be valued at costs of production.
- If the producer (or his or her banker) wants to know if all the bills associated with the heifer development enterprise can be paid, he or she would use the cash flow account for the replacement heifers.
- If a manager is trying to evaluate the future profitability of a proposed heifer development enterprise, he or she would use an economic cost analysis of the proposed heifer development enterprise.

The cost measure to use depends on the management question being addressed.

The rest of this article is devoted to the future profitability question associated with a proposed heifer development enterprise. This article lays out the recommended procedure for determining the economic cost of developing a proposed set of replacement heifers.

CONDUCTING AN ECONOMIC COST ANALYSIS

A manager's decision to add or not to add raised replacement heifers needs to be based on an economic cost analysis of the proposed heifer development enterprise, often better understood if referred to as a full cost analysis. Opportunity cost is the correct cost measure to use. Opportunity cost of each resource consumed is the value of that resource in its next best use.

The opportunity cost of resources that can be sold, like farm raised feeds, is defined as the local market prices for those feeds. Money tied up in heifer calf investment has an opportunity cost of the going interest rate on borrowed capital. Grass has an opportunity cost of the local rental rate. The rest of this article covers the recommended process for conducting an economic cost analysis of a raised replacement heifer enterprise.

INPUT NUMBERS USED

Table 1 presents the input numbers used to calculate the example economic cost of developing a pregnant replacement heifer. Once a heifer is diagnosed pregnant, she is assumed transferred into the breeding cow herd enterprise, and her future costs beyond pregnancy diagnosis become part of the beef cow enterprise's production

Table 1
Input figures used to calculate replacement heifer economic costs

		Year Heifers Born	2013
Average Weaning Weight of Heifers (lbs)			554
Weaning Date			01-Nov-13
Price of Heifer Calves at Weaning ($/hundredweight)			$159
Mature Weight of Cow Herd (lbs/cow)			1250
Spring Date to Grass			01-May-14
Target ADG on Grass (lbs)			1.5
Supplemental Feed While on Grass	lbs/d	0.19	
	Cost per lb of feed fed	$0.25	$0.05
Target Breeding Date			01-Jun-14
Heifer Wintering Costs: ($/Head)			$318
	Feed costs	$239.00	
	Lot costs	$37.00	
	Interest cost	$24.00	5.0%
	Veterinary visits & medicine	$7.00	
	Transportation costs	$0.00	
	Processing costs	$0.00	
	Death loss ($)	$11.00	
	Subtotal	$318.00	
Going Pasture Rents in Local Area ($/AUM)			$24
Date Pregnancy Diagnosis			01-Oct-14
Breeding Costs/Heifer:			$56
	Price of heifer bulls?	$4000	
	Servicing number of heifers?	20	
	For how many years?	4	
	Cull bull weight?	1900	
	Cull bull selling price ($/lb)?	$0.75	
	Annual bull feed costs?	$350	
Heifer Average Pregnancy Rate (%)			85%
Market Price of Cull Open Heifer ($/Hundredweight) (at Pregnancy Diagnosis)			$140
			Input

cost. Thus, the economic cost of developed heifers covers from conception of the heifer calf through pregnancy diagnosis of the developed heifer.

The input data in **Table 1** were compiled during the spring of 2013 and were designed to evaluate the economic cost of developing 2013 weaned heifer calves into pregnant heifers in the fall of 2014. More specifically, this analysis is for 2013 spring-born heifer calves weaned in November 2013, averaging 554 lbs. At that time, the price of weaned heifer calves was predicted to average $159 per hundredweight. The average mature weight of these heifer replacements was projected to be 1250 lbs.

These 2013 weaned replacement heifer calves are to be wintered in a drylot with a May 1, 2014, date to grass. A target average daily gain (ADG) for the wintered drylot period was calculated to allow these heifers to attain 65% of their average mature weight by breeding time, June 1, 2014, when these heifers will be exposed to a bull. Recent research suggests that heifers can be bred at 55% to 60% of mature weight without impacting the pregnancy rates. This might be a way to lower heifer development costs. These heifers' wintering costs will be discussed in more detail in a subsequent section.

Summer pasture costs will vary greatly from region to region. In my example (data for eastern Wyoming/western Nebraska), pasture rent was figured at $24 per animal unit month (AUM) and was adjusted to $19.20 per heifer month. AUM is a term typically used in western herds. For here, it is equivalent to cow–calf month. A growing heifer is assumed to consume 0.8 AUM per month on grass. Determination of pregnancy status for bred heifers is assumed to be performed on Oct. 1, 2014.

Heifer breeding costs were based on a $4000 heifer bull servicing 20 heifers annually. The bull was assumed to remain in the herd for 4 years. The average cull bull weight was assumed to be 1900 lbs, and the projected average cull bull selling price was $0.75 per pound. Annual bull feeding cost was projected at $350 per year. This calculates out to a breeding cost of $56 per heifer exposed. The salvage value of a bull is $1425. This makes the depreciation on a $4000 bull spread over 4 years equal $643 per year. Annual feed cost is $350. Interest on the average investment ([$4000 + 1425]/2 × 0.05) totals $136 per year. The total annual cost of a bull is projected at $1123. Divide the annual total by 20 heifers exposed, and the breeding cost comes to $56 per exposed heifer.

Finally, the heifer pregnancy rate was projected at 85%. With pregnancy diagnosis scheduled for Oct. 1, 2014, cull open heifers were projected sold at the time pregnancy examinations were performed for $140 per hundredweight.

RECOMMENDED 6 STEPS FOR CALCULATING RAISED REPLACEMENT HEIFER COSTS

The input numbers in **Table 1** were used in the recommended 6 steps for calculating the economic costs of developing replacement heifers:

1. Calculate costs from conception to weaning.
2. Calculate costs from weaning to breeding.
3. Calculate costs from breeding to pregnancy diagnosis.
4. Total the costs for all 3 periods.
5. Adjust for heifer pregnancy rate.
6. Adjust for cull heifer credit.

The following sections demonstrate how these 6 steps are executed utilizing the example input data.

Step 1: Pregnancy to Weaning

The single biggest opportunity cost of raising replacement heifers is the market value of not selling the heifer calf at weaning. It was projected that heifer calves weighing 554 lbs would bring $159 per hundredweight in November 2013, totaling $881 per head. This $881 market value is the opportunity cost for the pregnancy to weaning period.

Step 2A: Winter Feeding Costs

The winter feeding program needs to be developed around a target average daily gain (ADG) based on the average weaning weight, the target breeding weight, and the target breeding date. **Table 2** summarizes the calculated target ADG for these heifers.

The target breeding weight was set at 65% of the 1250 lbs mature weight or 813 lbs. The target breeding date was June 1, 2014. This calculates out to a 182-day winter drylot period and 31 days on grass before breeding.

The target weight to grass was 766 lbs, which requires a wintered drylot ADG of 1.2 lbs. These 1.2 lbs became the target ADG for the winter ration (see **Table 2**) and were used to formulate a ration for drylot feeding of a 554 lb heifer calf through the winter. The primary feed ingredient considered was $150 per ton of alfalfa hay. A small amount of grain was added, as well as salt and minerals.

Winter feed costs need to be based on the local market price of the feeds fed, not cash costs of production. As pointed out in **Table 3**, winter feed cost was predicted to total $239 per head. After including lot cost ($37), interest on the calf investment ($24, at 5%), and death loss ($11 with a 1% death loss), the total wintering costs was projected at $318 per head.

Step 2B: Wintering To Breeding

The $318 wintering costs in **Table 3** take the heifers up to grass on May 1, 2014. The cost of pasture and supplement while on grass brings the total wintering-to-breeding costs to $341 (**Table 4**).

Grass costs should be based on the going local rental rate in a producer's area. A 766 lb heifer was figured at 0.8 AU. In this case example, this calculates out to $19.20 per heifer month based on 80% of the local $24.00 per AUM rental rate.

Step 3: Breeding To Pregnancy Diagnosis

This period has 4.1 months of summer grazing ($70), supplement costs while on grass ($5.80), breeding costs ($56), and interest on animal investment costs ($21, at 5%), for an added total cost for this period of $153 per head (**Table 5**).

Table 2	
Beef replacement heifer template—calculation of the target ADG in winter grower phase	
Weaning weight	554
Weaning date	01-Nov-13
Mature weight of cows (lbs)	1250
Target breeding weight (lbs)	813
Weight to be added (lbs)	259
Date to grass	01-May-14
Target breeding date	01-Jun-14
Days on grass	31
Target ADG on grass (lbs)	1.5
Days on winter feed	181
Target winter gain (lbs)	212
Target weight to grass (lbs)	766
Target winter ADG (lbs)	1.2

Table 3
Drylot wintering costs of raising a replacement heifer

		Gain = 212 lbs
Item	Cost per Head	Cost per lb Gain
1 Feed cost	$239.00	$1.13
2 Lot cost	$37.00	$0.17
3 Interest	$24.00	$0.11
4 Veterinary visits and medicine	$7.00	$0.03
5 Hauling replacement	$0.00	$0.00
6 Processing	$0.00	$0.00
7 Death loss	$11.00	$0.05
Total	$318.00	$1.50
	Breakeven selling price =	$157.00/Cwt

Table 4
Wintering-to-breeding costs

Wintering costs		$318.00
Pasture costs to breeding	31 d	$17.86
$19.20/animal month		
Supplemental feed on pasture		$1.47
0.19 lbs/d @ $0.25/b.		
Interest on previous investment	5%	$3.74
	Total	$341/hd

Table 5
Costs from breeding to pregnancy diagnosis

					$19.20/mo	$70.27
Grazing costs						
Start date:	01-Jun-14	Ending:	01-Oct-14	= 4.1 mo		
Weight:	766 lbs		949 lbs			
Supplemental feeding on pasture						$5.80
0.19 lbs/d @ $0.25/lb						
Breeding costs						$56.00
$4000 Bull Serving: 20 females/year for 4 y						
Cull bull weights 1900 lbs @ $0.75 lb = $1425						
Feed cost = $350/y						
Interest costs = $136/y @ 5%						
Annual cost = $486						
Interest costs						$20
5% × $1222 for 122 d						
					Total	$153/hd

Step 4: Cost Summary for Developing a Replacement Heifer

Table 6 pulls all the different periods' costs into 1 subtotal. The pregnancy-to-weaning total was $881; weaning to breeding was $341, and breeding to pregnancy diagnosis was $153. This subtotals to $1375 per heifer entered into the development program.

Step 5: Adjust For Pregnancy Rate

Because not all heifers get pregnant, this $1375 needs to be divided by the pregnancy rate to calculate the total cost of a pregnant replacement heifer. This calculates out to $1618 ($1375/0.85) per pregnant replacement heifer.

Step 6: Adjust For Cull Heifer Credit

One still needs to adjust for the market value of the cull open heifers. These cull heifers are projected to average 949 lbs, with a projected price of $140 per hundred-weight, totaling $1328 per head. The cull heifer sales bring the average cost of developing a set of pregnant replacement heifers back down to $1418 per head. No labor cost has been included in this analysis. North Dakota's Farm Business Management Record Summaries for the 10-year period 2002 through 2011 indicate that those cooperators average 1.71 hours of labor per heifer developed. Using a conservative $10 per hour for labor, this would suggest a labor cost of $17 per replacement heifer exposed.

This 2013 heifer calf developed in 2014 is projected to be among the most expensive replacement heifers developed to date.

A MORE GENERALIZED APPROACH

The economic cost of developing replacement heifers will vary from year to year depending on a given year's feed prices. In addition, beef producers in different regions of the country will face different feed prices. Once a spreadsheet model is built to calculate the economic cost of raised replacement heifers, selected feed price input numbers can be changed, and the results recalculated. This is exactly what was done in the generation of the table values in **Table 7**.

Table 7 was designed to provide producers with an easy way to adjust the wintering feed costs to their own specific feed prices. This table allows a manager to pick a hay price and a corn price, and the intersection of that row and column provides an estimated feed cost for wintering heifer calves in a drylot.

Table 6
Projected cost summary for developing a raised replacement heifer

14-Feb-13			2013 Heifer
	Period 1: conception to weaning		$881
	Period 2: weaning to breeding		$341
	Period 3: breeding to pregnancy diagnosis		$153
		Subtotal	$1375
	Adjust for heifer pregnancy rate	85%	$1618
	Adjust for cull heifer credit	$140.00	$1418
		949 Lbs	
	Calculated heifer development costs	2013	$537
		Born	

Table 7
Alternative feed costs for wintering heifer calves (554–764 lbs)

Corn Price ($Bu.)	Price of Hay ($/Ton)									
	$75	$100	$125	$150	$175	$200	$225	$250	$275	$300
	Calculated Feed Costs of Winter Growing Replacement Heifers (181 d)									
$4.00	$127	$163	$199	$235	$271	$307	$343	$378	$414	$450
$5.00	$131	$167	$203	$239	$275	$310	$346	$382	$418	$454
$6.00	$135	$171	$207	$243	$278	$314	$350	$386	$422	$458
$7.00	$139	$175	$211	$246	$282	$318	$354	$390	$426	$461
$8.00	$143	$179	$214	$250	$286	$322	$358	$394	$440	$485

For example, assume that a producer's hay price is $250 per ton and that the corn price is $6 per bushel. Looking at the intersection of the $250 hay column and the $6 corn row gives a suggested feed cost of $386 for wintering heifer calves. This compares with the $239 feed cost used in the example discussed earlier in this article. This $386 feed cost is $147 higher than the earlier example.

This $147 added feed cost can be added to the previously calculated $1375 economic cost (see **Table 6**) of all exposed heifers, increasing the total cost to $1522. Adjusting for pregnancy rate ($1522/0.85 = $1791) and adjusting for cull open heifer sales comes to $1595 per pregnant heifer developed.

Table 8 builds on **Table 7** by incorporating the pregnancy rate adjustment and the cull heifer sales adjustments into the tabled values and presents the final projected economic cost of replacement heifers for alternative hay and corn prices.

The economic cost of raised replacement heifers can be generalized further. As discussed earlier in this article, the economic cost of a raised replacement heifer is comprised of 2 parts. The first part is the market value of the weaned heifer calf. The second part is the cost of growing and developing that heifer calf. **Table 9** allows a producer to select a weaned heifer calf price on the right and a hay price along the top, and where the specified row and column intersect is the projected total economic cost of a pregnant heifer.

For example, if one assumes that hay costs are $225 per ton and that the weaned heifer calf price is $150 per hundredweight, the intersection of this row and column in **Table 9** suggests a projected economic cost of $1487 for a pregnant heifer.

Table 8
Economic cost of replacement heifers (554–764 lbs.) for alternative winter feed costs (hay and corn prices)

Corn Price ($Bu.)	Price of Hay ($/Ton)									
	$75	$100	$125	$150	$175	$200	$225	$250	$275	$300
	Calculated Feed Costs of Winter Growing Replacement Heifers (181 d)									
$4.00	$1284	$1327	$1370	$1413	$1456	$1499	$1542	$1585	$1628	$1671
$5.00	$1289	$1332	$1375	$1418	$1461	$1504	$1547	$1590	$1633	$1676
$6.00	$1294	$1337	$1380	$1423	$1466	$1509	$1552	$1595	$1638	$1681
$7.00	$1299	$1342	$1385	$1428	$1471	$1514	$1557	$1600	$1643	$1686
$8.00	$1303	$1346	$1389	$1432	$1475	$1518	$1561	$1604	$1647	$1690

Table 9
Economic cost of replacement heifers based on alternative hay costs and weaned heifer prices (conception to pregnancy diagnosis)

Weaned Calf Price	Price of Hay ($/Ton) With $5/bu. Corn									
	$75	$100	$125	$150	$175	$200	$225	$250	$275	$300
	Calculated Economic Costs of Developing Replacement Heifers									
$140.00	$1163	$1206	$1249	$1292	$1335	$1378	$1421	$1464	$1507	$1550
$150.00	$1229	$1272	$1315	$1358	$1401	$1444	$1487	$1530	$1573	$1616
$160.00	$1296	$1339	$1382	$1425	$1468	$1511	$1554	$1597	$1640	$1683
$170.00	$1362	$1405	$1448	$1491	$1534	$1577	$1620	$1663	$1706	$1749
$180.0p	$1429	$1472	$1515	$1558	$1601	$1644	$1687	$1730	$1773	$1816

Not all producers will need to drylot the heifers as they grow them through the winter. Some producers can graze through the winter. **Table 10** allows a producer to estimate his or her winter feed costs from any heifer growing system by selecting a total wintering cost along the top of the table for his or her unique production system. Then, the producer can select a monthly cost for summer grazing of the heifers along the left side, and the intersection of the selected row and column gives a projected cost of developing a pregnant heifer.

An example might be a producer who can grow his or her replacement heifers on grass during the winter and estimates the total wintering cost to be $250 for the winter season. Total wintering costs should include feed, minerals and salt, grass, interest, veterinary visits, and medicine. If the going rate for grazing a growing heifer in his area is $12 per heifer month, the intersection of the $12 per heifer month row and $250 total winter feeding column projects the economic cost of developing a replacement heifer at $1298.

SUMMARY

The management decision to raise replacement heifers needs to be based on the economic costs of raising those replacement heifers. This article presented a

Table 10
Economic cost of replacement heifers based on alternative wintering costs and summer grazing costs (conception to pregnancy diagnosis)

Pasture Cost $Heifer Mo	Total Wintering Costs for 182-Day Season (85% Pregnancy Rate)[a]							
	$100	$150	$200	$250	$300	$350	$400	$450
	Calculated Feed Costs of Winter Growing Replacement Heifers (181 d)							
$10/AUM or 8/Heifer Mo	$1097	$1157	$1216	$1276	$1336	$1396	$1456	$1516
$15/AUM or $12/Heifer Mo	$1118	$1178	$1238	$1298	$1358	$1417	$1477	$1537
$20/AUM or $16/Heifer Mo	$1140	$1200	$1260	$1320	$1379	$1439	$1479	$1519
$25/AUM or $20/Heifer Mo	$1162	$1222	$1281	$1341	$1401	$1461	$1521	$1581
$30/AUM or $24/Heifer Mo	$1183	$1243	$1303	$1363	$1423	$1483	$1542	$1601

[a] This should include feed costs plus lot, interest, veterinary visits and medicine, transportation, processing, and death loss.

recommended 6-step process designed to calculate the economic cost of developing a raised pregnant replacement heifer. The 6 steps discussed were

1. Calculate costs from pregnancy to weaning.
2. Calculate costs from weaning to breeding.
3. Calculate costs from breeding to pregnancy diagnosis.
4. Total the costs for all 3 periods.
5. Adjust for the heifer pregnancy rate.
6. Adjust for the cull heifer credit.

The biggest cost associated with heifer development is the opportunity cost of not selling the heifer calf at weaning ($881 in this example). This is then augmented with the on-ranch development costs of another $494 per heifer exposed. This brings the total economic costs of raising replacement heifers to $1375 per heifer exposed. Adjusting for the 85% pregnancy rate and the sale of cull heifers makes this $1418 per pregnant heifer ready to be transferred into the beef cow herd.

Summarized another way, the opportunity cost of not selling a 2013 heifer calf at weaning is projected at $881. The on-ranch cost for developing this heifer calf into a November 2014 pregnant heifer, after adjustments for pregnancy rate and cull open heifer sales, is projected to be $537, for a total economic cost of $1418 per pregnant heifer developed.

REFERENCE

1. North Dakota's CHAPS benchmark data is available at: www.chaps2000.com/benchmarks.

Management Strategies for Adding Value to Replacement Beef Heifers: A Working Model

David J. Patterson, PhD[a],*, D. Scott Brown, PhD[b],
W. Justin Sexten, PhD[a], Jared E. Decker, PhD[a], Scott E. Poock, DVM[c]

KEYWORDS

- Beef heifer • Heifer development • Show-Me-Select Replacement Heifer Program

KEY POINTS

- Coordinated on-farm beef heifer development and marketing programs are designed to improve reproductive efficiency of beef herds and increase herd profitability.
- These programs expand working relationships among beef producers, extension specialists, and veterinarians to enhance information exchange and improve management of cow herds.
- Beef heifer development programs are improved through a Total Quality Management approach.
- Marketing opportunities for beef heifers that are developed according to established guidelines offer the potential to add value to heifers offered for sale.
- Over time, these programs are recognized for offering reliable sources of quality replacement beef heifers based on genetics and management.

INTRODUCTION

The advent of coordinated regional (Bourbon County Kentucky Elite Heifer Program) or statewide on-farm beef heifer development and marketing programs (Missouri Show-Me-Select Replacement Heifer Program and Sales) that focus on the collective management practices and procedures presented in this issue remove much of the risk of developing replacement beef heifers in comparison with situations whereby replacements are raised or purchased without these criteria being taken into consideration.[1–4]

Disclosures: The authors have nothing to disclose.
[a] Division of Animal Sciences, University of Missouri, Columbia, MO 65211, USA; [b] Department of Agricultural and Applied Economics, University of Missouri, Columbia, MO, USA; [c] Department of Medicine and Surgery, College of Veterinary Medicine, University of Missouri, Columbia, MO 65211, USA
* Corresponding author. University of Missouri, S132 Animal Sciences Research Center, Columbia, MO 65211.
E-mail address: pattersond@missouri.edu

Marketing heifers that are developed according to established guidelines, as in the Bourbon County Kentucky Elite Heifer Program (http://www.eliteheifer.com/) and the Missouri Show-Me-Select Replacement Heifer Program (http://agebb.missouri.edu/select/), are a viable means of rural economic development in the United States.[4] These programs are designed to: (1) improve reproductive outcomes resulting from heifer development programs through a total quality management approach; (2) increase marketing opportunities for, and add value to, the heifer portion of the calf crop; and (3) provide reliable sources of quality replacement females concerning genetics and management.

These programs require compliance with specific guidelines, and provisions for various management and reproductive practices and (or) procedures. The guidelines include provisions for ownership; health and vaccination schedules; parasite control; implant use; weight, pelvic measurement, and reproductive tract score; estrous synchronization and artificial insemination; service-sire requirements for birth-weight expected progeny difference (EPD) or calving-ease EPD; early pregnancy diagnosis and fetal aging; and body condition score.[3,4]

The Missouri Show-Me-Select Replacement Heifer Program was designed to improve reproductive efficiency of beef herds and increase herd profitability. The program was developed for beef producers in Missouri that are involved with the production and sale of beef cattle, and is dependent on active participation from University of Missouri Extension Regional Livestock Specialists and local veterinarians, each of which are critical components of the livestock sector of the state. The pilot effort of the Show-Me-Select Replacement Heifer Program began in 2 regions of Missouri in the fall of 1996, and involved 33 farms and 1873 heifers. Eldon Cole and Al Kennett, University of Missouri Extension Regional Livestock specialists in the southwest and northeast regions, respectively, led these pilot efforts. Since that time the program has grown statewide.

The Show-Me-Select Replacement Heifer Program draws on the fundamental basis on which Extension and the Land Grant System were founded: the use and application of what we know to create knowledge. Data collection is part of the delivery process, and reinforces the development of sound management practices on individual farms regardless of their size. Producers, along with their veterinarians and extension specialists, analyze data generated on their own farms to make decisions based on data collected from their herds. Dr Richard Randle developed the initial database for the program, and more recently funding from University of Missouri Extension was used to enhance the existing database to allow for more complete data capture and expanded use of data for research purposes. This use of data will be important in the long-term success and sustainability of the program.

Organization of the program depends in large part on University of Missouri Extension Regional Livestock Specialists, who serve as coordinators of the program locally and who work closely with veterinarians involved with the program statewide. State Extension Specialists from the University of Missouri provide program support to extension field staff and participating veterinarians. The reproductive goals for heifers enrolled in the program are aimed at improving the breeding performance of heifers during the first breeding period, minimizing the incidence and severity of dystocia at calving with the resulting delivery of healthy vigorous calves, and successful rebreeding of females during subsequent breeding seasons.

Outcomes from the program have met and, in many cases, exceeded the original program objectives, and include: (1) increased adoption by farmers in Missouri of management practices that offer potential to improve long-term reproductive efficiency of their herds and resulting profitability; (2) expanded working relationships among farmers, extension regional livestock specialists, and veterinarians that enhance information exchange and improve the management of cow herds across Missouri; (3) improved heifer development programs through a Total Quality Management approach; (4) increased marketing opportunities for and added value from Missouri-raised heifers; and (5) the creation of reliable sources of quality replacement heifers based on genetics and management.

PROGRAM RATIONALE

The profitability of cow-calf operations in Missouri and throughout the United States is influenced largely by pounds of calf weaned per cow exposed for breeding. Improvements in production efficiency are possible and can be expected to occur with improvements in reproductive management. Female replacement strategies have one of the greater long-term effects on profitability within a cowherd than any other decision made by a cow-calf producer. Producers must evaluate long-term and short-term effects of replacement choices, and the combined sensitivity of those choices to market price and long-term reproductive integrity of their herds. Decision-making systems that focus only on the short-term effects of female replacement strategies do not measure such factors as reproductive soundness, replacement rate, comparative productive capability between heifers and cows, death and morbidity rates, disease incidence, conception rates, comparative pregnancy distribution between heifers and cows, calving interval effects on weaning weight and prices, and effect of birth weight on dystocia and subsequent reproduction.

Selection and management of replacement beef heifers involves decisions that affect future productivity of an entire herd. Programs to develop heifers have therefore focused on the physiologic processes that influence puberty. Age at puberty is most important as a production trait when heifers are bred to calve as 2-year-olds and in systems that impose restricted breeding periods. The number of heifers that become pregnant during their first breeding season and within a defined time period is correlated with the number that exhibit estrus early in the breeding season. The decision to breed heifers as yearlings involves careful consideration of the economics of production, and the reproduction status and breed type or genetic makeup of the heifers involved. Several factors influence the ability of a cow to calve in a given year and successively over several years. Heifers that calve early during their first calving season have higher lifetime calf production than those that calve late. Because most calves are weaned at a particular time rather on a weight-constant or age-constant basis, calves born late in the calving season are usually lighter at sale time than those born early, thus tending to decrease the total lifetime profitability of their dams. In many cases subjective methods of selecting replacement heifers have not afforded suitable focus on reproductive traits. The ability to identify heifers with the greatest reproductive potential before the breeding season should result in increased reproductive efficiency, resulting in improvements in total cowherd productivity and profitability. Subsequently, culling opportunities are enhanced.

One of the largest problem areas for cow-calf operations is the developing phase of the replacement beef heifer, and related inadequacies or excesses in nutrition and management. Development of a fundamental understanding of basic principles regarding animal breeding, genetics, reproductive physiology, nutrition, animal health, and economics are essential in making informed management decisions that sustain long-term economic viability on a farm-to-farm basis. These considerations provide the foundation on which the Show-Me-Select Replacement Heifer Program was based.

The Show-Me-Select Replacement Heifer Program is unique in that it is first and foremost an educational program targeted at improving production efficiency through increased use of existing technology, coupled with a marketing component. Best Management Practices for replacement beef heifers, when collectively viewed as a "program," can assist beef producers in more effectively managing reproduction and production. These practices ensure that heifers entering a herd as raised or purchased replacements add value to the general performance and productivity of herds, both immediately and in the long-term.

The marketing aspect of the Show-Me-Select Replacement Heifer Program provides the opportunity for producers to develop and market programmed replacement heifers to herd owners who currently lack appropriate time, labor, facilities, or resources to develop their own herd replacements. Purchasers of programmed heifers benefit from the opportunity to more rapidly improve the genetic makeup of their herds, modify existing breeding programs, and ultimately enhance end-product quality and uniformity.

PROGRAM PRIVATIZATION
Show-Me-Select Replacement Heifers, Inc

Financial support from the University of Missouri Outreach Development Fund was used initially to underwrite costs of the Show-Me-Select Replacement Heifer Program. These funds were a catalyst in program development and implementation. Beginning June 30, 2004, University funding in support of the program ended, and the financial responsibility for continuation of the program transferred to program participants. At that point, individuals committed to the program and interested in the long-term benefits stemming from it came together to organize the program as a producer-owned and producer-managed business.

The statewide steering committee for the Show-Me-Select Replacement Heifer Program, comprising representatives from each region in Missouri, voted unanimously in August 2003 to move forward with the formation of a stand-alone, producer-owned business from which to operate the program over the long term. The Show-Me-Select Replacement Heifer Program was privatized in 2004 as a Not-for-Profit organization. Show-Me-Select Replacement Heifers, Inc now operates through official bylaws filed in the Office of the Missouri Secretary of State, and is officially declared "a body corporate, duly organized ... entitled to all rights and privileges granted corporations or organizations under the Missouri Nonprofit Corporation Law." Mike Kasten of the 4M Ranch, Millersville, Missouri was the organization's founding president.

Show-Me-Select Replacement Heifers, Inc continues to move forward as a corporation solely operated by beef producers in Missouri. The program is highly regarded nationally, and has been duplicated by other states and individuals to add value to replacement beef heifers. Missourians share great pride in the program's growth and success, and Show-Me-Select Replacement Heifer Sales have become the benchmark for replacement heifer sales across the country.

PROGRAM PARTICIPATION

Since the program's pilot effort in 1997 involving 2 regions of the state, 33 farms, and 1873 heifers, the Show-Me-Select Replacement Heifer Program has expanded statewide. Since 1997 and through the fall of 2012, 743 farms enrolled 104,918 heifers in the program. Regionally the program has been overseen by 10 extension regional coordinators and 17 extension regional livestock specialists, and 222 veterinarians have supported farms enrolled in the program in the 8 program regions. The marketing aspect of the program has involved 119 sales at 10 locations across Missouri, with the resulting sale of 25,276 heifers. Gross revenue generated from these sales amounted to $30,045,050. During the past 16 years, 8590 prospective buyers registered to buy heifers at Show-Me-Select Replacement Heifer Sales, and 2560 of these individuals successfully purchased heifers from the various sales. In addition, heifers have now been sold into 18 states, including Missouri. **Fig. 1** identifies counties in Missouri from which farms enrolled heifers in the Show-Me-Select Replacement Heifer Program. Producers from 103 counties in Missouri have now enrolled heifers in the program, accounting for 90% of Missouri's 114 counties.

Fig. **2** illustrates counties in Missouri from which producers registered to purchase heifers at one of the past 119 Show-Me-Select Replacement Heifer Sales. **Fig. 2** highlights that interested buyers from 113 of Missouri's 114 counties (99% of the counties in the state) attended sales intending to purchase heifers.

Fig. 3 illustrates counties in Missouri from which producers successfully purchased heifers in one of the past 119 Show-Me-Select Replacement Heifer Sales. **Fig. 3** highlights that heifers have now sold into 109 of Missouri's 114 counties, or 96% of the counties in the state.

Finally, **Fig. 4** illustrates the 18 states into which heifers have been sold from the past 119 Show-Me-Select Replacement Heifers sales. The map illustrates why the Show-Me-Select Replacement Heifer Program is now recognized as the "Midwest's source of replacement females."

SUPPORT FROM VETERINARIANS

The University of Missouri College of Veterinary Medicine and practitioners across the state play an integral role in success of the Show-Me-Select Replacement Heifer Program. Veterinarians who participate in the program are now more actively involved in supporting herd health on participating farms, along with their involvement in performing prebreeding examinations (reproductive tract scores [RTS] and pelvic examinations), early pregnancy diagnosis, and final pregnancy determination prior to sale. During this time participants in the program have seen the demand for pregnancy

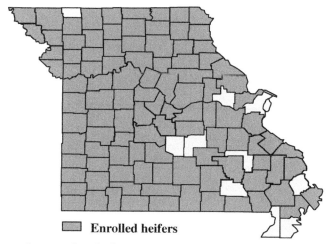

Fig. 1. Producers from 103 (90%) of Missouri's 114 counties enrolled heifers in the Show-Me-Select Replacement Heifer Program from 1997 to 2012.

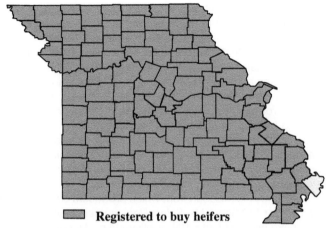

Fig. 2. Buyers from 113 (99%) of Missouri's 114 counties registered to purchase heifers from the Show-Me-Select Replacement Heifer Program from 1997 to 2012.

diagnosis via ultrasonography increase, because of improvements in accuracy of the diagnosis when comparing ultrasonography with palpation, and price differentials between natural service–sired and artificial insemination (AI)-sired calves. In addition, practitioners are becoming more involved with estrous synchronization programs on these farms as they relate to both heifers and cows. The demand for veterinary support of the program will continue, and likely will increase as adoption of technology expands and producers expect more in terms of the inputs they are provided and the types of information they seek to make better-informed decisions.

DEVELOPMENT OF TIER TWO

During the fall 2003 breeding season and under the leadership of Roger Eakins, Extension Regional Livestock Specialist in southeast Missouri, the first field trials involving

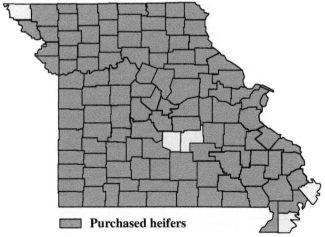

Fig. 3. Buyers from 109 (96%) of Missouri's 114 counties purchased heifers from the Show-Me-Select Replacement Heifer Program from 1997 to 2012.

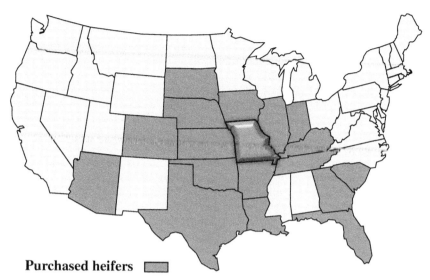

Purchased heifers

Fig. 4. Buyers from 18 states purchased heifers from the Show-Me-Select Replacement Heifer Program from 1997 to 2012.

fixed-time AI of postpartum beef cows were conducted in Missouri. Semen used in these trials was obtained from a high-accuracy Angus sire. The outcome of the field trials was successful from the standpoint of the numbers of cows that conceived to fixed-time AI, but what occurred subsequently resulted in a growing awareness of the power of stacking technologies that would add value to replacement females. Because a common sire was used in these trials, several half-sib progeny resulted, which led to the sale of 33 half-sisters in the spring 2005 Show-Me-Select Replacement Heifer Sale in Fruitland, Missouri. These commercial half-sisters, all sired by the same high-accuracy AI sire and bred back artificially to a high-accuracy calving-ease sire, sold for an average sale price of $1765, and the high-selling lot from this group of 33 sold for $2200 each. It should be noted that the overall sale average was $1515.

These results provided preliminary data for a subsequent project funded by the US Department of Agriculture (USDA) National Institute of Food and Agriculture (NIFA) and the National Research Initiative (NRI). The project was based on the premise that fixed-time AI using semen from high-accuracy sires could be used as a means to add value to replacement beef females and half-sib steer mates. On receipt of funding for the project, representatives from the American Angus Association and the Genetic Improvement Committee for Show-Me-Select Replacement Heifers, Inc met to draft requirements for what would become Tier Two of the Show-Me-Select Replacement Heifer Program. Given the level of awareness and general understanding of requirements for the program statewide, the logical addition to the program was to create a means by which genetic merit of heifers could be distinguished based on newly established guidelines. What resulted was the creation of Tier Two for the program, based on a defined set of traits and specific accuracies for those traits. The term Accuracy is defined as the reliability that can be placed on an EPD. Accuracy of close to 1.0 indicates higher reliability, and is affected by the number of progeny and ancestral records included in the analysis. Initially EPDs are derived from the average of an animal's parents (called a pedigree estimate); however, once an animal has its own measurement or performance record, the accuracy of the EPD increases and continues to do so as the animal has recorded progeny.

Heifers are now eligible to qualify as Tier Two replacements in the Show-Me-Select Program, based on the minimum accuracies of the heifer's sire at the time of sale for the respective traits listed in **Table 1**.

University of Missouri Extension, in support of this effort, funded the purchase of 8 double-box, portable AI breeding barns shown in **Fig. 5**. These barns are available to producers across Missouri to rent for a daily use fee of $50 that is paid to the respective region where they are used. The barns are also accessible to AI companies across Missouri. Extension Regional Livestock Specialists oversee the rental and maintenance of the barns at the local level. Purchase of the barns was intended to expand the use of AI in cow herds across the state by providing access to facilities that simplified fixed-time AI. Producers who have used the barns find that cattle typically enter the barns without hesitation; cattle stand quietly because of the absence of physical restraint except for being prevented from backing up; the barns can be used in all types of weather conditions, and are designed in such a way to ensure safety of technicians and cattle; and they provide an appropriate environment to process semen before insemination. In addition, the barns are being used extensively to perform ultrasonography on cattle at the time pregnancy examinations are performed.

PROGRAM SALES

The Show-Me-Select Replacement Heifer Program fosters the adoption of reproductive technologies focused on expanded use of estrous synchronization and AI, in addition to the use of high-accuracy AI sires. The program has fostered development of a production infrastructure for effective implementation of new reproductive technologies and economic feedback regarding their use. By-products of adoption of reproductive technologies in beef cattle include enhanced genetic merit of heifers and steers, and improvements in whole-herd reproductive management. The recent addition of the Tier Two classification now distinguishes heifers sired from high-accuracy AI sires.

Using data from the past 5 sales seasons (fall 2010 through fall 2012) in which Tier Two heifers were sold, we may begin to consider opportunities for producers to add value to their heifers as a result of improvements in genetic merit (**Table 2**). For example, if the average sales price of Show-Me-Select qualified heifers carrying a natural service–sired pregnancy is used as a baseline sale average for heifers, subsequent comparisons can be made to determine the relative added value that resulted from improvements in genetics of the heifer and/or the pregnancy she was carrying.

Although the numbers are at this point limited, the Tier Two program promises to provide significant economic incentives for producers to begin seriously considering expanded use of AI programs in their herds using semen from high-accuracy sires.

Table 1	
Tier Two requirements for the Missouri Show-Me-Select Replacement Heifer Program	
Trait	**Accuracy**
Calving ease (direct)	.65
Calving ease (maternal)	.30
Weaning weight	.75
Carcass weight	.20
Marbling	.20

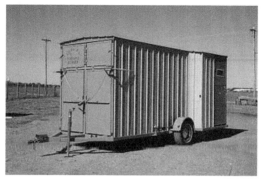

Fig. 5. The University of Missouri Extension funded the purchase of 8 large portable AI barns, available to rent for a daily-use fee, to support the expanded use of fixed-time AI programs in Missouri.

From these data, the economic incentive is clear; astute buyers understand the value of improved genetics and are willing to pay for it. Over time, the Tier Two program offers the potential for herd owners in Missouri to add significant value to heifers they retain as herd replacements or market through Show-Me-Select Replacement Heifer sales. Adoption of these technologies is building equity in cow herds across the state through improvements in genetics.

Economic impact stemming from the Show-Me-Select Replacement Heifer Program in Missouri is estimated at $3.5 million to $5 million on an annual basis. Impact on Missouri's economy from the first 16 years of the Show-Me-Select program now exceeds $65 million. **Table 3** provides a historical summary of program sales by season and year from the time the program began.

SHOW-ME-SELECT REPLACEMENT HEIFER PROGRAM REQUIREMENTS FOR 2013
Enrollment

Any person wishing to qualify heifers in the Show-Me-Select Replacement Heifer Program must be a member of Show-Me-Select Replacement Heifers, Inc, and officially enrolled. An annual membership fee of $25.00 is assessed from each producer. This membership fee is due at either one of two enrollment deadlines, February 1 or September 1 of each calendar year. Producers must enroll by notifying one of the Extension Regional Coordinators.

Ownership

Purchased heifers enrolled in the program must be owned a minimum of 60 days before breeding. All purchased heifers must be accompanied with an affidavit

Table 2
Sales averages for Show-Me-Select Replacement Heifers based on service-sire (natural service or AI) and Tier

	Tier One Show-Me-Select Heifer ($)	Tier Two Show-Me-Select Heifer ($)
Natural service–sired pregnancy	1549	1786 + 237
AI-sired pregnancy	1695 + 146	1906 + 357

Sales averages reflect sales of heifers from the fall of 2010 through the fall of 2012.

Table 3
Missouri Show-Me-Select Replacement Heifer Program sales averages by season and year

	Year	Average ($)
Fall sales (spring-calving bred heifers)	1997	826
	1998	767
	1999	824
	2000	1047
	2001	966
	2002	951
	2003	1122
	2004	1322
	2005	1349
	2006	1210
	2007	1323
	2008	1168
	2009	1177
	2010	1413
	2011	1706
	2012	2043
Spring sales (fall-calving bred heifers)	2000	1052
	2001	1110
	2002	1125
	2003	981
	2004	1403
	2005	1392
	2006	1378
	2007	1209
	2008	1294
	2009	1295
	2010	1332
	2011	1711
	2012	1948

indicating the name and address of the original breeder and approximate birth dates of the heifers. Heifers must be owned by residents of Missouri to sell in a sanctioned Show-Me-Select Replacement Heifer sale.

Prebreeding Evaluation

A prebreeding reproductive evaluation is required for all heifers. Individual animal identification, and pelvic area and reproductive tract scores are required. An enrollment fee of $3.00 per heifer is assessed at prebreeding on heifers entered into the program. All forms and fees for prebreeding must be submitted and paid before pregnancy examination. It is strongly encouraged that prebreeding examinations be performed 6 weeks before breeding. Heifers with a pelvic area less than 150 cm^2 at prebreeding may be remeasured at the initial pregnancy examination within 90 days from the start of the breeding season, and must have a minimum pelvic area of 180 cm^2 at this examination.

Minimum Vaccination Requirements

A comprehensive herd health vaccination program beginning at weaning age or before should be administered under the advice and guidance of a veterinarian in the context of a valid veterinary-client-patient relationship.

- Calfhood vaccination against brucellosis (Bangs) must be given in accordance with state and federal regulations by an accredited veterinarian.
- At weaning, heifers must be vaccinated and boostered for infectious bovine rhinotracheitis (IBR), bovine viral diarrhea (BVD), parainfluenza-3 (PI-3), bovine respiratory syncytial virus, leptospirosis (5-way), vibriosis, and 7-way clostridia. Heifers must be 5 months of age or older at the time vaccinations are administered.
- Before breeding and for the intended purpose of maximizing protection against reproductive loss, vaccinations against leptospirosis (5-way) and vibriosis must be administered between 60 and 30 days before breeding. A booster vaccination against IBR and BVD is required between 60 and 30 days before breeding. Modified live viral vaccines for IBR and BVD are recommended. If killed viral vaccine products are used, 2 boosters are strongly recommended.
- A booster vaccination against leptospirosis (5-way) is required at pregnancy examination.

Pregnancy Examination

An initial pregnancy examination must be performed within 90 days from the start of the breeding season. Individual animal identification, pregnancy status, and fetal age (in days) are required. Herds utilizing artificial insemination must report breeding dates. Any heifer that fails to become pregnant during, or loses a pregnancy following the original breeding season is no longer eligible for the program.

SALE ELIGIBILITY REQUIREMENTS FOR 2013

Heifers not enrolled at prebreeding are not considered to be eligible for sale.

Pelvic Measurement

Pelvic rechecks are to be done at the pregnancy check and cannot be done more than twice in the heifer's life to be qualified for sale.

Parasite Control

All heifers must be treated for internal and external parasites within 30 days of sale. Products for internal parasite control must have a label claim for immature stages of the parasite life cycle.

Surgery

Horns and scurs must be removed, and heifers must be completely healed by sale day.

Implants and Melengestrol Acetate

It is recommended that heifers not be implanted. If heifers are implanted, it is required that only products approved by the Food and Drug Administration (FDA) for replacement heifers be used and administered according to label guidelines. Long-term use of melengestrol acetate (MGA) is prohibited. Use of MGA for periods of up to 14 days to synchronize estrus is permitted.

Blemishes

Heifers with active cases of pinkeye or scars resulting from pinkeye are not eligible for sale. In addition, heifers with rat-tails, bob-tails, frozen ears, or other physical blemishes or deformities will not be eligible for sale. The regional sale committees reserve the right to refuse any heifer that does not meet the criteria for blemishes or any heifer deemed to have an undesirable disposition on sale day.

Weight and Body Condition

Bred heifers on the day of sale must weigh a minimum of 800 lb (363 kg) and receive a body condition score within a range of 5 through 8 using a 9-point scale. All bred heifers will be sold on a per-head basis.

BVD-PI

Heifers offered for sale must be tested and guaranteed negative for BVD-PI.

Inspection of Heifers

Heifers will be evaluated prior to sale by a certified USDA grader for frame, muscle, and body condition. All heifers must meet a minimum projected frame score of Medium using the USDA system for grades of cows, and a muscle score of 2.0 using the USDA feeder cattle scoring system.

Pregnancy

A confirmatory pregnancy examination must be performed within 30 days prior to sale. The consignor guarantees bred heifers to be safe in calf at the time of sale. If a heifer is proven by veterinary examination within 30 days after sale not to have been pregnant, the consignor will replace the heifer or make a financial settlement with the buyer. Spring-calving heifers must be bred to calve before May 1, and fall-calving heifers must be bred to calve before December 1. Heifers in individual sale lots are grouped to calve within approximately 45 days of each other, based on expected calving dates.

Tier Two Classification

Heifers are eligible to qualify for Tier Two in the Show-Me-Select Replacement Heifer Program based on minimum accuracies of the heifer's sire at the time of sale for the respective traits listed in **Table 1**.

Sire Requirements

Eligible sires must have known identification, be registered by their respective national breed registry, and have complete EPD information. Sires are evaluated for qualification in the program based on the EPD provided by their respective breed registry and not on EPD produced by progeny registration in any other breed or hybrid registry **Table 4**. Sires must meet calving-ease EPD requirements listed in **Table 5** for breeds reporting calving-ease EPD. For breeds not reporting calving-ease EPD, sires must meet birth-weight EPD requirements listed in **Table 5**. All sires used in conjunction with AI must have a minimum accuracy value of 0.6 on a scale of 0 to 1 for the respective EPDs.

- Bulls or semen purchased on or after February 1 of the current year must meet the requirements in **Table 5**. Bulls or semen purchased before February 1 must meet the previous year's requirements.
- Heifers that are bred artificially may not be exposed for natural service for a minimum of:
  - 14 days following a nonsynchronized, spontaneous estrus
  - 14 days after the administration of prostaglandin $F_{2\alpha}$ at the beginning of a synchronized period, when AI is performed on the basis of observed heat

Table 4
Active sire percentile rank requirements for 2013

Breed Group	Percentile Requirement
Angus	Upper 35%
American	Upper 20%
British	Upper 30%
Continental	Upper 15%
Hybrid	Upper 15%

- ○ 14 days after fixed-time AI when heifers are inseminated by appointment, following administration of an estrus synchronization protocol
- • All sires must be approved by the Regional Specialist before the planned breeding season.

CERTIFICATION FOR 2013

Only heifers that meet the aforementioned requirements with individual data entered in the official database for Show-Me-Select Replacement Heifers, Inc, are eligible to receive certification. Certification of heifers is publicly recognized by the Missouri "Show-Me-Select Replacement Heifer" ear tag. A certification fee of $10 per heifer is assessed and is due at the time Show-Me-Select qualified heifers receive their

Table 5
Service-sire expected progeny difference (EPD) requirements for birth weight and calving ease for 2013

Service-Sire Breed	Maximum Birth-Weight EPD	Minimum Calving-Ease EPD
Angus		7.0
Balancer		13.3
Beefmaster	−0.7	
Brangus		7.5
Braunvieh		8.0
Charolais		8.2
Gelbvieh		11.0
LimFlex		11.0
Limousin		12.0
Maine Anjou	0.6	
MaineTainer	0.0	
Polled & Horned Hereford		2.2
Red Angus		7.0
Red Poll	1.5	
Salers		0.9
Shorthorn		1.92
SimAngus		13.3
Simmental		11.0
South Devon	1.2	
Tarentaise		3.3

official tag. Misrepresentation, false advertisement, or use of the Missouri Show-Me-Select Replacement Heifer trademark for heifers that do not meet the aforementioned requirements is subject to penalty.

Regional coordinators working with producers in their respective regions have the flexibility to customize and/or broaden requirements for participation on a regional basis, as long as the basic minimum requirements of the program are met. Program requirements reflect these changes on a region-to-region basis.

SUMMARY

The Missouri Show-Me-Select Replacement Heifer Program is recognized nationally as being the first statewide, on-farm beef heifer development and marketing program in the United States. Technologies that producers are using for on-farm heifer development are now spilling over into cow herds across Missouri, largely evidenced by increased interest and adoption of estrous synchronization and AI programs. This expansion has occurred in part because of the more recent successful application of AI than in past years, but also financially encouraged by differentials in sales prices resulting from either heifers carrying AI-sired pregnancies or the heifers themselves being distinguished as Tier Two replacements. Whichever the case, an added spinoff has been a growing interest and appreciation for reproductive management and genetic improvement.

Today, names including Kleiboeker, Wheeler, Ladd Ranches, Trump, Keithley-Jackson, Kasten, Masters, Crooks Farm, Bennett, and many more have become household names across Missouri, based on reputations built from the Show-Me-Select Program. These farms and their herds are recognized not just for having been long-time participants in the Show-Me-Select program, but for the quality of heifers they produce and the repeat customers they have attracted. Each of these farms recognizes that the success they have enjoyed was supported by their Extension Regional Livestock Specialist along with their veterinarian.

Missouri's infrastructure to produce and supply more and better beef begins with the heifer portion of the calf crop and the state's significant beef cow inventory. In addition, the human resources enjoyed in Missouri are readily available to support this billion-dollar industry by adding value through programs such as Show-Me-Select.

REFERENCES

1. Patterson DJ. Adding value to replacement heifers with the Missouri Show-Me-Select Program. In: Proc. NCBA-IRM producer education seminars. Denver (CO); 1998. p. 103–9.
2. Randle RF. The Missouri Show-Me-Select Replacement Heifer Program: production summary from the first two years. In: Proc. reproductive tools and techniques. Columbia (MO): University of Missouri; 1999. p. 1–9.
3. Patterson DJ, Wood SL, Randle RF. Procedures that support reproductive management of replacement beef heifers. Proc Am Soc Anim Sci 1999. Available at: http://www.asas.org/jas/symposia/proceedings/0902.pdf. Accessed August 3, 2000.
4. Patterson DJ, Mallory DA, Parcell JL, et al. The Missouri Show-Me-Select Replacement Heifer Program. Joplin (MO), August 31–September 1. In: Proceedings, applied reproductive strategies in beef cattle. 2011. p. 237–51.

Incorporating Reproductive Management of Beef Heifers into a Veterinary Practice

Scott E. Poock, DVM*, Craig A. Payne, DVM, MS

KEYWORDS

- Reproductive tract score • Pelvic measurement • Ultrasound • Fetal age • Fetal sex

KEY POINTS

- Heifer development programs, such as the Missouri Show-Me-Select Replacement Heifer Program, are dependent upon veterinary involvement.
- Reproductive tract scores are a valuable tool in predicting success of a breeding program and/or culling heifers prior to the breeding season.
- Early pregnancy diagnosis is important to verify artificially inseminated-sired calves from cleanup natural-service sired calves when done at the appropriate gestational age.
- The use of ultrasound facilitates fetal aging and allows a veterinarian to determine fetal sex at the appropriate gestational age.

INTRODUCTION

Veterinarians have for some time played an important role in reproductive management of dairy herds across the United States; however, in many cases, the extent to which practitioners are involved in reproductive management of beef herds is limited.[1] The reasons for this vary; however, there are numerous ways in which practitioners are now able to become more actively involved in reproductive management of US beef herds.[1] Veterinarians can have an impact on producers' profits by implementing their skills and knowledge to beef heifer development programs, an area of production medicine.[2]

Disclosure: The authors have nothing to disclose regarding any relationship with a commercial company that has a direct financial interest in the subject matter or materials discussed in their article or with a company making a competing product.
Veterinary Extension and Continuing Education, College of Veterinary Medicine, University of Missouri, A331 Clydesdale Hall, Columbia, MO 65211, USA
* Corresponding author.
E-mail address: poocks@missouri.edu

Vet Clin Food Anim 29 (2013) 667–678
http://dx.doi.org/10.1016/j.cvfa.2013.07.010
0749-0720/13/$ – see front matter Published by Elsevier Inc.

This article provides an overview of the services veterinarians can provide to beef cattle producers that pertain to reproductive management of replacement beef heifers.

HEIFER DEVELOPMENT PROGRAMS

Veterinarians are able to become more actively involved in reproductive management of beef herds by encouraging beef producers to participate in beef heifer development programs patterned after the Missouri Show-Me-Select Replacement Heifer (SMS) Program. The SMS program began in 1997 as a cooperative effort between University of Missouri (MU) Extension, the MU Division of Animal Sciences, the MU College of Veterinary Medicine, and veterinary practitioners across Missouri.[3] The SMS program was designed to improve reproductive efficiency of beef herds beginning with heifers. Ultimately, when producers have success with their heifers, similar programs can be implemented in the cow herd.

The local veterinarian and MU extension livestock specialists are vital participants in this statewide program. Since 1997 and through the fall of 2012, producers on 722 farms enrolled 104,918 heifers in the SMS program. During this time, the program was supported by 27 regional extension livestock specialists and 222 veterinarians.[3] Veterinarians are certified in performing prebreeding reproductive examinations on heifers enrolled in the program that include reproductive tract scores and pelvic measurements. Veterinarians, in addition, are responsible for early pregnancy diagnosis and fetal aging, along with presale confirmation of pregnancy status. These services, along with careful tracking of data on heifers enrolled in the program, have been essential to the program's success.

The program has added value to replacement beef heifers and increased profits for participating producers. Added value for heifers enrolled in the program results from a list of factors, including proof of vaccination for reproductive diseases; proof of reproductive soundness, involving prebreeding examinations that include reproductive tract scores (RTS) and pelvic measurement (PM); estrous synchronization and artificial insemination; and determination of fetal age and guarantee of final pregnancy status.[3]

The following list provides a summary of requirements for heifers enrolled in the program that require veterinary intervention:

- Brucellosis vaccination by the veterinarian[3]
  - Veterinarian input on selection of other vaccines[3] (see article written by Paynne elsewhere in this issue)
- Prebreeding examinations (RTS and PM)
- Consultation regarding estrous synchronization programs
- Early and late pregnancy diagnosis[3] (early pregnancy diagnosis is required to be performed by at least 90 days from the start of the breeding season with the purpose of distinguishing heifers that conceived after artificial insemination [AI] versus those that conceived after natural service)
  - Ultrasound to determine gestational age and fetal sexing

Veterinarians involved in the SMS program become more actively involved with participating farms, and see an increase in demand for more specialized services, including ultrasound for early pregnancy diagnosis and fetal aging. In addition, some practitioners have begun offering expanded services that include estrous synchronization and AI.

In total, the SMS program has been a win–win for the producer and veterinarian. Other states either have or are beginning programs patterned after the SMS program, and veterinarians are encouraged to take advantage of the opportunities these programs provide.

REPRODUCTIVE TRACT SCORE

In order for a heifer to calve first at 2 years of age, it is important that she reach puberty in a timely manner. Early attainment of puberty increases the chance of a heifer experiencing multiple estrous cycles prior to the breeding season. This is an important consideration, because it was shown that heifers bred on their third estrous cycle after pubertal onset had a 23% improvement in pregnancy rate when compared with those that exhibited only 1 estrous cycle.[4] Therefore, heifers must be developed to reach puberty prior to the date the breeding season begins.

Age at puberty is defined as the age at which a heifer first exhibits estrus and ovulates.[5,6] Prebreeding examinations that include an RTS were standardized in 1991 by Anderson[7] and are used as an indirect measure of pubertal status.[5–8] The RTS scale ranges from a score of 1 to 5; a detailed description of these scores is found in **Table 1**. Although reproductive tract scoring requires experience in palpating bovine uteri and ovaries, it has been shown to be repeatable among experienced veterinarians.[5,9] RTS is correlated with age, body weight, and body condition score, whereas age at puberty is dependent on age, nutrition, and genetics.[5,6] Note the similarity in these determining factors.

RTS a good indicator of pubertal status and has been demonstrated to be a good predicator of which heifers will conceive.[6,10] Heifers assigned an RTS of 1 or 2 experience longer days to AI and reduced pregnancy rates.[5,6] In addition, there is a positive correlation between RTS and pregnancy rates within a 50-day AI season as well as reproductive success in the subsequent breeding season.[5,6,8,10,11] Heifers that conceive early in their first breeding season tend to follow that same early breeding and early calving pattern for the rest of their lives.[10]

Prebreeding examinations that include RTS should be performed 30 to 60 days prior to breeding,[3] and heifers with an RTS of 1 in most cases should be culled. If most heifers in a group are assigned an RTS below 4, it is highly recommended that the producer investigate the prepuberal status of the heifers to determine whether there were problems related to the development program.

Table 1					
Reproductive tract scoring system					
RTS	Uterine Horns	Ovarian Length (mm)	Ovarian Height (mm)	Ovarian Width (mm)	Ovarian Structures
1	Immature, <20 mm diameter, no tone	15	10	8	No palpable follicles
2	20–25 mm diameter, no tone	18	12	10	8 mm follicles
3	20–25 mm diameter, slight tone	22	15	10	8–10 mm follicles
4	30 mm diameter, good tone	30	16	12	10 mm follicles, CL possible
5	>30 mm diameter	>32	20	15	Corpus Luteum present

Data from Anderson KJ, Lefever DG, Brinks JS, et al. The use of reproductive tract scoring in beef heifers. Agri Pract 1991;12(4):123–8.

PELVIC MEASUREMENT

Until recent years, dystocia was a major problem in the beef cattle industry.[12–19] When analyzing the overall incidence of dystocia in beef cattle, primiparous cows experience an increased percentage of these problems.[15,18] The primary reason for this increased incidence is disproportion between calf size in relation to total pelvic area.[12,14,17–20]

First-calf heifers that experience dystocia are more likely to be culled due to subsequent reproductive problems (ie, days to pregnancy, or not becoming pregnant),[14,15,20] and calves born after a dystocia are more likely to develop health problems or die.[14,20] Thus, there has been an interest in obtaining pelvic measurements on replacement heifers to reduce the incidence and severity of these problems. However, it should be noted that this procedure is not without controversy.[21]

Pelvic width, height, and total pelvic area are moderately to highly heritable traits.[12,13] Some studies have reported a high correlation between pelvic area and calving ease; therefore measuring pelvic area should be beneficial.[17,19,22] Other studies have shown this correlation to be small.[12,13,18,21,22] In addition, the repeatability of pelvic measurements among veterinarians may vary.[21] For this reason, some authors suggest using a threshold value, in which heifers with abnormally small or abnormally shaped pelvises are culled. This may be the most effective use of pelvic measurements,[1,21] and it has been the approach taken in the Missouri SMS program.

Pelvic measurements on heifers should be obtained at 12 to 14 months of age.[14,18] Height and width of the pelvis are measured in centimeters; height is multiplied by width to obtain total pelvic area. Pelvic height is the vertical distance between the pubic symphysis and the sacral vertebrae.[18] The pelvic width is the horizontal distance between the shafts of the ileum at the widest point.[18]

Heifers enrolled in the SMS program are required to measure 150 cm^2 at the time prebreeding examinations are performed (30–60 days prior to breeding). Heifers not meeting this minimum pelvic area must be remeasured at the time of the first pregnancy examination (within 90 days from the start of the breeding season), and at this time must measure at least 180 cm^2 to qualify for the program sales.

Pelvic measurements should be used in addition to, not in place of, selection for size, weight, and above all fertility.[23] Producers should be aware that selection for pelvic area will not likely result in increased pelvic dimensions alone, but will result in increased size of the entire skeleton and animal.[24] Increased skeletal size of the dam will be reflected in higher birth weights and dimensions of the calf. Pelvic measurements, on the other hand, can be used successfully to identify abnormally small or abnormally shaped pelvises. These situations, left unidentified, often are associated with extreme dystocia, resulting in Cesarean delivery and even death of the calf or dam.[8] Selection of sires with low birth weight Expected Progeny Difference (BW-EPD) or high calving ease direct (CED) EPD (CED-EPD) mated to heifers that are screened for pelvic area contributes to a decrease in the incidence and (or) severity of calving problems and minimizes calf losses from dystocia.

Bullock and Patterson[25] reported that puberty exerts a positive influence on pelvic width and resulting pelvic area in yearling beef heifers; however, differences that were seen among heifers as yearlings did not carry through to calving as 2-year-olds. Therefore selection (culling) decisions based on pelvic measurements and contemporary grouping for genetic analysis of pelvic measurements should include consideration of pubertal status at the time of the examination. The data suggest that puberty plays a role in pelvic size as yearlings, but once heifers reach puberty, the effects may no longer be present. An independent culling level for pelvic size on heifers that are at different stages in their reproductive development appears to be more restrictive for those heifers that are peripubertal at the time of the examination.

The Rice Pelvimeter (Lane Manufacturing, Denver, Colorado) (**Fig. 1**) is the most commonly used pelvimeter the authors have observed while working with veterinarians involved with the SMS program. It is relatively inexpensive ($\sim$ \$200–\$250) and sturdy.

Using pelvic area as the sole predictor of calving ease has not been shown to be effective.[14,15,18,21,22] BW-EPDs, along with CED-EPDs were proven to be more effective than pelvic area alone for reduction in dystocia.[1,13] As stated previously, selection for pelvic area will not likely result in increased pelvic dimensions alone, but results in increased size of the entire skeleton and animal,[12,16,24] and is correlated with increased calf birth weight.[26] As birth weight increases, so does the incidence of dystocia.[18,20–22] Therefore, using pelvic measurements to screen heifers with abnormally small or abnormally structured pelvises in combination with service sire selection based on BW-CED and/or CED-EPD provides beef producers with the best possible scenario in managing dystocia.

ADDING VALUE TO PREGNANCY DIAGNOSIS

The importance of pregnancy diagnosis in a cow–calf operation should not be underestimated. For many years, rectal palpation was the mainstay of veterinarians for pregnancy diagnosis. Undoubtedly, rectal palpation will continue to be important.[27] However, alternative methods, such as ultrasound and blood tests for pregnancy, are available and may provide additional opportunities for veterinarians.

Using Ultrasound for Pregnancy Diagnosis

Pregnancy diagnosis in cattle has evolved over time. The simplest, and perhaps most definitive test for pregnancy, is to wait until the cow gives birth to the calf. However, this approach is of little use in intensively managed beef cattle operations. The desire for early pregnancy diagnosis led to the routine use of rectal palpation of the uterine contents for the purpose of detecting the pregnancy. Although traditionally practiced from 40 to 60 days after insemination, pregnancy diagnosis by rectal palpation has been pushed to the limit of detection (30–35 days after conception) in an effort to identify open cows sooner after insemination in the dairy industry. Earlier diagnosis by manual palpation clearly requires more precision in terms of sensitivity of the technique.

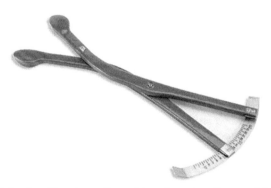

Fig. 1. The Rice Pelvimeter. (*Courtesy of* Lane Manufacturing, Denver, CO; with permission.)

The need for improved sensitivity led to the introduction of transrectal ultrasound for pregnancy detection. Transrectal ultrasound can be used as early as 25 days after insemination, but is more typically applied after 30 days.[28] Ultrasound provides a definitive test for pregnancy, and has become popular in some regions. However, this procedure requires specialized equipment, and the examination generally requires more time than rectal palpation. Regardless of whether rectal palpation or ultrasound is used, an individual with highly specialized training is needed to perform the diagnosis.

Ultrasound equipment

Ultrasound technology has been investigated now for nearly 25 years.[29–31] The use of ultrasound by bovine practitioners for reproductive purposes is the most common use of this technology.[32] Some of the earliest reports demonstrating use of ultrasound in bovine reproduction came from Ginther's laboratory at the University of Wisconsin. Ultrasound provides the practitioner with a way in which to gather more information than via rectal palpation.[33,34] Ultrasound was investigated and is used as a tool for use in early pregnancy diagnosis, evaluation of ovarian structures, fetal sexing, and fetal aging.[33,35–38] Initially, the high cost of ultrasound machines dissuaded their use. Yet, because of advances in technology over the past 15 years, use of ultrasound has increased due to the development of more inexpensive, portable equipment.[37]

There are now many types of ultrasound units available to the practitioner, including stationary and mobile units (goggles). Most ultrasound units used for reproductive purposes in cattle have transducers in the 5 to 9 MHz range. Transducers in the 5.0 to 7.5 MHz ranges are the most commonly used.[29,32] The 5 MHz transducer results in greater depth (1–3 in) but less detail compared with the 7.5 MHz transducer.[29,30] For detailed examination of the ovaries, a 7.5 to 10 MHz probe is preferred.[32] Crystals in the transducers create a sound wave that travels through the area being scanned. Tissues will cause the sound waves to echo back, but fluids are not echogenic.[30,37] Therefore, fetal fluids will appear black on an ultrasound monitor, whereas bones and tissue will appear white to shades of gray.

Ultrasound procedure

Prior to performing ultrasound, it is important to have proper facilities to conduct the procedure. Adequate restraint of the cattle is important, especially restraint that decreases lateral movement.[32] It is best to empty the rectum manually prior to the examination to obtain a quality image.[32] Veterinarians performing an examination should be systematic and methodical in their procedure, and it is recommended that ovaries always be examined first to help determine diagnostic precision.[32]

On average, an embryo with a visible heartbeat is first seen on or around day 20 to 28 of gestation, depending on experience of the technician and type of ultrasound probe being used.[39–41] Starting at day 30 of gestation, the amnion can be viewed.[32] Visualization of the embryo prior to day 30 can be more difficult, because the embryo may be hidden behind endometrial folds.[32] At around 45 days of gestation, the fetus will be active 60% of the time.[32]

The sensitivity and specificity in using ultrasound are described at various dates after insemination/breeding and begin as early as 9 to 10 days after breeding.[33,37,40] By 26 to 32 days after breeding, the sensitivity/specificity is such that it is acceptable to effectively diagnose a pregnancy/nonpregnancy at this time.[29,32–35,37,42]

One concern expressed with diagnosing pregnancy too early pertains to naturally occurring embryonic or fetal loss. The data suggest a 10% to 15% loss occurs between 28 and 42 days of gestation.[32] As the pregnancy progresses, the incidence of embryonic or fetal loss is reduced, with fetal mortality rates ranging between 6% and 3% for days 42 to 56 and 56 to 98, respectively.[32] For this reason, it is recommended that a follow-up pregnancy examination be performed.

Ultrasound vs manual palpation

Data collected from the Missouri SMS program have been used to compare breeding and calving dates of heifers and determine accuracy of fetal aging on the basis of whether pregnancy was diagnosed via rectal palpation or ultrasound. These data suggest that ultrasound improves accuracy in determining fetal age; however, several experienced practitioners were highly accurate in their determination of fetal age based on rectal palpation. This observation supports a recently published paper on the use of per rectum palpation; experienced palpators were shown to be highly accurate, while less experienced veterinarians were less accurate.[27] Another benefit observed among practitioners using ultrasound is that they often become more proficient at rectal palpation.[30,33,37]

Several studies appear in the literature regarding the low incidence of deleterious effects that result after rectal palpation by experienced veterinarians.[36,43,44] There are, however, some reports suggesting an increase in fetal loss after rectal palpation versus ultrasound. This problem arises in large part because of inexperienced palpators.[43] Likewise, there have been several reports that indicate potential problems in fetal development from palpation of early pregnancies.[34,37,45]

Using ultrasound in the beef cattle industry

The dairy industry embraced the use of ultrasound soon after it became available, making it possible for veterinarians to diagnose a cow as nonpregnant earlier than was possible based on palpation per rectum. This meant that cows could be resubmitted for insemination sooner, which enhanced reproduction and led to more profit for the dairy producer.

In contrast to dairy cattle, an ultrasound is used in beef cattle more for fetal aging and/or fetal sexing rather than the earliest pregnancy/open diagnosis.[34] Fetal aging is important to seedstock producers, because knowing the date of when a female conceives is important to determining the sire of the fetus in some instances.[34] Commercial producers who participate in value-added marketing programs may also need to know the identity of the sire, so fetal aging can prove beneficial for them as well.[34]

As was already mentioned, the Missouri SMS program requires pregnancy diagnosis by 90 days after the start of the breeding season. The 90-day time period is especially important when a breeding program utilizes fixed-time AI (FTAI) followed with a natural service cleanup period beginning 14 days after FTAI. Using ultrasound, the veterinarian can accurately determine age of the fetus and therefore determine if the pregnancy resulted from the FTAI or the cleanup bull. Likewise, the veterinarian can determine sex of the fetus from FTAI and most likely the first round of cleanup bull matings (~70 days), if the ultrasound is performed 90 days after FTAI.

FETAL AGING

In order to accurately determine fetal age, various measurements of anatomic structures of the fetus may be taken. The most accurate estimate of gestational age is derived from obtaining an actual anatomic measurement.[37,38,46] Early in gestation (20–55 days of gestation), it is recommended that the crown-to-rump length be used.[33,37] Later, the head or body circumference and length of the head are used to determine gestational age of the fetus (**Table 2**).[37] Using these measurements, the actual date of calving can be predicted within an average of 4.5 days (crown to

Table 2
Embryonic or fetal measurements used to determine gestational age

Days Pregnant	Primary Structure	Size	Secondary Structure	Size	Tertiary Structure	
<30	Crown to rump	0.9 cm				
35	**Crown to rump**	**1 cm**				
40	**Crown to rump**	**2 cm**				
45	**Crown to rump**	**3 cm**				
50	**Crown to rump**	**4 cm**	Head diameter	0.7 cm		
55	**Crown to rump**	**5 cm**	Head diameter	1.1 cm		
60	Head Length	2.5 cm	Head diameter	1.5 cm		
70	**Head Length**	**3 cm**	Head diameter	2 cm		
75	**Head Length**	**3.5 cm**	Head diameter	2.3 cm	Trunk diameter	2.5 cm
80	**Head Length**	**4 cm**	Head diameter	2.5 cm	Trunk diameter	3 cm
85	**Head Length**	**4.5 cm**	Head diameter	2.8 cm	Trunk diameter	3.5 cm
90	**Head Length**	**5 cm**	Head diameter	3.1 cm	Trunk diameter	4 cm
95	Head Length	5.5 cm	Head diameter	3.5 cm	Trunk diameter	4.5 cm
100	Head Length	6 cm	Head diameter	4 cm	Trunk diameter	5 cm
105	Head Length	7 cm	Head diameter	4.5 cm	Trunk diameter	6 cm
110	Head Length	8 cm	Head diameter	5 cm	Trunk diameter	7 cm

Data from Refs.[30,31,47]

rump), 6.9 days (head), or 7.8 days (trunk).[37] Thus, the earlier the measurements are taken, the more accurate the veterinarian will be.

The authors use a simplified rule of thumb for determining fetal age in teaching or training students to perform an ultrasound. Most ultrasounds will have a scale or grid on the monitor; these grids may be used to estimate the length of various structures. For early pregnancies (35–55 days of gestation), the rule is 1 to 2, 2 to 3, 3 to 4, and 4 to 5 cm, crown-to-rump length is correlated to 35 to 40, 40 to 45, 45 to 50, 50 to 55 days of gestation, respectively (highlighted in bold on **Table 2**). For later pregnancies (70–90 days of gestation), the rule is 3.0 to 3.5, 3.5 to 4.0, 4.0 to 4.5, 45 to 5.0 cm, head length is correlated to 70 to 75, 75 to 80, 80 to 85, 85 to 90 days of gestation, respectively (highlighted in bold on **Table 2**). These guidelines are easy for students to remember and utilize.

FETAL SEXING

Fetal sexing was first described in 1989 by Curran.[31,47] She discovered that around day 53 to 56 of gestation, the genital tubercles have migrated to their proper positions.[29,31,37,38,47] Therefore, the earliest date at which veterinary practitioners are able to realistically determine fetal sex is 55 days.[32,35,46]

The latest fetal sex can be determined varies, but may be performed as late as 100 days of gestation in dairy cattle and 110 days in beef cattle. At this time, the gravid uterus becomes more difficult to scan. It is generally concluded that sex determination is most practical between 60 and 85 days of gestation.[32,33,37,38] For teaching purposes, the authors prefer that cattle be 70 to 85 days of gestation. Remarkably, fetal sexing can predict the sex of the resulting calf by 92% to 100%.[29,31,33,38] However, this level of accuracy takes time and practice to achieve.

There are 2 keys in learning to determine fetal sex. The first is to identify the genital tubercle, which is relatively easy[31] to locate. The genital tubercles of the female and male will appear as oval, hyperechogenic, bilobed structures.[31,47] The male genital tubercle (MGT) will be found just caudal to the umbilicus, and the female genital tubercle (FGT) is located ventral to the tail.[31] At approximately 80 to 90 days of gestation, secondary anatomic structures can improve diagnosis.[31] In the bull, the scrotum is visible, and in the heifer, the teats become distinctive.[31]

The second step, which is more difficult, is to produce an image that is of high enough quality so that the tubercles are visualized.[31] Cross-sectional views appear to be more useful for fetal sexing as opposed to saggital views.[47]

An additional item that is important to understand when learning to determine fetal sex is which direction is cranial/caudal and ventral/dorsal on the fetus. Proper orientation helps the ultrasonographer create a higher-quality image. There are 3 specific anatomic references: the head, beating heart, and umbilicus.[31,47] These sites help direct the practitioner to the correct orientation when manipulating the transducer. Also, the front and rear legs can be difficult to differentiate at times, and proper orientation will make the determination of which is front or back[31] much easier.

In conclusion, taking time to learn the art of pregnancy diagnosis in cattle by ultrasound has many benefits. Early detection of pregnancy, fetal sexing, fetal aging, and ovarian and uterine pathology all aid the cattleman to increase profits.

Important steps to fetal sexing include

- Identify the genital tubercles (relatively easy)[31]
- Determine anatomic directions: dorsal, ventral, cranial, and caudal
- Find the umbilicus, as it is the focal point for determining fetal sex; the male genital tubercle will be immediately caudal to the umbilicus, and if not seen, the practitioner then proceeds to verify the female genital tubercle
- Learn to produce an image that is of high quality, which is the most difficult step[31]

SUMMARY

In conclusion, veterinarians are able to assist beef producers with heifer development programs in areas related to reproductive health and management. Incorporating a reproductive examination at the time prebreeding vaccinations are administered that includes RTS and pelvic measurements helps to predict potential reproductive success (RTS) and/or possible problems at calving. The advent of the use of ultrasound for reproductive purposes focused on early pregnancy diagnosis may be enhanced by adding fetal aging and fetal sexing to the menu of services a practitioner provides. Additionally, as value-added programs gain strides into the industry, verifying AI-sired from natural service-sired calves, and determination of fetal sex will become more common and in many cases expected.

REFERENCES

1. Caldow G, Lowman B, Riddell I. Veterinary intervention in the reproductive management of beef cow herds. Practice 2005;27:406–11.
2. Larson RL. Heifer development: reproduction and nutrition. Vet Clin North Am Food Anim Pract 2007;23:53–68.
3. Patterson DJ, Mallory DA, Parcell JL, et al. The Missouri show-me-select replacement heifer program. In: Patterson D, editor. Proceedings, applied reproductive strategies in beef cattle. Joplin (MO): University of Misssouri; 2011. p. 237–51.

4. Bylerley DF, Stagmiller RB, Betrardinelli JG, et al. Pregnancy rates of beef heifers bred either on puberal or third estrus. J Anim Sci 1987;65:645–50.
5. Holm DE, Thompson PN, Irons PC. The value of reproductive tract scoring as a predictor of fertility and production outcomes in beef heifers. J Anim Sci 2009; 87:1934–40.
6. Pence M, Ensley D, Berghaus R, et al. Improving reproductive efficiency through the use of reproductive tract scoring in a group of beef replacement heifers. Bov Pract 2007;41:35–40.
7. Anderson KJ, Lefever DG, Brinks JS, et al. The use of reproductive tract scoring in beef heifers. Agri Pract 1991;12(4):123–8.
8. Patterson DJ, Perry RC, Kiracofe GH, et al. Management considerations in heifer development and puberty. J Anim Sci 1992;70:4018–35.
9. Rosenkrans KS, Hardin DK. Repeatability and accuracy of reproductive tract scoring to determine pubertal status in beef heifers. Theriogenology 2003;59: 1087–92.
10. Pence M, BreDahl R, Thomson JU. Clinical use of reproductive tract scoring to predict pregnancy outcome. Beef Research Report. Ames: Iowa State University; 1999. A.S. Leaflet R1656.
11. Stevenson JL, Rodrigues JA, Braga FA, et al. Effect of breeding protocols and reproductive tract score on reproductive performance of dairy heifers and economic outcome of breeding programs. J Dairy Sci 2007;91:3424–38.
12. Kriese LA, Van Vleck LD, Gregory KE, et al. Estimates of genetic parameters for 320-day pelvic measurements of males and females and calving ease of 2-year-old females. J Anim Sci 1994;72:1954–63.
13. Cook BR, Tess MW, Kress DD. Effects of selection strategies using heifer pelvic area and sire birth weight expected progeny difference on dystocia in first-calf heifers. J Anim Sci 1993;71:602–7.
14. Basarab JA, Rutter LM, Day PA. The efficacy of predicting dystocia in yearling beef heifers: I. Using ratios of pelvic area to birth weight or pelvic area to heifer weight. J Anim Sci 1993;71:1359–71.
15. Dargatz DA, Dewell GA, Mortimer RG. Calving and calving management of beef cows and heifers on cow–calf operations in the United States. Theriogenology 2004;997–1007.
16. Bellows RA, Genho PC, Moore SA, et al. Factors affecting dystocia in brahman-cross heifers in subtropical southeastern United States. J Anim Sci 1996;74: 1451–6.
17. Naazie A, Makarechian M, Berg RT. Genetic, phenotypic, and environmental parameter estimates of calving difficulty, weight, and measures of pelvic size in beef heifers. J Anim Sci 1991;69:4793–800.
18. VanDonkersgoed J, Ribble CS, Townsend HG, et al. The usefulness of pelvic area measurements as an on-farm test for predicting calving difficulty in beef heifers. Can Vet J 1990;31:190–3.
19. Colburn DJ, Deutscher GH, Nielsen MK, et al. Effects of sire, dam traits, calf traits, and environment on dystocia and subsequent reproduction of two-year-old heifers. J Anim Sci 1997;75:1452–60.
20. Hickson RE, Morris ST, Kenyon PR, et al. Dystocia in beef heifers: a review of genetic and nutritional influences. N Z Vet J 2006;54:256–64.
21. VanDonkersgoed J, Ribble CS, Booker CW, et al. The predictive value of pelvimetry in beef cattle. Can J Vet Res 1993;57:170–5.
22. Micke GC, Sullivan TM, Rolls PJ, et al. Dystocia in 3-year-old beef heifers: relationship to maternal nutrient intake during early- and mid-gestation, pelvic area

and hormonal indicators of placental function. Anim Reprod Sci 2010;118: 163–70.

23. Bellows RA, Staigmiller RB. Selection for fertility. In: Proceedings of the 39th Annual Beef Cattle Short Course. Gainesville (FL): University of Florida; 1990. p. 172–89.

24. Morrison DG, Williamson WD, Humes PE. Estimates of heritabilities and correlations of traits associated with pelvic area in beef cattle. J Anim Sci 1986;63:432–7.

25. Bullock KD, Patterson DJ. Pelvic growth in beef heifers and the effects of puberty. In: Proc. Beef Improvement Federation. Raleigh (NC): 1995. p. 171–3.

26. Benyshek LL, Little DE. Estimates of genetic and phenotypic parameters associated with pelvic area in simmental cattle. J Anim Sci 1982;54:258–63.

27. Kasimanickam R, Whittier WD, Tibary A, et al. Error in pregnancy diagnosis by pre-rectal palpation in beef cows. Clin Ther 2011;3(1):43–7.

28. Fricke PM. Scanning the future-ultrasonography as a reproductive management tool for dairy cattle. J Dairy Sci 2002;85:1918–26.

29. Fricke PM, Lamb GC. Potential applications and pitfalls of reproductive ultrasonography in bovine practice. Vet Clin Food Anim 2005;21:419–36.

30. Stroud B. The use of ultrasound in cow/calf applications. In: Smith R, editor. AABP Proceedings. Auburn (AL): 2006. p. 3–7.

31. Stroud B. Guidelines for ultrasound fetal sexing in a cow/calf operation. In: Smith R, editor. AABP Proceedings. Auburn (AL): 2006. p. 66–9.

32. DesCoteaux L, Gnemmi G, Colloton J. Ultrasonography of the bovine female genital tract. Vet Clin Food Anim 2009;25:733–52.

33. Lamb GC, Fricke PM. Ultrasound—early pregnancy diagnosis and fetal sexing. In: Funston R, Meyer TL, editors. Proceedings of Applied Reproductive Strategies in Beef Cattle. North Platte (NE): University of Nebraska; 2004. p. 219–29.

34. Ramano JE, Thompson JA, Forrest DW, et al. Early pregnancy diagnosis by palpation per rectum: influence on embryo/fetal viability in dairy cattle. Theriogenology 2007;67:486–93.

35. Beal WE, Perry RC, Corah LR. The use of ultrasound in monitoring reproductive physiology of beef cattle. J Anim Sci 1992;70:924–9.

36. Fricke PM. Sync programs and ultrasound: are we getting in there too early? In: Proceedings of the American Association of Bovine Practitioners. Auburn (AL): 2006. p. 173–80.

37. Jones AL, Beal WE. Reproductive applications of ultrasounds in the cow. Bov Pract 2003;37:1.

38. Ribadu AY, Nakao T. Bovine reproductive ultrasonography: a review. J Reprod Dev 1999;45:13–28.

39. Baxter SJ, Ward WR. Short communications–incidence of fetal loss in dairy cattle after pregnancy diagnosis using an ultrasound scanner. Vet Rec 1997;3:287–8.

40. Nation DP, Malmo J, Davis GM, et al. Accuracy of bovine pregnancy detection using transrectal ultrasonography at 28 to 35 days after insemination. Aust Vet J 2003;81:63–5.

41. Kastelic JP, Curran S, Pierson RA, et al. Ultrasonic evaluation of the bovine conceptus. Theriogenology 1988;29:39–54.

42. Mohamed SM, Abd El-Aty AM. Advances in ultrasonography and its applications in domestic ruminants and other farm animals reproduction. J Advanc Res 2010; 1:123–8.

43. Richardson RD, Mortimer RG, Whittier JC. Comparison of fetal losses from diagnosis of pregnancy using ultrasonography or rectal palpation in beef heifers by novice or experienced technicians. The Prof Anim Scientist 2010;26:341–6.

44. Thurmond MC, Picanso JP. Fetal loss associated with palpation per rectum to diagnose in cows. J Am Vet Med Assoc 1993;203:432–5.

45. Ramano JE, Thompson JA, Forrest DW, et al. Early pregnancy diagnosis by transrectal ultrasonography in dairy cattle. Theriogenology 2006;66:1034–41.

46. Mortimer R, Hansen T. The future of pregnancy testing in beef cattle. In: Perry G, editor. Applied Reproductive Strategies in Beef Cattle Proceedings. Brookings (SD): South Dakota State University; 2006. p. 281–8.

47. Curran S, Kastelic JP, Ginther OJ. Determining sex of the bovine fetus by ultrasonic assessment of the relative location of the genital tubercle. Anim Reprod Sci 1989;19:217–27.

Index

Note: Page numbers of article titles are in **boldface** type.

A

B

Vet Clin Food Anim 29 (2013) 679–689
http://dx.doi.org/10.1016/S0749-0720(13)00075-3
0749-0720/13/$ – see front matter © 2013 Elsevier Inc. All rights reserved.

Moving?

Make sure your subscription moves with you!

To notify us of your new address, find your **Clinics Account Number** (located on your mailing label above your name), and contact customer service at:

Email: journalscustomerservice-usa@elsevier.com

800-654-2452 (subscribers in the U.S. & Canada)
314-447-8871 (subscribers outside of the U.S. & Canada)

Fax number: 314-447-8029

Elsevier Health Sciences Division
Subscription Customer Service
3251 Riverport Lane
Maryland Heights, MO 63043

*To ensure uninterrupted delivery of your subscription, please notify us at least 4 weeks in advance of move.

Printed and bound by CPI Group (UK) Ltd, Croydon, CR0 4YY

03/10/2024

01040478-0003